Handbook of Esophageal Disorders

Handbook of Esophageal Disorders

Editor: Freya Owen

MURPHY & MOORE
www.murphy-moorepublishing.com

www.murphy-moorepublishing.com

MURPHY & MOORE

Cataloging-in-Publication Data

Handbook of esophageal disorders / edited by Freya Owen.
p. cm.
Includes bibliographical references and index.
ISBN 978-1-63987-279-4
1. Esophagus--Diseases. 2. Esophagus--Diseases--Diagnosis. 3. Esophagus--Diseases--Treatment.
4. Gastroenterology. I. Owen, Freya.
RC815.7 .H36 2022
616.32--dc23

Murphy & Moore Publishing,
1 Rockefeller Plaza,
New York City, NY 10020, USA

ISBN 978-1-63987-279-4 (Hardback)

Contents

Preface

Every book is a source of knowledge and this one is no exception. The idea that led to the conceptualization of this book was the fact that the world is advancing rapidly; which makes it crucial to document the progress in every field. I am aware that a lot of data is already available, yet, there is a lot more to learn. Hence, I accepted the responsibility of editing this book and contributing my knowledge to the community.

Esophagus, also known as the food pipe, is the organ through which food and liquid passes from pharynx to the stomach through peristaltic contractions. It can be affected by cancer, gastric reflux, constrictions, prominent dilated blood vessels called varices, tears and disorders of motility. Disorders can cause difficulty in swallowing, chest pain, painful swallowing or cause no symptoms at all. Most common disorder of esophagus is gastroesophageal reflux disease. In this disease, a muscle at the end of the esophagus doesn't close properly and the contents of the stomach leak back into the esophagus and irritate it. The diagnosis of esophageal disorders can be done through techniques and procedures such as endoscopy, CT scans and X-rays. The objective of this book is to give a general view of the various esophageal disorders. It provides significant information of this discipline to help develop a good understanding of their diagnosis and treatment. This book is a vital tool for all researching and studying this field.

While editing this book, I had multiple visions for it. Then I finally narrowed down to make every chapter a sole standing text explaining a particular topic, so that they can be used independently. However, the umbrella subject sinews them into a common theme. This makes the book a unique platform of knowledge.

I would like to give the major credit of this book to the experts from every corner of the world, who took the time to share their expertise with us. Also, I owe the completion of this book to the never-ending support of my family, who supported me throughout the project.

Editor

1

Radiation Therapy for Esophageal Cancer

Ivan M. Buzurovic, Borbala Daroczi,
Desmond A. O'Farrell, Mandar S. Bhagwat and
Phillip M. Devlin

Abstract

Esophageal cancer develops in the mucosa of the esophagus and spreads toward the muscle layer. The nonsurgical treatment for localized, deeply invasive esophageal cancer has been external beam radiation therapy (EBRT) and concurrent chemotherapy. Recently, intraluminal brachytherapy showed a strong potential for the improvement of the therapeutic ratio. It was found that the fractionated high dose rate (HDR) brachytherapy offered beneficial palliation for a longer period of time with more durable symptom control. A similar was concluded for advanced unresectable esophageal cancer in previously irradiated patients. HDR brachytherapy may be a useful salvage treatment option for inoperable patients diagnosed with local esophageal cancer. Although better local control can be achieved with higher brachytherapy dose, this increases the risk of acute morbidity and late morbidity, especially in the setting of recurrence cancer. It was found that the moderate dose of EBRT and HDR brachytherapy could give a better local response than EBRT alone.

Keywords: esophageal cancer, radiation therapy, brachytherapy

1. Introduction

Esophageal cancer is the eighth most common cancer worldwide, besides being the sixth most common cause of cancer death. There were 456,000 new cases in the world in 2012 [1]. It is four times more common in men than in women; it occurs more frequently among people above 45 years of age and reaches its plateau among people at 65–74 years of age. Its mortality is high; it can be as high as 84%. For the locally advanced disease, the 5-year survival is 15–34%. The cornerstone of treatment remains surgery; however, there is evidence that survival is favorably influenced when additional therapies, such as chemotherapy or radiation therapy or their combination, or targeted therapies are used for lymph node-positive or cT2 or tumors that are larger than cT2. The clinical studies assessing treatment modalities for esophageal cancer are diverse: the modalities (chemotherapy, radiation therapy and surgery) have been evaluated in various orders and combinations. The number of study subjects has rarely been over 100 per study. The study populations have not always been homogeneous; different portions of the esophagus were affected, and the study population is sometimes mixed, regarding staging and histology.

1.1. Histology

Histology is usually based on the histologic analysis of an endoscopic sample. There are two main types of esophageal cancer: squamous cell carcinoma (SCC) and adenocarcinoma. Squamous cell carcinoma mostly occurs in the lining in the upper portion of the esophagus. Adenocarcinoma develops at the junction between the esophagus and the stomach. Most of the tumors are squamous cell carcinoma, but the incidence of adenocarcinoma has been increasing.

1.2. Predisposing factors

Intraepithelial neoplasias, such as epithelial dysplasias and in situ carcinoma, are the most significant precursor lesions for the development of esophageal cancer. Generally, it occurs a decade prior to carcinoma. The classification of dysplasias is based on the extent of the epithelial involvement. Some of the dysplasias show spontaneous regression. Nearly 30% of the severe dysplasias become invasive cancer. Tobacco use and/or consuming alcohol predominantly increase the risk of esophageal squamous cell carcinoma. Being overweight and/or reflux disease can primarily increase the risk of esophageal adenocarcinoma.

The multifocal appearance and intramural spread are common characteristics of esophageal cancer. It often spreads through the lymphatic system. Tumors involving the proximal portion of the esophagus may give metastases to the cervical lymph nodes, and tumors involving the lower portion may also give metastasis to the vicinity of the celiac artery. Cancer can infiltrate its surroundings, the pars membranacea of the trachea and the prevertebral fascia.

2. Treatment options

From a surgical point of view, early cancer means that the lesion only involves the mucosa and/or submucosa. The treatment option remains surgery for very early cancers (up to stage pT1b) while it is palliative in the case of metastatic esophageal cancer. For other cases, additional therapies, such as chemotherapy and/or radiation therapy may result in improved survival.

Regarding epidemiology, tumor biology, pathogenesis, and prognosis, the two main histological types of esophageal cancer, SCC and adenocarcinoma, are different from each other.

The perioperative mortality is higher for squamous cell cancer. It might be due to comorbidities and the localization of cancer since SCC mostly involves the upper third of the esophagus, and the postoperative mortality is significantly higher for esophageal cancer involving the proximal third. Esophageal cancer affecting the upper third and/or middle third of the esophagus recurs in a locoregional manner whereas adenocarcinoma can more often metastasize to distant sites. However, the prognosis of adenocarcinoma in an early stage is more favorable than that of SCC.

2.1. Chemoradiotherapy

The results of several randomized, phase III studies have been reported so far. Practically, a platinum-based medication is used in combination with radiation.

Morbidity and mortality are unclear regarding the use of neoadjuvant chemoradiotherapy. Some authors reported an increase in the anastomosis insufficiency and an increase in mortality, whereas others did not find an increase in mortality. A recent US study analyzed the data obtained from 1939 patients who had undergone esophagectomy. Seven hundred and eight patients received neoadjuvant therapy. They found no differences in mortality or morbidity [2]. The studies are unclear about the stage in which neoadjuvant therapy can be safely omitted. The American recommendation [3] states that neoadjuvant therapy is reasonable in the case of pT1b (>2 cm in size or dedifferentiated) whereas the European recommendation finds it reasonable only in stage T3-4 or lymph node-positive disease [4]. Chemoradiotherapy can be used

- Definitively: in inoperable cases or if the disease involves the upper third portion of the esophagus, with or without preventive, induction chemotherapy;
- In an adjuvant manner; or
- For a neoadjuvant purpose: if the patient is eligible for surgery (chemoradiotherapy, followed by surgery).

In a prospective multicenter study [5] with 186 patients with esophageal squamous cell carcinoma, three-year survival was significantly higher in patients receiving either pre-operative radiation or pre-operative chemotherapy, radiotherapy and surgery. Definitive chemoradiotherapy can be used in patients who are not surgical candidates or if the disease involves the proximal third portion of the esophagus. The main aims of care are to improve the quality of life and to maintain the patient's ability to swallow. The RTOG 8501 [6] study evaluated the benefits of concurrent chemotherapy compared to radiation therapy alone. The randomized portion of the study included 121 patients, and 61 were enrolled in the chemoradiation arm. No one had any distant metastases. Chemotherapy included the combination of continuous 5-fluorouracil (5-FU) and cisplatin. 1000 mg/m^2 of 5-FU was administered daily over 4 days during Week 1 and Week 5 of radiation treatment, as well as cisplatin at 75 mg/m^2 during the first day of Week 1 and Week 5 in combination with 50 Gy irradiation. After completion of radiation therapy, another two cycles were administered at unchanged doses. By contrast, 64 Gy irradiation was delivered as monotherapy in the other arm. Most of the patients (82%) had squamous cell carcinoma. The study proved the superiority of chemoradiotherapy over radiation therapy alone, regarding both median survival (12.5 vs. 8.9 months) and the 5-year survival (26 vs. 0%). A PRODIGE-5/ACCORD-17 study [7] included 267 patients with up to IV/A stage esophageal cancer. Cisplatin and 5-FU used in the RTOG 8501 study were compared with the administration of six cycles of FOLFOX. FOLFOX + radiation yielded results similar to those of the regimen used in the RTOG study (median PFS: 9.7 vs. 9.4 months), but it was significantly less toxic.

Primarily, the combination of taxane and platinum was assessed in the neoadjuvant setup. The most commonly used paclitaxel (50 mg/m^2) and carboplatin (AUC2, weekly over 5 weeks) were at least as efficient as the combination of platinum and 5-FU [8]; therefore, it is accepted as definitive treatment. In general, definitive chemoradiation is a choice of treatment for those patients who are not suitable for surgery or who do not consent to surgery.

Since distant metastases are present nearly in 75% of patients with locally advanced esophageal cancer, induction chemotherapy prior to chemoradiotherapy would be a rational choice. Usually, patients with locally advanced but resectable esophageal cancer were enrolled in the studies. Since there are no phase III study results, these regimens have not become recommendations. Seventy-two patients participated in the phase II, RTOG 0113 study [9]. The induction treatment included 5-FU (5 × 700 mg/m^2), cisplatin (5 × 15 mg/m^2) and paclitaxel (200 mg/m^2) or cisplatin (75 mg/m^2) and paclitaxel (175 mg/m^2), which was followed by a similar combination (5-FU + paclitaxel or cisplatin + paclitaxel) administered simultaneously with a total radiation dose of 50.4 Gy. Median survival showed no significant differences, and the toxicity was similar in both arms.

Neoadjuvant chemoradiotherapy can be used in those patients who are suitable for surgery. The method of treatment is practically identical to that of the definitive chemoradiotherapy. The aim of the treatment of inoperable patients is palliative, and the aim is to improve the proportion of operability or recovery. The studies frequently yielded contradictory results. However, based on several clinical trials and meta-analyses, neoadjuvant chemoradiotherapy proved to be superior to surgery alone in patients with locally advanced esophageal cancer. A significant survival benefit was found in the CROSS study [10] in which 366 patients with potentially resectable esophageal or gastroesophageal junction cancer were randomized to get either preoperative chemoradiotherapy (50 mg/m^2 paclitaxel a week + carboplatin AUC2, concurrent radiotherapy with a total dose of 41.4 Gy over 5 weeks) or surgery alone. Patients tolerated the combined treatment well. There were no significant differences in mortality or morbidity. The complete resection rate was 92 vs. 69% in favor of the combined treatment, and the complete pathological remission (pCR) ratio was 29% in patients receiving chemoradiotherapy. There was a significant difference in median overall survival (preoperative chemoradiotherapy followed by surgery vs. surgery alone: 49.4 vs. 24.0 months).

In the FFCD 9901 study [11], the efficacy of preoperative chemoradiotherapy was evaluated in patients with small-sized, resectable tumors. 195 patients with stage I or II disease were randomized into the preoperative chemoradiation arm (two cycles of 5-FU at 800 m/m^2 daily at Days 1–4 and 29–32, plus cisplatin at 75 mg/m^2 at Day 1 or Day 2 of the cycle, in both cycles, plus a total dose of 45 Gy concurrent radiation) or the surgery alone arm. During this study with a median follow-up of 93.6 months, there were no significant differences in the 3-year survival. No significant survival benefits were noted in any of the subgroups. Based on these data, the combined treatment may not result in any survival benefit.

Numerous meta-analyses have dealt with the comparison of the effects on survival regarding the trimodal treatment or surgery alone. One of the latest studies was published by Sjoquist and his colleagues [12]. It includes the twelve most significant neoadjuvant chemoradiation studies. The reducing effect of neoadjuvant chemoradiotherapy on mortality proved to be significant, which led to an absolute survival benefit of 8.7% after two years. It was independent of the histologic type of the tumor, and it was not associated with increased perioperative mortality, either.

In addition to the conventional cisplatin + 5-FU therapy, adding paclitaxel to platinum has become more popular lately. Results of ten studies were analyzed in another meta-analysis, and a comparison was made between the efficacy of paclitaxel together with platinum and the efficacy of platinum together with 5-FU. The analysis proved the benefit provided by neoadjuvant chemoradiation therapy over both combinations. The risk of mortality was significantly reduced with both chemotherapy combinations, but the benefit was more pronounced in the taxane arm. However, it was only statistically significant in the case of squamous cell cancer [8]. Some small-sized studies have found the combination of docetaxel and platinum effective [13, 14].

Based on the consequent results of several clinical studies, the response to perioperative treatment, especially the pCR, is an important indicator of better overall survival. Thus, intensification of the perioperative treatment could be a potential approach. Based on the results of 22 studies, survival of those patients who achieved pCR as a result of treatment was 2–3 times longer compared to those patients who had residual cancer in the resection specimen obtained via surgery following neoadjuvant chemoradiotherapy. During the intensification of neoadjuvant treatments, the employments of chemotherapy prior to chemoradiation, as well as the increase of the number of the agents have been studied. According to the INT0123 study, radiation dose intensification resulted in no improvement in either the survival or the local control [15].

Some work was conducted in relation to the non-surgical treatment options of patients with squamous cell carcinoma of the esophagus. Trimodal therapy (chemoradiotherapy followed by surgery) was compared with chemoradiotherapy by Stahl et al. and in the FFCD 9102 study. Stahl et al. [16] enrolled 172 patients. Patients received three cycles of bolus 5-FU, leucovorin, etoposide, cisplatin (FLEP) followed by chemoradiotherapy including a total dose of 40 Gy irradiation and cisplatin and etoposide chemotherapy. Patients then underwent either observation or surgery. In the surgery arm, 62 out of 86 patients underwent surgery. However, there were no significant differences in overall survival. The two-year progression-free survival was more beneficial for those patients who had undergone surgery (64.3 vs. 40.7%). Notably, both the radiation dose and the intensity of chemotherapy were lower than those used in conventional treatments. In the FFCD 9102 study [17], 259 patients with locally advanced, resectable SCC were randomized into two arms following low-dose chemoradiotherapy. If a therapeutic response was noted after the induction treatment, surgery was performed or chemoradiotherapy was completed. No significant differences were found in overall survival between the two treatment groups. However, the 3-month mortality was significantly higher ($p = 0.002$) in the surgery arm (9.3 vs. 0.8%).

Little is known about the results of the nonsurgical treatment of patients with adenocarcinoma. Based on a retrospective analysis of the results of 276 patients treated with definitive chemoradiotherapy for esophageal adenocarcinoma at the university of texas MD Anderson cancer center [18]. After a median follow-up of 54.3 months, 33.3% of the patients never had a relapse. Local relapse was present in 51% of the patients, and distant dissemination was detected in 43.5% of the patients.

There are not enough phase III results in relation to adjuvant chemoradiation. In a retrospective study by Bedard et al. [19], data of 38 patients who had undergone surgery for node-positive esophageal cancer, had received postoperative adjuvant chemoradiation (concurrent or sequential radiation therapy plus cisplatin and 5-FU ± epirubicin) were compared with data of patients who had undergone surgery only. Both the local control and median survival proved to be better in patients receiving adjuvant treatment, and so did overall survival. In another retrospective analysis [20], benefits of adjuvant chemoradiation were evaluated in 304 patients who had undergone surgery for node-positive esophageal squamous cell cancer. Based on the data, both the 5-year overall survival and the disease control proved significantly better in patients who had also received chemotherapy in addition to radiotherapy. According to a prospective study [21] that evaluated chemoradiation vs. chemotherapy and included 45 patients, neither survival benefit nor improved locoregional control was shown in the chemoradiation treatment arm relative to chemotherapy alone (cisplatin + 5-FU over 5 weeks plus 50 Gy of irradiation over 5 weeks vs. cisplatin + 5-FU over 5 weeks).

2.1.1. *Neoadjuvant chemotherapy*

Eight hundred and two patients with either SCC or adenocarcinoma were randomized in the MRC OEO2 study [22]. Patients received either two cycles of cisplatin + 5-FU preoperatively or underwent surgery primarily. The 5-year overall survival was 23 vs. 17% in favor of the neoadjuvant treatment regimen. In Sjoquist's meta-analysis, data of 1981 patients were assessed. Nine neoadjuvant chemotherapies were compared to surgery alone [12]. Chemotherapy reduced mortality in the entire patient population receiving neoadjuvant chemotherapy. It was significant in patients with adenocarcinoma. Based on these, neoadjuvant chemotherapy seems to be superior to surgery alone.

It is unclear whether neoadjuvant chemotherapy can be an alternative to neoadjuvant chemoradiation therapy. Stahl et al. [23] enrolled 119 patients with adenocarcinoma involving the lower third portion of the esophagus or the gastroesophageal junction. In one of the arms, patients received 15 weeks of chemotherapy (cisplatin + leucovorin + continuous 5-FU) followed by surgery. In the other arm, 12 weeks of chemotherapy were followed by concurrent chemoradiation therapy (low-dose radiation therapy and concurrent cisplatin + etoposide) over 3 weeks, and surgery was then performed. The ratio of pCR was significantly higher in the arm that included chemoradiation therapy (2 vs. 15.6%). However, there were no significant differences in median survival and the 3-year overall survival between the two treatment arms. Burmeister et al. [24] received similar results when they evaluated 75 patients with adenocarcinoma. Regarding pCR and R1 resection, chemoradiotherapy was significantly more beneficial, but there were no significant differences in median survival.

Briefly, chemotherapy can be employed as part of chemoradiation, in a neoadjuvant manner, in an adjuvant manner, or as palliation in metastatic disease.

3. Brachytherapy of esophageal cancer

The results in a large cohort of patients indicated that HDR brachytherapy alone was an effective method for the palliation of advanced esophageal cancer [25]. Similar long-term results were reported in favor of treatments involving concurrent chemoradiotherapy followed by HDR brachytherapy [26]. Although brachytherapy was found to be preferable, there are studies (such as Refs. [27, 28]) suggesting the stent placement may play an important role for the palliation of disease. In that case, the prognostic models were used as evidence-based tools in decision making. However, the health-related life quality was reported to be improved in patients treated with the HDR brachytherapy. Recent studies suggested the usage of Californium-252 neutron brachytherapy combined with EBRT for esophageal cancer. The treatment resulted in favorable local control and long-term survival rates with tolerable side effects [29]. Patient selection, timing of brachytherapy and dose specifications were well documented [30–32]. Clinicians continue to urge caution in using brachytherapy treatment techniques since severe toxicity can occur post treatment [15, 26, 30]. Therefore, the addition of brachytherapy, with consequently high surface doses, should be limited to well-selected patients [33].

For that reason, the clinical implementation and accuracy in dose delivery is crucial for favorable treatment outcomes. The radiation dose is delivered using esophageal transoral or transnasal applicators with an external diameter of 0.6–1 cm. Ideally, the single channel applicator needs to be placed centrally in the lumen of the esophagus; however, there exists a possibility that the applicator will be closer to one side of the lumen, delivering a larger dose to the epithelium, lamina propria and muscularis mucosa, resulting in local esophageal complications. In those cases, stricture formation, fistula and esophageal ulceration are the common late toxicities of HDR brachytherapy [34]. A possible difference in the delivered dose is caused by disagreements in the choice of the dose point (i.e. mucosal surface or certain distance from the central line of the applicator) in various institutions, as reported in Ref. [35]. For instance, it was reported in the long-term experience with esophageal brachytherapy treatment [36] that radiation was delivered at a level of 5 mm below the surface of the mucosa. However, no correlation was found between the post-treatment complications and the diameter of the brachytherapy applicator [37]. In most of the HDR brachytherapy treatments, 3D treatment plans were generated using computed tomography (CT) images; however, magnetic resonance imaging (MRI) can be used to assist the localization of the tumor and the applicator [38]. The treatment planning for the esophageal cancer patient is performed using the TG-43 formalism [39], since the dose calculation accuracy of the TPS was confirmed in a homogeneous medium [40].

Overall, this HDR treatment is demonstrated to be well-tolerated and effective for superficial primary and recurrent esophageal cancer in inoperable patients [41, 42]. The authors concluded that dose escalation with larger diameter applicators may allow for improved therapeutic coverage without exceeding the organs ate risk tolerances [43]. The latest research in the combined approach (EBRT and HDR) to palliation in esophageal cancer together with the review of the current techniques is reported in Refs. [44, 45].

3.1. Clinical implementation

To decrease the dose to the organs at risk in the upper gastrointestinal region a novel disposable brachytherapy transoral balloon centering esophageal applicator (BCEA) with five independently inflatable balloons was developed [44]. The complete treatment process for this applicator consisted of three principal steps: pre-treatment preparation, treatment planning and treatment delivery (**Figure 1**). This applicator allows for the central placement of the radioactive source during treatment. The BCEA allows for the treatments outside the balloon region with the constraint where the BCEA becomes similar to the standard esophageal applicator (EA).

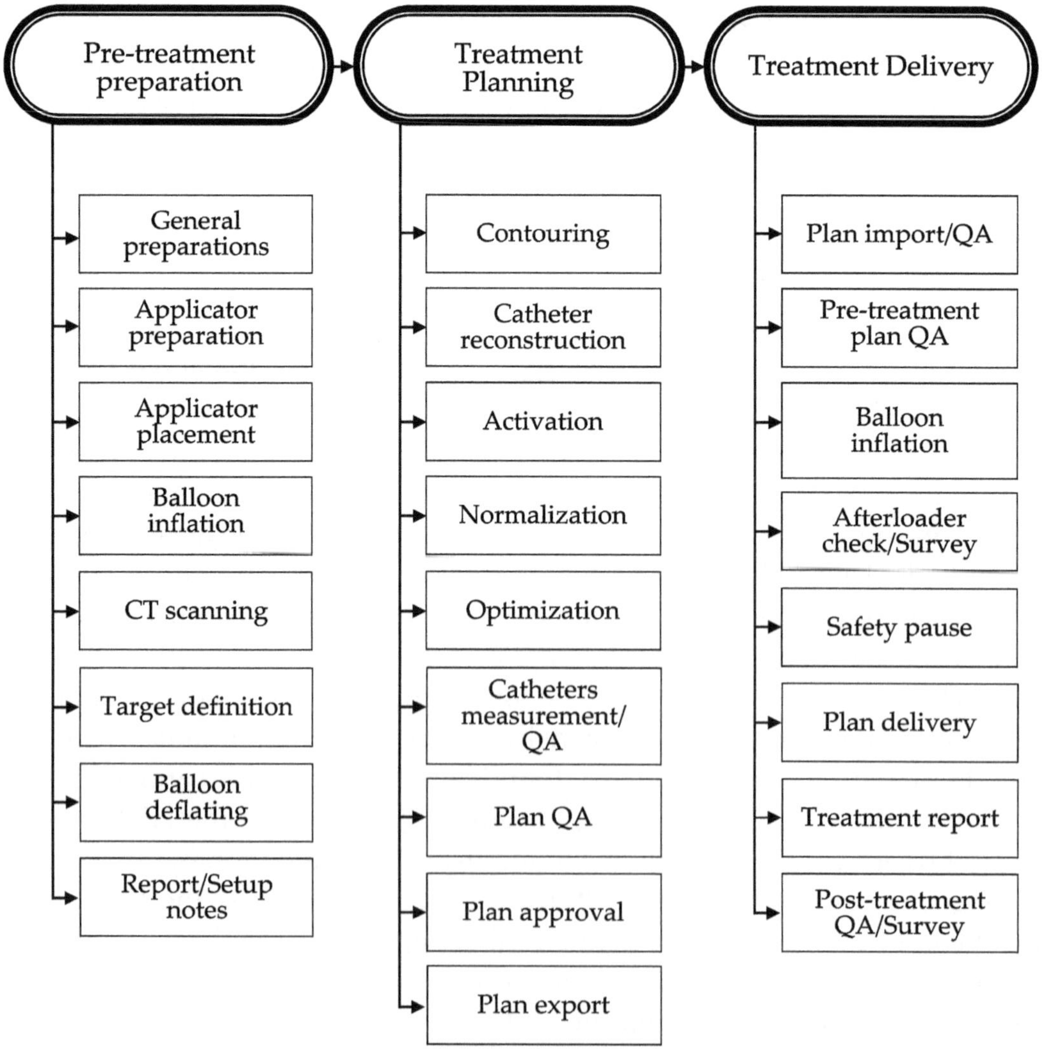

Figure 1. The detailed process map of the treatment was developed for improved treatment plan generation and quality assurance of the process.

The experience in the treatment of esophageal cancer using a standard intraluminal esophageal applicator (EA) was summarized in Ref. [45]. Unlike with the transnasal insertion (EA) where the endoscope would be placed via the anesthetized nose past turbinates and nasopharynx behind the larynx and into the esophagus, the BCEA is placed transorally.

3.2. Treatment planning and delivery

The BCEA positions the catheter centrally when the balloons are inflated. Due to that fact, the treatment plan can be additionally optimized (not the case for the standard EA) for improved dose distribution and conformality. The treatment length was defined as a pretreatment tumor length with 1–2 cm distal and proximal margin determined by pretreatment imaging and confirmed by the CT images.

The prescription dose is usually planned to be delivered to the diameter of 1 cm with respect to the central catheter with an additional optimization to avoid the critical anatomical structures such as the heart, lung, pharyngeal constrictor and spine. The dose calculation is performed using the TG-43 formalism that includes the anisotropy corrections. With the standard EA, the dose point is defined at the mucosal surface or a certain distance from the central line of the applicator with identical dwell times along the treatment length. This was mostly done to minimize the uncertainties in dose delivery related to the positioning of the EA inside the esophagus. In standard approach when EA is used the dose optimization outside the balloon region should be avoided due to the complicated position reproducibility. **Figure 2** shows the differences in the treatment plans between the EA and BCEA.

The centrally placed catheter inside the esophagus lumen resulted in enhanced dose distribution and reproducibility in multi fractional treatment (**Figure 2**). The position of the applicator and the balloon diameters can be verified before the treatments using the planning CT images and the CT images obtained prior to each fraction. Three methods can be used to verify the

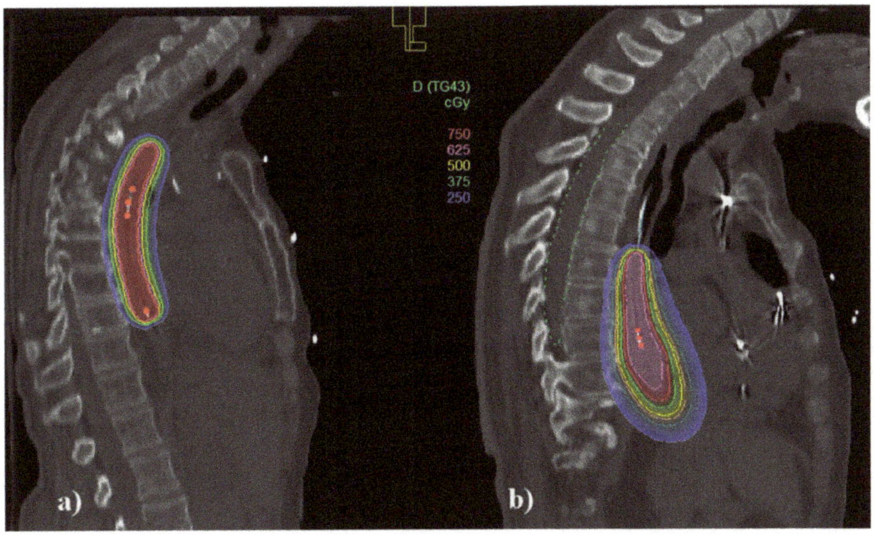

Figure 2. Sagittal images show: (a) the non-optimized plan using the EA and (b) optimized dose distribution achieved with the BCEA.

proper positioning of the BCEA prior to each treatment: (a) using an external marker to verify the length of the catheter in the patient, (b) evaluation of the position of 12 radio-opaque markers on the exterior side of the catheter in the CT images, and (c) measurements of the diameters of the balloons on CT images after inflation to confirm that they were properly inflated.

4. Conclusion

In this chapter, various aspects of esophageal cancers were disused such as histology, predisposing factors and treatment options. It was found that the moderate dose of EBRT and HDR brachytherapy could give a better local response than EBRT alone. Therefore, the brachytherapy of esophageal cancer was elaborated in more detail.

Classically, one of the limitations for the deployment of esophageal brachytherapy has been the difficulties associated with the placement and tolerance of the transnasal applicator [44]. The common adverse effects included significant pain on placement and for the duration of its indwelling. Nasal bleeding, often significant, can be seen from both the scope and catheter placement. There is often the need of significant pain medicine to tolerate this procedure. These effects are pronounced if the applicator is kept in place for an extended period of time.

Long-term toxicities and the correlation between the formation of a fistula or ulceration and the novel design of the BCEA are the topics that can be additionally investigated using the data of more patients treated with the novel BCEA and longer follow-up. Due to the limited number of patients, it is not yet possible to conclude if the patients benefit from the treatment using the centrally placed applicator. Furthermore, due to the provision to additionally optimize the dose, there exists a possibility of dose escalations for certain patients, depending on their anatomy and the spread of disease. The initial implementation of this applicator required strict and careful testing, especially in the determination of the accurate treatment length that would allow the radioactive source to be sent to the most distal position (first dwell position). Multiple tests and an interobserver agreement are required since the inaccurate results of this test can potentially offset the whole treatment, causing adverse events. Therefore, the treatment length and BCEA applicator positioning should be evaluated before each fraction.

Author details

Ivan M. Buzurovic[1*], Borbala Daroczi[2], Desmond A. O'Farrell[1], Mandar S. Bhagwat[1] and Phillip M. Devlin[1]

*Address all correspondence to: ibuzurovic@lroc.harvard.edu

1 Department of Radiation Oncology, Dana-Farber/Brigham and Women's Cancer Center, Harvard Medical School, Boston, MA, USA

2 Department of Radiology, Brigham and Women's Hospital, Harvard Medical School, Boston, MA, USA

References

[1] World Cancer Research Fund International. Oesophageal Cancer Statistics [Internet]. Available from: http://www.wcrf.org/int/cancer-facts-figures/data-specific-cancers/oesophageal-cancer-statistics [Accessed: April 17, 2017]

[2] Mungo B, Molena D, Stem M, Yang SC, Battafarano RJ, Brock MV, Lidor AO. Does neoadjuvant therapy for esophageal cancer increase postoperative morbidity or mortality? Diseases of the Esophagus. 2015;**28**(7):644-651

[3] The National Comprehensive Cancer Network. NCCN Clinical Practice Guidelines in Oncology: Esophageal Cancer [Internet]. Available from: www.nccn.org/professionals/physician_gls/pdf/esophageal.pdf [Accessed: April 17, 2017]

[4] European Society for Medical Oncology. Oesophageal Cancer: ESMO Clinical Practice Guidelines [Internet]. Available from: www.esmo.org/Guidelines/Gastrointestinal-Cancers/Oesophageal-Cancer [Accessed: April 17, 2017]

[5] Nygaard K, Hagen S, Hansen HS, Hatlevoll R, Hultborn, R, Jakobsen A, Mäntyla M, Modig H, Munck-Wikland E, Rosengren B, Tausjø J. Pre-operative radiotherapy prolongs survival in operable esophageal carcinoma: A randomized, multicenter study of pre-operative radiotherapy and chemotherapy. The second Scandinavian trial in esophageal cancer. World Journal of Surgery. 1992;**16**(6):1104-1109

[6] Herskovic A, Martz K, Al-Sarraf M, Leichman L, Brindle J, Vaitkevicius V, Cooper J, Byhardt R, Davis L, Emami B. Combined chemotherapy and radiotherapy compared with radiotherapy alone in patients with cancer of the esophagus. New England Journal of Medicine. 1992;**326**(24):1593-1598

[7] Conroy T, Galais MP, Raoul JL, Bouché O, Gourgou-Bourgade S, Douillard JY, Etienne PL, Boige V, Martel-Lafay I, Michel P, Llacer-Moscardo C. Definitive chemoradiotherapy with FOLFOX versus fluorouracil and cisplatin in patients with oesophageal cancer (PRODIGE5/ACCORD17): Final results of a randomised, phase 2/3 trial. The Lancet Oncology. 2014;**15**(3):305-314

[8] Huang TC, Hsu CH, Lin CC, Tu YK. Systematic review and network meta-analysis: Neoadjuvant chemoradiotherapy for locoregional esophageal cancer. Japanese Journal of Clinical Oncology. 2015;**45**:1023-1028

[9] Ajani A, Winter K, Komaki R, Kelsen DP, Minsky BD, Liao Z, Bradley J, Fromm M, Hornback D, Willett CG. Phase II randomized trial of two nonoperative regimens of induction chemotherapy followed by chemoradiation in patients with localized carcinoma of the esophagus: RTOG 0113. Journal of Clinical Oncology. 2008;**26**(28):4551-4556

[10] van Hagen P, Hulshof MC, Van Lanschot JJB, Steyerberg EW, Henegouwen MVB, Wijnhoven BPL, Richel DJ, Nieuwenhuijzen GAP, Hospers GAP, Bonenkamp JJ, Cuesta MA. Preoperative chemoradiotherapy for esophageal or junctional cancer. New England Journal of Medicine. 2012;**366**(22):2074-2084

[11] Mariette C, Dahan L, Mornex F, Maillard E, Thomas PA, Meunier B, Boige V, Pezet D, Robb WB, Le Brun-Ly V, Bosset JF. Surgery alone versus chemoradiotherapy followed by surgery for stage I and II esophageal cancer: Final analysis of randomized controlled phase III trial FFCD 9901. Journal of Clinical Oncology. 2014;**32**(23):2416-2422

[12] Sjoquist KM, Burmeister BH, Smithers BM, Zalcberg JR, Simes RJ, Barbour A, Gebski V, and Australasian Gastro-Intestinal Trials Group. Survival after neoadjuvant chemotherapy or chemoradiotherapy for resectable oesophageal carcinoma: An updated meta-analysis. The Lancet Oncology. 2011;**12**(7):681-692

[13] Li QQ, Liu MZ, Hu YH, Liu H, He ZY, Lin HX. Definitive concomitant chemoradiotherapy with docetaxel and cisplatin in squamous esophageal carcinoma. Diseases of the Esophagus. 2010;**23**(3):253-259

[14] Ma HB, Di ZL, Wen J, Ke Y, Sun X, Ren J. Prospective, open, multicentre Phase I/II trial to assess safety and efficacy of neoadjuvant radiochemotherapy with docetaxel and cisplatin for esophageal carcinoma. Japanese Journal of Clinical Oncology. 2015;**45**(2):169-175

[15] Minsky BD, Pajak TF, Ginsberg RJ, Pisansky TM, Martenson J, Komaki R, Okawara G, Rosenthal SA, Kelsen DP. INT 0123 (Radiation Therapy Oncology Group 94-05) phase III trial of combined-modality therapy for esophageal cancer: High-dose versus standard-dose radiation therapy. Journal of Clinical Oncology. 2002;**20**(5):1167-1174

[16] Stahl M, Stuschke M, Lehmann N, Meyer HJ, Walz MK, Seeber S, Klump B, Budach W, Teichmann R, Schmitt M, Schmitt G. Chemoradiation with and without surgery in patients with locally advanced squamous cell carcinoma of the esophagus. Journal of Clinical Oncology. 2005;**23**(10):2310-2317

[17] Bedenne L, Michel P, Bouché O, Milan C, Mariette C, Conroy T, Pezet D, Roullet B, Seitz JF, Herr JP, Paillot B. Chemoradiation followed by surgery compared with chemoradiation alone in squamous cancer of the esophagus: FFCD 9102. Journal of Clinical Oncology. 2007;**25**(10):1160-1168

[18] Sudo K, Xiao L, Wadhwa R, Shiozaki H, Elimova E, Taketa T, Blum MA, Lee JH, Bhutani MS, Weston B, Ross WA. Importance of surveillance and success of salvage strategies after definitive chemoradiation in patients with esophageal cancer. Journal of Clinical Oncology. 2014;**32**(30):3400-3405

[19] Bedard EL, Inculet RI, Malthaner RA, Brecevic E, Vincent M, Dar R. The role of surgery and postoperative chemoradiation therapy in patients with lymph node positive esophageal carcinoma. Cancer. 2001;**91**(12):2423-2430

[20] Chen J, Pan J, Liu J, Li J, Zhu K, Zheng X, Chen M, Chen M, Liao Z. Postoperative radiation therapy with or without concurrent chemotherapy for node-positive thoracic esophageal squamous cell carcinoma. International Journal of Radiation Oncology Biology Physics. 2013;**86**(4):671-677

[21] Tachibana M, Yoshimura H, Kinugasa S, Shibakita M, Dhar DK, Ueda S, Fujii T, Nagasue N. Postoperative chemotherapy vs. chemoradiotherapy for thoracic esophageal cancer:

A prospective randomized clinical trial. European Journal of Surgical Oncology. 2003;**29**(7):580-587

[22] Swisher SG, Hofstetter W, Komaki R, Correa AM, Erasmus J, Lee JH, Liao Z, Maru D, Mehran R, Patel S, Rice DC. Improved long-term outcome with chemoradiotherapy strategies in esophageal cancer. The Annals of Thoracic Surgery. 2010;**90**(3):892-899

[23] Stahl M, Walz MK, Stuschke M, Lehmann N, Meyer HJ, Riera-Knorrenschild J, Langer P, Engenhart-Cabillic R, Bitzer M, Königsrainer A, Budach W. Phase III comparison of preoperative chemotherapy compared with chemoradiotherapy in patients with locally advanced adenocarcinoma of the esophagogastric junction. Journal of Clinical Oncology. 2009;**27**(6):851-856

[24] Burmeister BH, Thomas JM, Burmeister EA, Walpole ET, Harvey JA, Thomson DB, Barbour AP, Gotley DC, Smithers BM. Is concurrent radiation therapy required in patients receiving preoperative chemotherapy for adenocarcinoma of the oesophagus? A randomised phase II trial. European Journal of Cancer.2011;**47**(3):354-360

[25] Sur RK, Levin CV, Donde B et al. Prospective randomized trial of HDR brachytherapy as a sole modality in palliation of advanced esophageal carcinoma—An International Atomic Energy Agency study. International Journal of Radiation Oncology Biology Physics. 2002;**53**(1):127-133

[26] Yorozu A, Toya K, Dokiya T. Long-term results of concurrent chemoradiotherapy followed by high dose rate brachytherapy for T2-3 N0-1 M0 esophageal carcinoma. Esophagus. 2006;**3**(1):1-5

[27] Steyerberg EW, Homs MY, Stokvis A et al. SIREC Study Group. Stent placement or brachytherapy for palliation of dysphagia from esophageal cancer: A prognostic model to guide treatment selection. Gastrointestinal endoscopy. 2005;**62**(3):333-340

[28] Bergquist H, Wenger U, Johnsson E et al. Stent insertion or endoluminal brachytherapy as palliation of patients with advanced cancer of the esophagus and gastroesophageal junction. Results of a randomized controlled clinical trial. Diseases of the Esophagus. 2005;**18**(3):131-139

[29] Liu H, Wang Q, Wan X et al. Californium-252 neutron brachytherapy combined with external beam radiotherapy for esophageal cancer: Long-term treatment results. Brachytherapy. 2014;**13**(5):514-521

[30] Gaspar LE, Nag S, Herskovic A et al. Clinical Research Committee. American Brachytherapy Society (ABS) consensus guidelines for brachytherapy of esophageal cancer. International Journal of Radiation Oncology Biology Physics. 1997;**38**(1):127-132

[31] Gaspar LE. Radiation therapy for esophageal cancer: Improving the therapeutic ratio. Seminars in Radiation Oncology. 1994;**4**(1):192-201

[32] Gaspar LE, Winter K, Kocha WI et al. A phase I/II study of external beam radiation, brachytherapy, and concurrent chemotherapy for patients with localized carcinoma of the esophagus (Radiation Therapy Oncology Group Study 9207). Cancer. 2000;**88**(5):988-995

[33] Muijs CT, Beukema JC, Mul VE et al. External beam radiotherapy combined with intraluminal brachytherapy in esophageal carcinoma. Radiotherapy and Oncology. 2012;**102**(2):303-308

[34] Chauhan A, Kaur P, Annex E. Radical external beam radiotherapy with intraluminal high rate dose brachytherapy in patients with carcinoma esophagus. The International Journal of Gastroenterology. 2009;**8**(1):1-7

[35] Okawa T, Dokiya T, Nishio M et al. Multi-institutional randomized trial of external radiotherapy with and without intraluminal brachytherapy for esophageal cancer in Japan. International Journal of Radiation Oncology Biology Physics. 1999;**45**(3):623-628

[36] Gaspar LE, Qian C, Kocha WI et al. A phase III study of external beam radiation, brachytherapy and concurrent chemotherapy in localized cancer of the esophagus (RTOG 92-07): Preliminary toxicity report. International Journal of Radiation Oncology Biology Physics. 1997;**37**(3):593-599

[37] Hishikawa Y, Kurisu K, Taniguchi M et al. High-dose-rate intraluminal brachytherapy for esophageal cancer: 10 years experience in Hyogo College of Medicine. Radiotherapy and Oncology. 1991;**21**(2):107-114

[38] Prott FJ, Pötter R, Kovacs G et al. Magnetic resonance imaging assisted localization of tumor and applicator for brachytherapy of cancer of the esophagus. Tumor Response Monitoring and Treatment Planning. 1992;**1**:607-612

[39] Rivard MJ, Coursey BM, DeWerd LA et al. Update of AAPM Task Group No. 43 Report: A revised AAPM protocol for brachytherapy dose calculations. Medical Physics. 2004;**31**(3):633-674

[40] Uniyal SC, Sharma SD, Naithani UC. Dosimetric verification of a high dose rate brachytherapy treatment planning system in homogeneous and heterogeneous media. Physica Medica. 2013;**29**(2):171-177

[41] Folkert MR, Cohen GM, Wu AJ et al. Endoluminal high-dose-rate brachytherapy for early stage and recurrent esophageal cancer in medically inoperable patients. Brachytherapy. 2013;**12**(5):463-470

[42] Bhatt L, Tirmazy S, Sothi S. Intraluminal high dose rate brachytherapy for palliation of dysphagia in cancer of the esophagus: Initial experience at a single UK center. Diseases of the Esophagus. 2013;**26**(1):57-60

[43] Laskar SG, Lewis S, Agarwal JP, Mishra S, Mehta S, Patil P. Combined brachytherapy and external beam radiation: An effective approach for palliation in esophageal cancer. Journal of Contemporary Brachytherapy. 2015;**6**:453-461

[44] Buzurovic IM, Hansen JL, Bhagwat MS, O'Farrell DA, Friesen S, Harris TC, Damato AL, Cormack RA, Martin NE, Devlin PM. Clinical implementation of a novel applicator in high-dose-rate brachytherapy treatment of esophageal cancer. Journal of Contemporary Brachytherapy. 2016;**8**(4):319-325

[45] Stewart AJ, Tselis N, Albert M et al. Gastrointestinal brachytherapy. In: Brachytherapy: Applications and Techniques. Springer Publishing Company, New York, NY, USA; 2015. pp. 319-354

2

Prescription of Proton Pump Inhibitors in Elderly Subjects in Real Life: A Retrospective Study in a Gastroenterology Department

Mona Boudabous, Héla Gdoura, Leila Mnif, Lassad Chtourou, Amal Grati, Ali Amouri and Nabil Tahri

Abstract

The proton-pump inhibitor (PPI) is an effective and widely used treatment but may cause side effects, especially for the elderly. Materials and methods: this is a cross-sectional study including 45 patients older than 65 years, followed at our outpatient and treated with PPIs for at least a year. The indication for PPI, the results of any endoscopy, and the quality of the tolerance of these molecules is specified by the data folder. During the consultation, we conducted an interrogation to an update of the history and medications to our patients and a type checking of the molecule, the dose, and the quality of the observance. Results: patients were divided into 32 women and 13 men with a mean age of 75 ± 7 years (65–92). The average length of PPI use was 6 ± 4 years (1–16) with a consumption of a double dose for at least 1 year in 28.8% of cases. The prescribed dose was higher than the recommended dose in at least 15.5% of cases. PPIs were well tolerated. One patient had presented a microscopic colitis, revealed by diarrhea regressed after discontinuation of PPIs. Conclusion: PPIs were prescribed in elderly subjects by gastroenterologists, in a university center, with a high dose and long. In our series, this treatment is well tolerated in the elderly.

Keywords: aged person, drug interactions, drug-related side effects, drug utilization, proton pump inhibitors

1. Introduction

Proton pump inhibitors (PPI) constitute a very effective and used treatment at present [1–3]. Previously, they would seem to cause undesirable effects and medicinal interactions probably serious and badly known, especially for the elderly person often fragile and exposed to a polypharmacy [4]. On the other hand, it is a very expensive therapeutic class and frequently used in an inappropriate way [2–4]. In Tunisia, the use of these medicines to the old subject, in the public structures, by specialists, was not studied. So, we have led this study to realize an evaluation of the professional practices concerning the prescription of these molecules, by gastroenterologists, in a teaching hospital (CHU) of the Tunisian South, to the geriatric population.

The objectives of our study were:

1. Specify the main indications and the modalities of the long-term prescription of the PPI to the old subjects and compare them with the international recommendations.
2. Evaluate the observance, the tolerance, and the possible medicinal interactions of the prescribed PPI in the long term to the elderly subjects.
3. Specify, through our results and review of the literature, the difficulties were met and the risks incurred during the prescription of these medicines to the elderly and proposed strategies to overcome them in our current practice.

2. Material and methods

It was about a retrospective study including 45 subjects of more than 65 years old followed in the external consultation of the gastroenterology department of Hédi Chaker hospital of Sfax, having consulting between July 01st, 2015 and December 31st, 2015. The PPI indication, the results of a possible initial endoscopic exploration, and their tolerance were specified by the data of the file. During the consultation, we realized an interrogation with the aim of checking the molecule's type, the dose, and the quality of the PPI observance. The criteria of inclusion were as follows: an upper age or equal to 65-year-old during the beginning of PPI treatment and PPI consumption at least three times a week during a duration of more than 12 months. The criteria of noninclusion were represented by the absence of an exhaustive list of the personal histories of patients and their medicines. The evaluation of the best use of the PPI was realized by referring to the current recommendations of the High Authority of Health and the French Agency of sanitary safety of the products of health (Afssaps) in 2007 [5]. The data were analyzed by using the statistical software SPSS 20.0.

3. Results

The average age of our patients was of ±75 7 years (65–92). About 1/3 of the patients were less than 70 years old (**Figure 1**). In our study, a clear feminine predominance was noted with a sex ratio H/F of 0.4 (**Figure 2**). The majority of our patients were of urban origin (60%) (**Figure 3**). The distribution of the patients according to antecedent is specified as in **Table 1**. Excepting the pathology that justifies the PPI use, 25 patients (55.4%) had at least 3 medical antecedent with a daily average number of medicine consumption of 4.8 ± 4.3 (0–17). Six patients had osteoporosis, diagnosed before the establishment of the PPI in a case and after the establishment of the PPI in the five remaining cases. The average deadline separating the beginning of taking the PPI and the discovery of the osteoporosis was of 2.5 years (1–4). No control of the bone densitometry was asked during the follow-up of our patients who have a normal initial examination. Two patients (4.4%), with antecedent of ischemic heart disorder with angioplasty, were treated by clopidogrel (Plavix®) neither with any precaution's closed view to the type of the molecule nor with the schedule of taking PPI. During our interview, we recommended them to keep an interval of 12 hours between the consumption of the PPI and that of the clopidogrel. The main indication of the PPI at our patients was the gastroesophageal reflux (GER) (75.6%) (**Figure 4**). Before the prescription of the PPI, 41 patients (91%) underwent upper digestive endoscopy FOGD. The results of this examination were dominated by the association of a peptic esophagitis and a hiatal hernia (**Table 2**). Among the four remaining patients:

- The FOGD was refused by two patients having abdominal pain
- The FOGD was made after a deadline of using of the PPI (2 years and 6 months respectively) in two patients having typical clinical signs of GER.

Five patients having a normal FOGD had:

- Typical symptoms of GER in three cases
- Abdominal pain in a case
- A long-term treatment by nonsteroidal anti-inflammatory drug (NSAID) in a case.

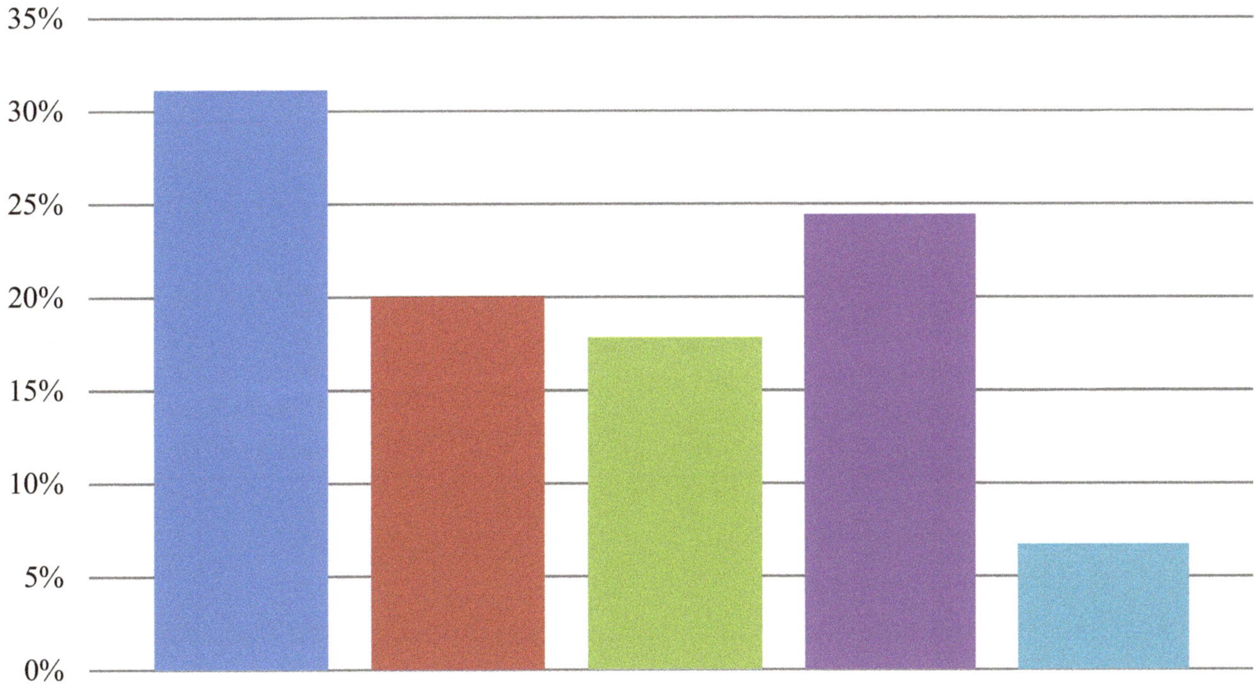

Figure 1. Dividing patients according to the age.

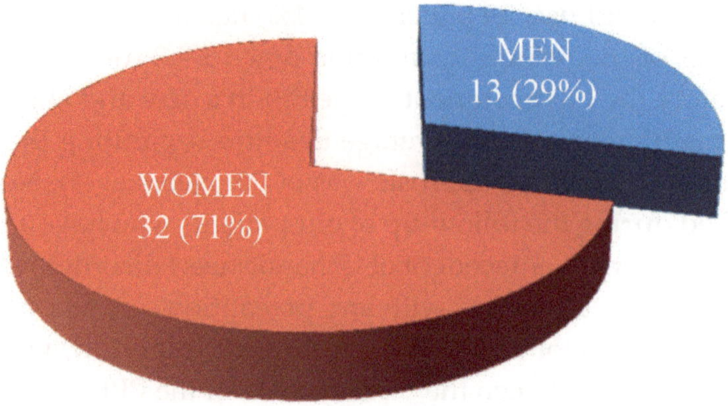

Figure 2. Dividing patients according to sex.

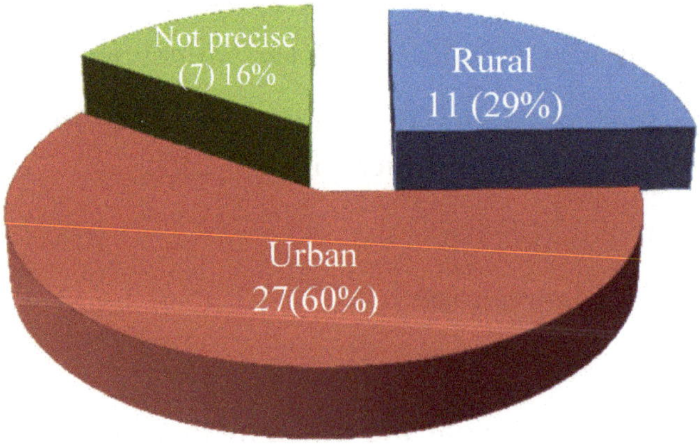

Figure 3. Dividing patients according to their geographic origin.

Antecedents	N (%)
HTA	24 (53.3)
Rheumatologic pathology	16 (35.6)
Dyslipidemia	11 (24.4)
Heart disease	9 (20)
Diabetes	8 (17.7)
Osteoporosis	6 (13.3)
Anemia	2 (4.4)

Table 1. Dividing patients according to antecedents.

The FOGD data at five patients who had abdominal pain motivating the endoscopy were the following ones:

- A bulbar ulcer in one patient
- Bulbar ulcerations in one patient

- Ulcerated antral gastropathy associated with a bulbar ulcer in one patient
- A congestive gastropathy in one patient
- Normal FOGD in one patient

Gastric biopsies were realized in all the patients who had a bulbar ulcer or bulbar ulcerations. These biopsies were concluded with the absence of the helicobacter pylori in all cases. It was probably caused by the intermittent consumption of AINS in these patients. During the follow-up, only three patients had undergone an endoscopic control, having two peptic stenosis and one Barrett esophagus (BO). It revealed the disappearance of the stenosis in both patients and the absence of dysplasia in the third.

During the period of study (in July 01st, 2015–December 31st, 2015), the PPI availability in the pharmacy of the hospital and in the health centers was omeprazole in the form of 20 mg capsules. Concerning the years preceding the study's period, the molecules availability in the hospital list were either the omeprazole in the form of tablets or 20 mg capsules, or the lansoprazole in the form of 30 mg capsules.

However, these medicines were not always available in this pharmacy and\or in the pharmacies of health centers (frequent breaks of the stock). As a result, some patients would have used other molecules, which they had bought from nearby pharmacies. The interrogation of the patients and their parents was not able to specify the type of these molecules. The average duration of the PPI treatment was of 6 ± 4 years (1–16) with a duration of more than 2 years in 34 cases (75.6%). The PPI was prescribed at the rate of a simple daily dose for 29 patients (64.4%) and of a double daily dose for 5 patients (11.1%). For the rest of the patients, the treatment was prescribed:

- At first, in simple daily dose, during an average duration of 39.1 months (2–96) and then in double daily dose for 9 patients (20%) during an average duration of 4.5 years (1–10).
- At first in double daily dose and then in simple daily dose for two patients (4.4%). The duration of taking the simple dose was of 2 months for a patient and 9 months for the second and that of the double dose was of 6 years and 18 months respectively.

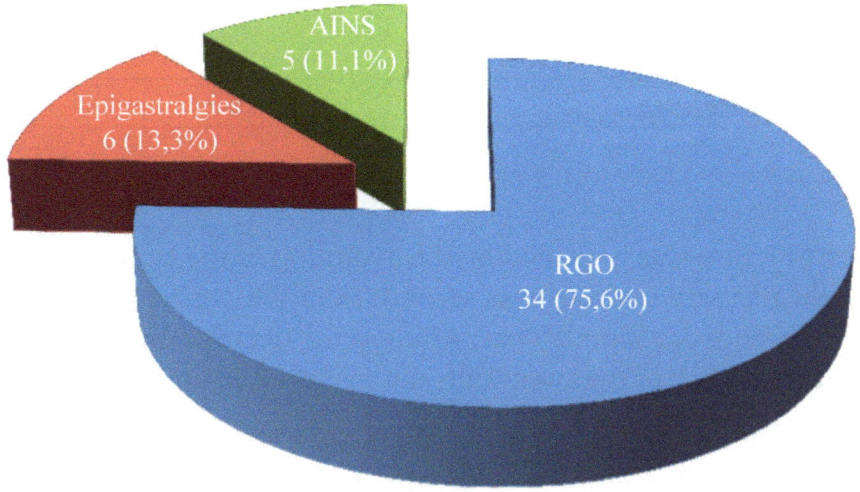

Figure 4. Dividing patients according to PPI indications.

Localization and types of lesions	N (%)
Isolated esophageal lesions	8 (19.5)
Peptic esophagitis OP	4
Peptic stenosis	2
Mycosic esophagitis	1
Barrett esophagus	1
HH/G isolated	1 (2.4)
OP + HH	10 (24.4)
Isolated gastric lesions:	7 (17.1)
Congestive antral gastropathy	3
Ulcerated antral gastropathy	2
Nodular antral gastropathy	1
Pyloric big folds	1
Isolated duodenal infringement:	2 (4.9)
UB	1
Bulbar ulcerations	1
Multiple locations of the lesions:	8 (19.5)
HH + congestive antral gastropathy + bulbar ulcer	1
OP + HH+ bulbar ulcerations	2
OP + HH+ congestive antral gastropathy	1
OP + bulbar ulcerations	1
Ulcerated antral gastropathy + UB	2
HH + bulbar ulcerations	1
FOGD normal	5 (12.2)
Total	41 (100)

OP: peptic esophagitis; HH: hiatal hernia.

Table 2. Dividing patients according to the data of initial FOGD.

The change of the PPI dose was indicated by the evolution of the symptoms motivating their prescription. So, the increase in doses was secondary in the persistence of the symptoms in spite of a good observance of a simple dose, whereas the decrease in doses was motivated by the decrease in the frequency of the symptoms under a double dose of treatment.

The characteristics of seven patients treated straightaway by an PPI double dose are detailed in **Table 3**. The recommendations of the HAS were not respected within the frameworks of:

- The indication of the FOGD in four cases (9%): because of the absence of realizing an FOGD before prescribing the PPI for four patients having abdominal pain or symptoms of GER with an age > 60 years.
- The PPI indication in two other cases (4.4%): having a prescription of the PPI in front of abdominal pain with a normal FOGD, for one case and a congestive gastropathy in another case, without prescribing long-term AINS in two cases. These two situations do not establish an indication for a treatment by a PPI according to the HAS recommendations.
- the PPI posology:
  - Seven cases (15.5%) were treated straightaway by an PPI double dose. Indeed, according to the HAS recommendations, the interest of a double dose was not even demonstrated in RGO case with a severe esophagitis (except in not healing case and subject to a good observance of the treatment, where an increase in the posology can be proposed). So, no indication, among those of our patients, justifies an IPP treatment with one double dose straightaway. For the other cases, it was difficult to judge the concordance of posology with the recommendations against the difficulties of specifying the molecule's type of the prescribed IPP (omeprazole or lansoprazole), because the recommended posology, within the framework of our study's indications, is the full dose (or simple dose) for the omeprazole and the half-dose for the other molecules. The average duration of using PPI with our patients was of 6 ± 4 years (1–16). During the follow-up of our patients, the evaluation of PPI tolerance and the efficiency of the PPI, realized every 6 months, were based on anamneses data without any complementary examination. Furthermore, updating the antecedent list and the patients' treatments was not realized in a systematic way at every consultation. Among our patients, 31 (75.6%) had a good observance for the PPI. The nonavailability of the PPI in the public sanitary structures was the cause of the limited observance.

No.	Age (years)	Sex	Indication of the IPP	Duration of the DD of the PPI (months)	Endoscopic data
1	72	F	Abdominal pain	12	Congestive antral gastropathy
2	84	M	+ NSAID GER	2	Ulcerated antral gastropathy
3	76	F	Abdominal pain	9	+ bulbar ulcer
4	78	F	GER	60	Congestive antral gastropathy
5	82	M	GER	48	HH/G, OP type 2
6	78	F	GER	24	Peptic stenosis
7	68	M	GER	12	Normal

HH: hiatal hernia, GER: gastroesophageal reflux, NSAID: regular consumption of non steroidal anti inflammatory drugs
OP type 2: peptic esophagitis type 2.

Table 3. Characteristics of patients treated by double dose (DD) of PPI.

The PPI did not cause any symptoms in 44 patients (97.7%). The remaining patients were presented after the consumption of lansoprazole double dose during 1 year (in front of a refractory GER) with profuse diarrhea. The colonoscopy revealed a normal colonic mucous membrane, but the colonic biopsies had revealed a microscopic colitis of colitis collagen type. Stopping the use of PPI has entrained the disappearance of the diarrhea. Because of the absence of treating the GER by famotidine in the dose of 40 mg/d, the patient was treated by the omeprazole in the dose of 20 mg/d). A few days after the beginning of the treatment, the evolution was marked by the reappearance of the diarrhea. So, the PPI was stopped. For the GER treatment, the patient was treated by a double dose of famotidine associated with the sodium alginate with a satisfying control of symptoms without diarrhea.

4. Discussion

The PPI are an expensive medicinal class and widely prescribed in the world. Indeed, they represented more than 16 million of prescriptions in France in 2008 and about 101 million prescriptions in the United States in 2006 [5, 7]. A recent study, led in Denmark, has revealed a greater increase in the prescription of the PPI during the last decade [8]. In Tunisia, the PPI prescription was not evaluated on the national scale, but the development of several generic medicines since 2013 (10 for omeprazole, 6 for esomeprazole, 4 for lansoprazole, and 1 for pantoprazole) suggests an increasing in the prescription during these last years [9].

The overuse of the PPI is a notorious problem in the world. Numerous studies were interested in the evaluation of the good use of this therapeutic class by basing itself on the recommendations. In the United States, in 2007, a study showed that 54% of the prescriptions of IPP were not adapted [10]. In France, a report from the accounts commission of the Social Security in October, 2009 reported that 15% of the IPP would prescribe out the planned indications. According to this report, 65% of the IPP prescriptions for GER in 2008 were concerned with patients more than 65 years old [11]. Furthermore, in retirement homes, this medicinal class was prescribed for the old subjects in 21.8–37.8% of cases according to the studies [3, 12] However, few studies were interested in the harmlessness of the PPI in the long term, and particularly to the elderly [13].

In spite of its retrospective and monocentric character, with a limited number of patients and impossibility to study the effect of every PPI molecule alone, this study has allowed us to evaluate, for the first time in Tunisia, the tolerance of these medicines, in short and medium terms, as well as the current modalities of their prescription, to old subjects, by gastroenterologists, in a Tunisian CHU.

In our study, the PPI indications were not in agreement with the recommendations in 4.4% of the cases. This percentage was lower than that found in a study led in an American urban geriatric university health center, which was 29% [2]. This fact could be related to the more limited number of patients in our study (45 vs. 100 in the American study) and to the use of different recommendations concerning the good use of the PPI.

Concerning the PPI dose prescribed in our study, it was higher than the dose recommended in at least 15.5% of the cases. This fact could be partially explained by the unavailability, in our public sanitary structures, of some PPI molecule dosages (such as tablets or capsules of lansoprazole of 15 mg), which could impose to the prescriber an increase in doses, because of the economic problems of patients who cannot get themselves treated on their own responsibility in the private pharmacies. However, the increase in the PPI doses was found in a prospective French study evaluating the practices in general medicine to the patients of 75 years old and more, where the full dose represented 53% of the prescriptions in prevention of the gastroduodenal lesions or for the EGR without esophagitis, whereas the recommended dose, in these indications, was half of the dose [14].

In our study, the duration of the prescribed PPI was more than 2 years in 34 cases (75.6%). This result was found in another study where two-third of the old subjects was treated by PPI during more than 2 years [14]. However, the indications of the extended treatment by IPP are limited in the symptomatic periods of EGR or in case of treatment by long-term AINS after 65 years, or in case of a bulbar ulcer Hp (−). This prolonged duration was related to a strong adherence of the patients who felt a bounce effect of the symptoms while stopping the PPI and insisting by consequence on extending the prescription in near the prescribers.

According to our study, the PPI was tolerated well, during an average follow-up of 6 years, with a single unwanted effect (2.3%), a type of diarrhea was related to a microscopic colitis. The well-tolerated character of PPI with long term, to the elderly, was found in other studies [15]. In a study, a type of case witness, by comparing old subjects treated by PPI versus others without PPI, the diarrhea was independently related to the PPI use with an odds ratio of 1.60 [1.20–2.15] [12]. The PPI incrimination in the induction of microscopic colitis is also well documented in the literature with an odds ratio of 6.4 for the collagenous colitis [16]. Other potential unwanted effects of the PPI were described in the literature, in particularly the elderly, such as:

- The consequences of the malabsorption: hyponatremia [17, 18], deficiency in vitamin B12 [19] and hypomagnesemia [20, 21] (which could have serious consequences such as confusion [22, 23])
- The infections, particularly, the bacterial pneumopathies [24] and the intestinal infections, especially to *Clostridium difficilae* [25]
- Osteoporotic fractures [26, 27]
- On the other hand, medicines decreasing the acid gastric secretion such as the long-term PPI would be theoretically capable of leading the genesis of gastric tumors, and even colorectal; in fact, the hypergastrinemia is led by these treatments [28, 29].

In our study, six patients (13.3%) had an osteoporosis without arisen pathological fracture during the follow-up. The PPI incrimination in the genesis of this disease cannot be realized in this study, caused by the absence of a comparison with a witness group, especially that the osteoporosis is frequent in the Tunisian old subject with 23.4% prevalence in Tunisian woman aged more than 50 years old [30]. No control of the densitometry bone and no supplementation by the association vitamin D + calcium were realized during the follow-up of our patients. This decision could be explained by the controversial character of the results of the studies. Indeed, several observational studies and meta-analyses evaluated the PPI effect, alone or in association with biphosphonates, concerning the risk of fractures. In these studies, the PPI use was associated with a higher risk of pathological fractures (particularly of the hip and the vertebras) favored by an osteoporosis, but the association strength was low most of the time. The PPI impact would be higher in case of a good adhesion to high daily doses [31]. In fact, the role of the multiple confusing factors (represented by the age, the female, body mass indexes, the alcoholism, the smoking, the antecedent of falls or previous fractures, the neurological and hematological diseases and the use of antidepression, anxiolytics, antipsychotics, antiepileptics, diuretics, and antidiabetics) could explain the weak character of this association. Moreover, Kaye et al. showed the absence of PPI association at a higher risk of pathological fractures, to a population of 1098 patients having no risk factor of osteoporosis [32]. Also, the supervision results in the long-term tolerance of treated patients by PPI, within the framework of two clinical trials (followed forward looking until 12 years), and hazardous pathological fractures [33] did not appear. Finally, only 1–5% of fractures on osteoprotic bone would be attributed for the PPI use [31].

So, in the United States, the administration of food and medicine (FDA) considered the low clinical impact, neither justifying a calcium supplementation nor a regular supervision of the osseous density [34]. The mechanisms at the origin of changing of the osseous density by PPI are represented by the decrease in the ionization and the absorption of the calcium and the inhibition of the osteoclastic activity, compulsory for the norm progress of the physiological osseous reshaping [13]. Concerning hypomagnesemia risk, no patient in our study benefited from a magnesium plasmatic dosage. This attitude is debated in the literature, due to the absence of a forward-looking study with a long-term follow-up. However, in 2012, after a literature review, Hess et al. recommended a dosage of magnesemia plasmatic rate before the introduction of an PPI long-term treatment, particularly with the patients treated with other hypomagnesemiants medicine (such as the digoxine, the diuretics), with a regular follow-up. In case of discovering a hypomagnesemia, these authors recommended a stop of PPI with an addition of calcium and magnesium [35]. In this case, according to these authors, the substitution of the PPI by the anti- histaminic receptor (anti-H2), which does not lead to a hypomagnesemia risk, could not be recommended. If the symptoms related to the hypersecretion acid were not controlled by the anti-H2, occasional cures by PPI can be prescribed by a biological supervision [35]. In front of the potentially serious complications of the hypomagnesemie, especially with elderly (vomiting, diarrhea, hypokalemia, hypocalcemia, muscular tetanizes, rhythm disorders, the extension of the interval QT, the convulsions, the confusion) and through the frequent undesirable effects, which is considered rare if the PPI was prescribed by recommended doses, the FDA recommended a magnesemia dosage before the introduction of a PPI treatment:

- If the treatment duration would be extended.
- Or in case of association with other hypomagnesemiants medicine.

A regular supervision of the magnesemia was also recommended by the FDA in the quoted situations, without specifying the monitoring methods [34]. In a recent literature review, besides the authors had recommended this conduct to the elderly or those having chronic diseases (diabetics, kidney insufficiency, or having a cardiovascular pathology) [31].

No patient of our series presented an intestinal or lung infection during the follow-up, but the retrospective character of our study does not eliminate this fact, because the patients could forget or neglect to mention these infections to the consultant physician of the IPP, during the various consultations. The PPI was different in the increase of infectious risk that caused the decrease in the gastric acidity, which is considered as an antimicrobial natural barrier. A meta-analysis demonstrated the PPI association with an increasing risk of Salmonella infection, Campylobacter, and other bacteria except *Clostridium difficilae* (CD) (odds ratio = 3.33 [1.84–6.02]) [36].

The increasing risk of the infection by the CD was demonstrated by three meta-analyses published in 2012 (odds ratio between 1.48 and 2.31) [37–39] with an increase of this risk in case of IPP association with an antibiotic treatment [37]. However, the other confusing factors such as the elderly and the comorbidity were not specified in most of these studies [31]. On the other hand, a recent retrospective study recommended avoiding the PPI use with the patients having antecedent of repeated infections with CD [40].

Because of these data, the FDA recommended considering the infection diagnosis with CD in case of persistent diarrhea under PPI and limiting the use of these molecules to the effective minimal dose during the shortest possible duration, to avoid this risk [41]. The upper age to 65 years constitutes an individual factor risk for the infections with CD [42]. Furthermore, the consequences of this infection (diarrhea, colitis, megacolon, colonic perforation) are more serious in the elderly. Moreover, in England and in WALES, the death rate related to these infections is concerned mainly with elderly more than 65 years old [43]. So, this risk justifies the limitation of the IPP prescription, particularly to the elderly.

Concerning the pneumonia's risk under PPI, the pathophysiological mechanisms of this association were not clearly established, but they are essentially represented by the gastric bacterial colonization, the change of the bacterial oropharyngeal flora, and the lung microinhalation of these bacteria [31]. The results of the case-witness studies and meta-analysis suggest a moderate increase in the arising out of community-acquired pneumonia by using the PPI [31]. The odds ratio found in a recent literature review was 1.49 (1.16–1.92) [44]. The community-acquired pneumonia risk by using the PPI is related to the treatment duration with a more important risk after a month of starting the treatment (odds ratio = 2.1 (1, 39–3, 16)) independently of the posology and of the patient's age [31]. Though there is the absence of forward-looking studies and the intervention possibility of confusing factors, these data suggest the importance to limit the IPP prescriptions to the validated indications.

In conclusion, the responsibility of the PPI in the happening of events, which is unwanted and sometimes serious, was demonstrated, but the studies were often retrospective and sometimes biased and the strength of the association was low most of the time with an odds ratio 2 [31]. However, you should not consider these medicines as simple "gastric defenders" without any risk and to limit their prescription to the validated indications, to the recommended posology, during a well-determined duration, especially to the fragile elderly subject treated by a lot of drugs.

The PPI use may increase the risk of medicinal interactions (by modifying the absorption of medicine by acting on the gastric pH or by competition on the cytochrome P450 (CYP)) being able to make tilt the balance profit/risk negatively, at the elderly person. Indeed, by increasing the gastric pH, the PPI decreases the dissolution and the solubilization of some administered medicines per bone, such as antifungals (for example, the itraconazole [45]) or the immunosuppressors (such as the mycophenolate mofetil [46]). On the contrary, they can increase the reduction of some medicines such as the saquinavir [47]. On the other hand, the taking of a PPI could theoretically improve the bioavailability of medicines for which an important part of the ingested dose is normally hydrolyzed in acid area (such as penicillin) [48]. Finally, it was demonstrated that the omeprazole increased the bioavailability of the digoxine [49] and the nifedipine [50] by inhibiting at the intestinal level of the isoenzyme 3A4 of the CYP450 and the glycoprotein P.

On the other hand, all the PPIs, except the rabeprazole, are mainly metabolized by isoenzymes 2C19 and 3A4 of the CYP, [51]. At the same time, the PPI inhibit these enzymes. The omeprazole is also a moderate inductor of the CYP 1A2 [52]. Thus, pharmacokinetics interaction risk exists with medicines that are major substrata of these isoforms. The particular case of the interaction between the IPP and the clopidogrel, a platelet antiaggregant in which the efficiency depends on its bioactivation by the CYP 2C19, was widely studied, without formal proof of its clinical impact. The clopidogrel belongs to the class of thienopyridines. It is a prodrug, absorbed by the intestine and then transformed into an active metabolite by the liver via two successive reactions of oxidation by cytochromes P450, and more exact isoforms CYP2C19, CYP3A4/5, CYP2C9, and CYP2B6. By inhibiting the CYP 2C19, the PPI (except for a very weak action for the pantoprazole) decreases the clopidogrel activation and thus its efficiency, hence exposing the patients to ischemic accidents. Numerous retrospective studies confirmed this interaction [53]. According to the FDA's to the healthcare professionals of November 17th, 2009, the association of the omeprazole with the clopidogrel is not advisable. The FDA, presented the pantoprazole as a possible alternative in case of necessary association of an IPP with clopidogrel, because of its slightest inhibitive potential on the CYP 2C19 [54]. As far as the inhibition of the CYP 2C19 by the PPI is reversible and considering the short half-life of the PPI, some authors suggested minimizing the clinical consequences of this interaction by prescribing the PPI in the morning and the clopidogrel in the evening with an interval of 12 hours by separating both the takings [55]. However, the published randomized forward-looking studies did not find this interaction and confirmed the beneficial effects of the PPI on the digestive bleedings [31, 56, 57, 58]. In 2012, these data allowed Afssaps (become ANSM: National agency of Safety of the Medicine) to remove, the PPI-clopidogrel interaction from the thesaurus of the medicinal interactions [59].

However, the ANSM has issued a reserve in its recommendations of 2012 advising to avoid the clopidogrel-omeprazole and clopidogrel-esomeprazole associations [60]. In our series, two patients were treated with the clopidogrel in association with the PPI and they did not receive any information concerning the possibility of a medicinal interaction. Though a formal proof of the clinical impact of this association was absent, we preferred to recommend our patients to space out the taking of both medicines for 12 hours, because of the pantoprazole's unavailability in our public pharmacies.

By taking into account the data of our series, which confirms the concomitant use of several medicines by elderly besides the IPP with the possibility of medicinal interactions, it is important to update the medicines' list taken by the patient at every consultation as well as to recommend him stopping the PPI if this treatment is not anymore indicated. Indeed, one of the main obstacles in stopping the PPI is the rebound effect that is generated. It is established from now on that the stop of a treatment by PPI can lead relapses by rebound effect on the gastric acidity. So, since 1996, an increase of 50% of the gastric acid secretion has been highlighted at nine patients for 14 days after the stop of a three-month treatment by omeprazole to the 40 mg/d posology [61]. In 2009, a randomized trial, with double blind versus placebo, realized at 120 asymptomatic healthy volunteers, confirmed the clinical impact of this rebound effect by showing that only after 8 weeks of a treatment with esomeprazole to the 40 mg/d posology, 44% of the exposed subjects presented the symptoms of rebound effect (heartburns, gastroenteritis ebb: esophageal or dyspepsia) against 15% in the witness group [62] These symptoms arose from the second week following the PPI stop, and they were still described till the end of the follow-up period, that is 4 weeks after the stop. Other studies showed that the rebound effect on the acid secretion lasts beyond 8 weeks after the stop [63, 64]. To the naive subjects for the pylori helicobacter, this effect rebound seems to be proportional in the rise of pH during the treatment, while it tends to be masked by the persistent hypochlorhydria observed at the infected patients by the pylori helicobacter [63]. Other multicentral trials, randomized, in double blind showed that less than a third of patients receiving a long-term IPP, succeeded to stop the treatment without an effect on the control of the symptoms and the quality of life, whereas another third passed to a treatment "in the request" [65, 66]. Several pathophysiological hypotheses were envisaged to explain this rebound effect on the acid gastric secretion, such as a hypergastrinemia [61] or a hypertrophy and a hyperplasia of the cells of the gastric wall [63].

Author details

Mona Boudabous*, Héla Gdoura, Leila Mnif, Lassad Chtourou, Amal Grati, Ali Amouri and Nabil Tahri

*Address all correspondence to: boudabousmona@yahoo.fr

Gastroenterology Department, Hedi Chaker Hospital, Sfax, Tunisia

References

[1] Robinson M. Proton pump inhibitors: Update on their role in acid-related gastrointestinal diseases. International Journal of Clinical Practice. 2005;**59**:709-715

[2] George CJ, Korc B, Ross JS. Appropriate proton pump inhibitor use among older adults: A retrospective chart review. The American Journal of Geriatric Pharmacotherapy. 2008;**6**(5):249-254

[3] De Souto Barreto P, Lapeyre-Mestre M, Mathieu C, Piau C, Bouget C, Cayla F, Vellas B, Rolland Y. Prevalence and associations of the use of proton-pump inhibitors in nursing homes: A cross-sectional study. Journal of the American Medical Directors Association. 2013;**14**(4):265-269

[4] Sheen E, Triadafilopoulos G. Adverse effects of long-term proton pump inhibitor therapy. Digestive Diseases and Sciences. 2011;**56**:931-950

[5] Agence française de sécurité sanitaire des produits de santé. Les anti-sécrétoires gastriques chez l'adulte. In: Recommandations de bonne pratique. AFSSAPS: Saint-Denis; 2007

[6] Haute Autorité de Santé. Proton-pump inhibitors drugs in adults. Reevaluation. 2009

[7] IMS Health, IMS National Sales Perspectives 3/2007. Top 10 therapeutic classes by US sales. http://www.imshealth.com/ims/portaljfront/articleC/0,2777,6599_80408854_8041855,00.html

[8] P1 H, Paulsen MS, Zwisler JE, Begtrup LM, Hansen JM, Rasmussen S, Jarbøl DE. Rapidly increasing prescribing of proton pump inhibitors in primary care despite interventions: A nationwide observational study. The European Journal of General Practice. 2014;**20**(4):290-293

[9] Site de la pharmacie centrale de Tunisie. www.phct.com.tn/index.php#b

[10] Batuwitage BT, Kingham JGC, Morgan NE, et al. Inappropriate prescribing of proton pump inhibitors in primary care. Postgraduate Medical Journal. 2007;**83**(975):66-68

[11] Sécurité Sociale. Rapport à la commission aux comptes de la Sécurité Sociale. In: Les prescriptions des IPP. 2009

[12] Teramura-Grönblad M, Hosia-Randell H, Muurinen S, Pitkala K. Use of protonpump inhibitors and their associated risks among frail elderly nursing home residents. Scandinavian Journal of Primary Health Care. 2010;**28**:154-159

[13] Schuler A. Risks versus benefits of long-term proton pump inhibitor therapy in the elderly. Geriatric Nursing. 2007;**28**(4):225

[14] Micheaux SLD. Inhibiteurs de la pompe à proton chez les sujets âgés, évaluation des pratiques professionnelles en médecine générale. Human Health and Pathology. 2014

[15] Pilotto A, Franceschi M, Paris F. Recent advances in the treatment of GERD in the elderly: Focus on proton pump inhibitors. International Journal of Clinical Practice. 2005;**59**:1204-1209

[16] T1 P, D1 C, C1 M. Microscopic colitis: A review of etiology, treatment and refractory disease. World Journal of Gastroenterology. 2015;**21**(29):8804-8810

[17] Buon M, Gaillard C, Martin J, Fedrizzi S, Mosquet B, Coquerel A, et al. Risk of proton pump inhibitor induced mild hyponatremia in older adults. Journal of the American Geriatrics Society. 2013;**61**(11):2052-2054

[18] Fenoglio I, Guy C, Beyens M-N, Mounier G, Marsille F, Mismetti P. Drug induced hyponatremia. About a series of 54 cases notified to the regional center of pharmacovigilance of Saint-Etienne. Thérapie. 2011;**66**(2):139-148

[19] Rozgony NR, Fang C, Kuczmarski MF, Bob H. Vitamin B(12) deficiency is linked with long-term use of proton pump inhibitors in institutionalized older adults: Could a cyanocobalamin nasal spray be beneficial? Journal of Nutrition for the Elderly. 2010;**29**(1):87-99

[20] Luk CP, Parsons R, Lee YP, Hughes JD. Proton pump inhibitor-associated hypomagnesemia: What do FDA data tell us? The Annals of Pharmacotherapy. 2013;**47**(6):773-780

[21] William JH1, Danziger J. Proton-pump inhibitor-induced hypomagnesemia: Current research and proposed mechanisms. World Journal of Nephrology. 2016;**65**(2):152-157

[22] Delgado MG, Calleja S, Suarez L, Pascual J. Recurrent confusional episodes associated with hypomagnesaemia due to esomeprazol. BML Case Reports. 2013

[23] Kim S, Lee H, Park CH, Shim CN, Lee HJ, Park JC, Shin SK, Lee SK, Lee YC, Kim HY, Kang DR. Clinical predictors associated with proton pump inhibitor-induced hypomagnesemia. American Journal of Therapeutics. 2015;**22**(1):14-21

[24] Eom C-S, Jeon CY, Lim J-W, Cho E-G, Park SM, Lee K-S. Use of acid-suppressive drugs and risk of pneumonia: A systematic review and meta-analysis. Canadian Medical Association Journal. 2011;**183**(3):310-319

[25] Kwok CS, Arthur AK, Anibueze CI, Singh S, Cavallazzi R, Loke YK. Risk of *Clostridium difficile* infection with acid suppressing drugs and antibiotics: Meta-analysis. The American Journal of Gastroenterology. 2012;**107**(7):1011-1019

[26] Geller JL, Adams JS. Proton pump inhibitor therapy and hip fracture risk. JAMA. 2007; **297**(13):1429-1430

[27] Khalili H, Huang ES, Jacobson BC, Camargo CA Jr, Feskanich D, Chan AT. Use of proton pump inhibitors and risk of hip fracture in relation to dietary and lifestyle factors: A prospective cohort study. BMJ. 2012:344-372

[28] Ahn JS, Eom CS, Jeon CY, Park SM. Acid suppressive drugs and gastric cancer: A meta-analysis of observational studies. World Journal of Gastroenterology. 2013;**28; 19**(16):2560-2568

[29] Lai SW, Liao KF, Lai HC, Lin CL, Sung FC. Use of proton pumps inhibitors correlates with increased risk of colorectal cancer in Taiwan. Asia-Pacific Journal of Clinical Oncology. 2013;**9**(2):192-193

[30] Sahli H, Testouri N, Ben Chihaouia M, et al. Bone mineral density in healthy Tunisian women. Maturitas. 2009;**63**:227-232

[31] De la Coba Ortiz C, Argüelles Arias F, Martín de Argila de Prados C, Júdez Gutiérrez J, Linares Rodríguez A, Ortega Alonso A, Rodríguez de Santiago E, Rodríguez-Téllez M, Vera Mendoza MI, Aguilera Castro L, Álvarez Sánchez Á, Andrade Bellido RJ, Bao Pérez F, Castro Fernández M, Giganto Tomé F. Proton-pump inhibitors adverse effects: A review of the evidence and position statement by the Sociedad Española de Patología Digestiva. Revista Española de Enfermedades Digestivas. 2016;**108**(4):207-224

[32] Kaye JA, Jick H. Proton pump inhibitor use and risk of hip fractures in patients without major risk factors. Pharmacotherapy. 2008;**28**:951-959

[33] Attwood SE, Ell C, Galmiche JP, Fiocca R, Hatlebakk JG, Hasselgren B, Långström G, Jahreskog M, Eklund S, Lind T, Lundell L. Long-term safety of proton pump inhibitor therapy assessed under controlled, randomised clinical trial conditions: Data from the SOPRAN and LOTUS studies. Alimentary Pharmacology & Therapeutics. 2015;**41**:1162-1174

[34] FDA Drug Safety Communication. Possible Increased Risk of Fractures of the Hip, Wrist, and Spine with the Use of Proton Pump Inhibitors. Washington, DC, US: Food and Drug Administration; 2011 Accessible en: http://www.fda.gov/Drugs/DrugSafety/ucm213206.htm

[35] MW1 H, Hoenderop JG, Bindels RJ, Drenth JP. Systematic review: Hypomagnesaemia induced by proton pump inhibition. Alimentary Pharmacology & Therapeutics. 2012 Sep;**36**(5):405-413

[36] Leonard J, Marshall JK, Moayyedi P. Systematic review of the risk of enteric infection in patients taking acid suppression. The American Journal of Gastroenterology. 2007;**102**:2047-2056

[37] Kwok CS, Arthur AK, Anibueze CI, Singh S, Cavallazzi R, Loke YK. Risk of *Clostridium difficile* infection with acid suppressing drugs and antibiotics: Meta-analysis. The American Journal of Gastroenterology. 2012;**107**:1011-1019

[38] Janarthanan S, Ditah I, Adler DG, Ehrinpreis MN. *Clostridium difficile*-associated diarrhea and proton pump inhibitor therapy: A meta-analysis. The American Journal of Gastroenterology. 2012;**107**:1001-1010

[39] Deshpande A, Pant C, Pasupuleti V, Rolston DD, Jain A, Deshpande N, Thota P, Sferra TJ, Hernandez AV. Association between proton pump inhibitor therapy and *Clostridium difficile* infection in a meta analysis. Clinical Gastroenterology and Hepatology. 2012;**10**:225-233

[40] McDonald EG, Milligan J, Frenette C, Lee TC. Continuous proton pump inhibitor therapy and the associated risk of recurrent *Clostridium difficile* infection. JAMA Internal Medicine. 2015;**175**:784-791

[41] FDA Drug Safety Communication. *Clostridium difficile*-associated Diarrhea can be Associated with Stomach Acid Drugs Known as Proton Pump Inhibitors (PPIs). Washington, DC: US Food and Drug Administration; 2012

[42] Bignardi GE. Risk factors for *Clostridium difficile* infection. The Journal of Hospital Infection. 1998;**40**(1):1-15

[43] Office for National Statistics. Deaths involving *Clostridium difficile*: England and Wales, 1999-2004. London: Crown; 2006

[44] Lambert AA, Lam JO, Paik JJ, C4 U-G, MB1 D, Crowell TA. Risk of community-acquired pneumonia with outpatient proton-pump inhibitor therapy: A systematic review and meta-analysis. PLoS One. 2015;**10**:e0128004

[45] Johnson MD, Hamilton CD, Drew RH, Sanders LL, Pennick GJ, Perfect JR. A randomized comparative study to determine the effect of omeprazole on the peak serum concentration of itraconazole oral solution. The Journal of Antimicrobial Chemotherapy. 2003;**51**:453-457

[46] Kofler S, Deutsch MA, Bigdeli AK, Shvets N, Vogeser M, Mueller TH, Meiser B, Steinbeck G, Reichart B, Kaczmarek I. Proton pump inhibitor co-medication reduces mycophenolate acid drug exposure in heart transplant recipients. The Journal of Heart and Lung Transplantation. 2009;**28**:605-611

[47] Winston A, Back D, Fletcher C, Robinson L, Unsworth J, Tolowinska I, Schutz M, Pozniak AL, Gazzard B, Boffito M. Effect of omeprazole on the pharmacokinetics of saquinavir-500 mg formulation with ritonavir in healthy male and female volunteers. AIDS. 2006;**20**:1401-1406

[48] Ogawa R, Echizen H. Drug-drug interaction profiles of proton pump inhibitors. Clinical Pharmacokinetics. 2010;**49**:509-533

[49] Oosterhuis B, Jonkman JH, Andersson T, Zuiderwijk PB, Jedema JN. Minor effect of multiple dose omeprazole on the pharmacokinetics of digoxin after a single oral dose. British Journal of Clinical Pharmacology. 1991;**32**:569-572

[50] Soons PA, van den Berg G, Danhof M, van Brummelen P, Jansen JB, Lamers CB et al. Influence of single- and multipledose omeprazole treatment on nifedipine pharmacokinetics and effects in healthy subjects. European Journal of Clinical Pharmacology 1992;**42**:319-324.

[51] Li XQ, Andersson TB, Ahlström M, Weidolf L. Comparison of inhibitory effects of the proton pump-inhibiting drugs omeprazole, esomeprazole, lansoprazole, pantoprazole, and rabeprazole on human cytochrome P450 activities. Drug Metabolism and Disposition. 2004;**32**:821-827

[52] Diaz D, Fabre I, Daujat M, Saint Aubert B, Bories P, Michel H, Maurel P. Omeprazole is an aryl hydrocarbon-like inducer of human hepatic cytochrome P450. Gastroenterology. 1990;**99**:737-747

[53] J1 S, Gaussem P. Proton pump inhibitors and clopidogrel: A hazardous association? La Revue de Médecine Interne. 2013;**34**(2):99-104

[54] Information for Healthcare Professionals: Update to the labeling of Clopidogrel Bisulfate (marketed as Plavix) to alert healthcare professionals about a drug interaction with omeprazole (marketed as Prilosec and Prilosec OTC). 2009. Available at http://www.fda.gov/Drugs/DrugSafety/PostmarketDrugSafetyInformationforPatientsandProviders/DrugSafetyInformationforHeathcareProfessionals/ucm190787.htm

[55] Chyrchel B, Surdacki A, Chyrchel M, Dudek D, Dubiel JS. Separate dosing of clopidogrel and omeprazole may improve platelet inhibition on dual antiplatelet therapy. International Journal of Cardiology. 2011;**149**:124-125

[56] Ho PM1, Maddox TM, Wang L, Fihn SD, Jesse RL, Peterson ED, Rumsfeld JS. Risk of adverse outcomes associated with concomitant use of clopidogrel and proton pump inhibitors following acute coronary syndrome. JAMA J Am Med Assoc. 2009;**301**(9):937-944

[57] Hsu P-I, Lai K-H, Liu C-P. Esomeprazole with clopidogrel reduces peptic ulcer recurrence, compared with clopidogrel alone, in patients with atherosclerosis. Gastroenterology. 2011;**140**(3):791-798

[58] Melloni C, Washam JB, Jones WS, Halim SA, Hasselblad V, Mayer SB, Heidenfelder BL, Dolor RJ. Conflicting results between randomized trials and observational studies on the impact of proton pump inhibitors on cardiovascular events when coadministered with dual antiplatelet therapy: Systematic review. Circulation. Cardiovascular Quality and Outcomes. 2015;**8**:47-55

[59] Thesaurus des interactions médicamenteuses [site Internet]. ANSM: Agence nationale de sécurité du médicament et des produits de santé; 2012 Consultable sur: http://ansm.sante.fr/Dossiers-thematiques/Interactionsmedicamenteuses/Interactionsmedicamenteuses/(offset)/0

[60] Agence Nationale de la Sécurité du Médicament. Bon usage des antiplaquettaires—Recommandations (26/06/2012). http://ansm.sante.fr/var/ansm_site/storage/original/application/31f541bfa5cbe1460f1a25ce11ba6550.pdf

[61] Waldum HL, Arnestad JS, Brenna E, Eide I, Syversen U, Sandvik AK. Marked increase in gastric acid secretory capacity after omeprazole treatment. Gut. 1996;**39**:649-653

[62] Reimer C, Søndergaard B, Hilsted L, Bytzer P. Proton-pump inhibitor therapy induces acid-related symptoms in healthy volunteers after withdrawal of therapy. Gastroenterology. 2009;**137**:80-87

[63] Gillen D, Wirz AA, Ardill JE, McColl KE. Rebound hypersecretion after omeprazole and its relation to on-treatment acid suppression and Helicobacter pylori status. Gastroenterology. 1999;**116**:239-247

[64] Fossmark R, Johnsen G, Johanessen E, Waldum HL. Rebound acid hypersecretionafter long-term inhibition of gastric acid secretion. Alimentary Pharmacology & Therapeutics. 2005;**21**:149-154

[65] Björnsson E, Abrahamsson H, Simrén M, Mattsson N, Jensen C, Agerforz P, Kilander A. Discontinuation of proton pump inhibitors in patients on long-term therapy: A double-blind, placebo-controlled trial. Alimentary Pharmacology & Therapeutics. 2006;**24**:945-954

[66] Van der Velden AW, de Wit NJ, Quartero AO, Grobbee DE, Numans ME. Pharmacological dependency in chronic treatment of gastroesophageal reflux disease: A randomized controlled clinical trial. Digestion 2010;**81**:43-52

3

Immunotherapy for Esophageal Cancer

Tian Wang and Yi Zhang

Abstract

As the third most common cancer of the gastrointestinal tract, esophageal cancer has a rather worse prognosis treated with current therapy strategies, and a poor 5-year survival rate lower than 15%. Recent years, emerging immunotherapy has showed a gratifying effect in treating other solid tumors which illuminates its usage for esophageal cancers. Immunotherapy for esophageal cancer basically includes adoptive-cell-therapy-based, antibody-based and vaccine-based therapies, and all of which have shown preliminary favorable results in treating esophageal cancer. However, due to the rather lower mutation rate and a tough microenvironment inside the cancer, promising immunotherapies like immune checkpoint blockade drugs, gene-modified-T cell therapies are hindered by the immunosuppressive factors from microenvironment. Future endeavors will be focusing on targeting immunosuppressive factors, combining immunotherapies with classical treatments to create a satisfying effect.

Keywords: esophageal cancer, tumor microenvironment, immunotherapy, immune checkpoint blockade drugs, CAR-T cell therapy

1. Introduction

Esophageal cancer is one of the leading culprits of mortality worldwide and is responsible for a total number of 746,000 [1] new cases and 439,000 [2] deaths every year. A large number of these cancers are diagnosed at an advanced stage and the metastasis causes bad outcomes. Endoscopic surgery, cytotoxic chemotherapy and radiotherapy remain to be the active and essential clinical treatment but only provide modest benefits, with median overall survival (OS) only in the range of 8–10 months [3]. After nearly 20 years of fast development, immunotherapy turned to be a promising method for treating esophageal cancer. Recent advances have brought some therapeutic regimens to be approved by Food and Drug Administration (FDA) then coming to clinical practice in first- and second-line settings (**Table 1**). The future

Treatment	Cancer type	Treating method	Phase	Study number
ACT				
	EC	CIK	II	NCT02490735
	Multiple cancer types (including EC)	CTL	I	NCT00004178
	EC	NY-ESO-1-TCR T cells	II	NCT01795976
Tumor vaccine				
Cell vaccine	Multiple cancer types (including EC)	Tumor cell vaccine	I	NCT01258868
	Multiple cancer types (including EC)	H1299 lysate vaccine	I/II	NCT02054104
	Multiple cancer types (including EC)	Allogeneic tumor vaccine	I	NCT01143545
Peptide vaccine	EC	IMF-001	I	NCT01003808
	EC	LY6K, VEGFR1, VEGFR2	I	NCT00561275
	EC	URLC10, TTK, KOC1, VEGFR1, VEGFR2, cisplatin, fluorouracil	I	NCT00632333
	EC	URLC10	I	NCT00753844
	EC, GC	G17DT, cisplatin, fluorouracil	III	NCT00020787
Immune checkpoints therapies	EC + GEJC + GC	Nivolumab/placebo	III	NCT02743494
	EC + GEJC Siewert I	Pembrolizumab vs. investigator's choice	III	NCT02564263
	EC	Pembrolizumab + brachytherapy	I	NCT02642809
	EC	Nivolumab vs. paclitaxel/docetaxel	III	NCT02569242
	EC + GEJC Siewert I	Pembrolizumab	II	NCT02971956
	EC + GC	Pembrolizumab + trastuzumab	II	NCT02318901
	EC	Durvalumab (anti-PD-L1) + chemoradiotherapy	I/II	NCT02735239
	Solid tumors (including ESCC)	LAG525 (anti-LAG3) + PD001 (anti-PD-1)	I/II	NCT02460224
	Solid tumors (including ESCC)	Nivolumab + ipilimumab	I	NCT02834013

ACT: adoptive cell therapy; CIK: cytokine-induced killer cells; CTL: cytotoxic T-cells; VEGFR: vascular endothelial growth factor receptors; PD: programmed cell death receptor; EC: esophageal cancer; ESCC: esophageal squamous cell carcinoma; GEJC: gastroesophageal junction carcinoma.

Table 1. Recent or completed clinical trials of potential therapeutic approaches for immunotherapy of esophageal cancer.

of immunotherapy is promising in treating solid tumors, yet still there is a desperate need for more effective and less toxic treatment options for patients with advanced esophageal cancer.

In recent years, emergence of immunotherapy towards cancer has improved the management of several malignancies dramatically, especially melanoma, renal cell carcinoma, non-small cell lung cancer and so on, shedding light on its usage on esophageal cancer as well. Identification of more suppressive factors in tumor microenvironment and insights into the biology of T cell functioning yielded a large number of diverse and novel anti-tumor regimens. Global efforts continue to explore how and when to integrate these agents in treatment of esophageal cancer. Immune checkpoint inhibition through antibodies that block cytotoxic T-lymphocyte antigen 4 (CTLA-4) and programmed cell death protein 1 (PD-1) has led to meaningful improvements in survival [4]. Vaccine adjuvant administration has also reduced tumor recurrence to some degree. CAR-T (chimeric antigen receptor T-cell) immunotherapy is a typical example of recent advances in synthetic biology, genome engineering, and cell manufacturing that has made it possible to develop highly specific and potent tumor-reactive T cells and offer many opportunities for experimentation and broader clinical translation. Combined regimens of immunotherapy with other classical esophageal treating procedures will illuminate the future of clinical oncotherapy. Recent achievements, which are illustrated below, including finished or ongoing clinical trials and laboratory findings of immunotherapy for esophageal cancer, bringing optimism for meaningful changes in treatment algorithms and for better outcomes in this fatal disease.

2. Immunotherapy regimens for esophageal cancer

2.1. History of immunotherapy

A few decades ago, several rare clinical regression of advanced cancer in response to immune stimulation aroused interests in the area of cancer treatment. A passionate handful of immunologists, oncologists and surgeons carried out forward-looking researches into the relations between tumor progress and body immune system. Their respectable efforts turned the seemingly insignificant clinical phenomenon into reproducible concrete success by revealing the hidden mechanisms of tumor response.

At the earliest period of cancer immunotherapies, the exact mechanism remained unknown and the anti-tumor growth effect was limited yet providing impetus for in-depth study. The first effective immunotherapies aiming at directly modulating cell function using well-characterized recombinant cytokines including interleukin-2 (IL-2) and interferon alpha (IFNα), yet the safety was lowered associated with substantial toxicity. Other cytokines, including IFNγ, IL-4, IL-7, IL-10, IL-12, IL-15, IL-18, IL-25, etc., failed to provide substantive benefit. The following breakthrough was the emerging conception of monoclonal antibodies (mAbs) targeting tumor cell surface receptor proteins (human epidermal growth factor receptor 2 (HER2)/Neu, epidermal growth factor receptor (EGFR), etc.) and were integrated into cancer care. Vaccination therapies using the modified peptide, whole tumor, recombinant proteins, dendritic cells (DCs), and adjuvants were only modestly successful. With researching deeper into the cross-talk happening in the tumor microenvironment between tumor cells and immune cells, the modern era of immunotherapy launched with the extraordinary novel efficacy (and toxicities) of mAbs targeting immune checkpoints in patients with various cancer types in order to decrease the suppressive potential that would prevent immune cells from functioning. Current alternative approach to overcoming the suppressive tumor microenvironment was the administration of genetically modified autologous T cells targeting specific cancer-related antigens [5]. This could be done in the form of T cells in which modified specific T cell receptors (TCR) were inserted for a shared tumor antigen or a tumor-specific neoantigen accompanied by co-transduction of stimulatory cytokines such as IL-12 or could co-administrate with PD-1 pathway blockers to sustain the capability before being expanded in large numbers *in vitro* following lymphodepleting chemotherapy. These approaches have produced dramatic responses in a few patients with a variety of individual tumor types, especially hematological malignancies [6]. Further improvement of adoptive cell transfer therapy came from the modified T cells expressing chimeric antigen receptors (CAR) targeting tumor-specific binding domains. After several generations of amelioration, CAR-T therapy showed extraordinary effect in treating hematological malignancies yet treatment of patients with solid tumors using CAR-T cells had been less fruitful and had troubled clinicians much through the off-tumor/on-target toxicity. Given the virtually limitless possibility of *ex vivo* engineering of T cells, many of these potential hurdles will likely be resolved by the additional modification of T cell products prior to treatment.

Immunotherapy showed great potential in the treatment of esophageal cancer. Modern treatments of patients with esophageal cancer integrated immunotherapy with conventional surgical, chemotherapeutic, and radiation oncologic strategies. In spite of the seemingly gratifying results, the 5-year survival rate of patients with esophageal cancer in the middle and late stages is still lower than 15%, the 5-year survival rate of patients with locally advanced surgery alone is only 20–25% [7]. Postoperative chemotherapy or neoadjuvant chemoradiation only turns the 5-year survival rate up to only 30–35% [8]. One of the causes to blame of the rather poor prognosis of esophageal cancer is the rapid disease progression. More than 50% of patients already have visible metastases at the time of diagnosis [7]. Therefore, further investigation of esophageal cancer microenvironment and its impact on disease progression will lay a solid theoretical foundation for early diagnosis and treatment improvement of esophageal cancer.

In this chapter, we tried to converge concepts relevant to the complicated relationship between the host and the neoplastic tissue.

2.2. Immune microenvironment and molecular correlations in esophageal cancer

As early as 100 years ago, Paget [9] had put forward the hypothesis of "seeds and soil", which laid the foundation for the concept of tumor microenvironment. Numerous data indicate that many immune-related cells, factors and immune-related signaling pathways in the tumor microenvironment play an important role in the occurrence, metastasis, recurrence, angiogenesis, and drug resistance of tumors. The in-depth study of the tumor immune microenvironment is to search for molecular pathogenesis and new therapeutic models of esophageal cancer.

Tumor microenvironment is constituted by various immune cells, endothelial cells, adipocytes, paravascular cells, nerve cells, fibroblasts, and extracellular matrix components around the cancer cells [10]. Some stromal cells in the tumor microenvironment have immunosuppressive potential to inhibit the function of immune effector cells and promote tumor progression. Thus inhibiting cancer cell apoptosis and promoting mechanisms such as proliferation, angiogenesis, drug resistance, and immune escape to promote tumorigenesis [11]. Chemokines CCL17 and CCL22 secreted by tumor cells or tumor-associated macrophages (TAMs) recruit CCR4+ regulatory T cells (Treg), which then inhibit immune effector cells by contacting directly or secretion of cytokines (IL-10 and IL-35). Th17 cells can be transformed into Treg cells stimulated by IL-6 and transforming growth factor-β (TGF-β). Inflammation and tumor-derived factors stimulate the activation of myeloid-derived suppressor cells (MDSCs). Activated MDSCs can directly inhibit the expression of CD8 + T cells. Activation and induction of Treg cells and other mechanisms contribute to immune escape of cancer cells. TAM cells and CAF cells promote the growth, invasion, metastasis, and angiogenesis of tumor cells through the secretion of cytokines, chemokines, and various growth factors. In addition, tumor cells and TAM cells can express programmed cell death ligand (PD)-L1/2 inhibiting T cell activation after binding to PD-1.

MDSCs have been shown to play an important role in promoting tumor immune escape, activating CAF cells and angiogenesis [12]. The presence of proinflammatory cytokines such as IL-1, IL-6 and prostaglandins in esophageal cancer microenvironment can activate MDSC [13]. MDSC inhibits activation of T cells by direct inhibition [14], cytotoxicity of natural killer cells (NK) [15], depletion of arginine and cysteine, induction of Treg cells, etc. to achieve immune escape [16]. Another group of immunosuppressive cells that exert similar functions are Treg cells. Under physiological conditions, Treg cells can regulate the activation and proliferation of T cells, B cells, and cytotoxicity of NK cells. But in tumor microenvironment, Treg cells can promote the occurrence and progression of tumor cells by secreting immunosuppressive related factors, secreting tumor-associated antigens (TAAs), and suppressing the cellular adverse reactions of immune effector cells and the release of granzymes [17]. Studies have shown that tumor cells and TAMs can recruit CCR4+ Treg cells to tumor sites by secreting CCL17 and CCL22 and other chemokines [18]. Treg cells are highly aggregated in tumor cites, promoting tumor invasion and metastasis, and are associated with disease severity, survival after chemotherapy, and prognosis [17]. Additionally, Th17 cells can secrete IL-17 and IL-22 and activate STAT3 related signaling pathways to promote angiogenesis and tumor growth [23]. However, the role of Th17 cells is still controversial. What factors affect the function of Th17 have not yet been well defined [18]. Therefore, we still have to know more about Th17 cells in esophageal cancer to explore potential therapeutic targets.

The tumorigenic mechanisms of TAMs are varied. Phenotype spectrum of macrophage ranges from M1 to M2: M1 macrophages represent the classical activated macrophages, with functions of cytokines secretion, antigen presentation, resistance to infection and anti-tumor ability, etc., while M2 macrophages secrete type II cytokines and induce activation of COX2/prostaglandin E and other mechanisms that cause tumorigenesis [19]. The presence of cancer associated fibroblasts (CAFs) in patients with esophageal cancer is associated with microvessel density, and can also promote tumor progression and metastasis through epithelial mesenchymal transition (EMT). CAFs are also associated with 3-year survival rates and disease recurrence after radiotherapy and chemotherapy [20].

PD-1 is a member of the CD28 superfamily and is an important immunosuppressive molecule that inhibits the activation of T cells after binding to its ligand PD-L1/PD-L2 [4]. Multiple experiments confirmed that PD-L1 and PD-L2 are highly expressed in esophageal cancer [21], in which PD-L1 expression is closely related to tumor invasion depth and poor prognosis, whereas PD-L2 expression is associated with decreased CD8+ T cell infiltration [21]. The increasing PD-L2 expression can promote the secretion of Th2 cytokines such as IL-4/IL-13 [22]. These pieces of evidence suggest that blockers targeting PD-1 are of great significance in the treatment of esophageal cancer [23].

In the early stages of esophageal cancer, TGF-β signaling suppresses tumor growth by downregulating the expression of Smad4 and c-Myc genes, while promoting growth and EMT in advanced esophageal cancer [24]. This "switching" effect is thought to be caused by the loss of adaptor proteins. For instance, an important adaptor protein, β2-spectrin, plays an important part in cell–cell interactions and maintenance of epithelial cell polarity. In esophageal adenocarcinoma, decreasing β2-spectrin in tumor cells results in increased expression of SOX9 and c-Myc, but it also reduces other TGF-β targets such as E-cadherin and cell cycle-regulated p21 and p27 genes [25]. In summary, these changes make TGF-β promote the progression and metastasis of the tumor by inducing EMT, especially in epithelial tumors like esophageal cancer.

In addition to growth factors, chemokines in the tumor microenvironment also play an important role in the development of tumors. Mainly, there is stromal cell derived factor-1 (CXCL12/SDF-1) secreted by fibroblasts [26], binding to its corresponding receptor CXCR4 or CXCR7 thus inducing tumor growth, promoting angiogenesis, stimulating tumor movement, invasion and metastasis [26]. SDF-1/CXCR4/CXCR7 axis is closely related to tumor invasion, metastasis and survival. However, the use of these separate components as indicators of prognostic analysis has yielded inconsistent results [27]. Nonetheless, CXCL12 has been shown to regulate the migration of CXCR4-positive tumor cells in esophageal adenocarcinoma *in vitro* and *in vivo*. Knockout of CXCR4 expression in KYSE-150 and TE-13 esophageal cancer cells by small interfering RNA can inhibit the proliferation, invasion and metastasis of tumor cells. Local CCL5 and CXCL10 in esophageal squamous cell carcinoma can recruit CD8+ T cells to the tumor site [28].

Further researches showed that remodeling body immune state by various means in esophageal cancer patients will be the main research direction of immunotherapy for esophageal cancer.

2.3. Checkpoint inhibitor regimens

Immune system has sophisticated regulatory mechanisms. Several checkpoints are involved to maintain the balance between effective immune-responses fighting against infection or cancer state yet won't activate excessively to prevent damaging healthy cells. Cytotoxic T lymphocyte antigen-4 (CTLA-4) and PD-1 are among the major inhibitory receptors expressed by Tregs which downregulate immune responses [29]. Inhibitory antibodies modulating these immune checkpoints have been most frequently used in immune-oncology trials in esophageal cancers.

PD-1/PD-L1 blockers have achieved encouraging clinical results in treating melanoma, lung cancer and other cancer types [30, 31]. The potential role of PD-1 blockers in treatment of esophageal cancer can be predicted by genomic map of the tumor immune microenvironment. The expression of PD-L1 on MDSCs isolated from esophageal cancer tissue was higher obviously, and PD-1 expression was detected in approximately 60% of the tumor infiltrating lymphocytes (TILs) from esophageal cancer tissues [32]. Therefore, inhibition of the PD-1/ PD-L1 pathway for esophageal cancer treatment cannot be ignored.

Preliminary results of ongoing studies indicated that PD-1 blocker Pembrolizumab had acceptable safety in PD-L1 positive esophageal cancer patients. The objective response rate for mid-term analysis was approximately 30% with a sustained response period of up to 40 weeks [33]. These results laid the foundation for the continued completion of checkpoint inhibitor regimens pivotal study in esophageal cancer patients.

CTLA-4, also known as CD152, belongs to the immunoglobulin superfamily and serves as an immunological checkpoint. When activated CD4+ helper T cells express CTLA-4, this kind of cells sends inhibitory signals to T cells [34]. High CTLA-4 expressing CD4+ Treg cells block T cells by reducing IL-2 secretion and downregulating IL-2 receptor expression then retard T cells in G1 phase of the cell cycle [35]. Ipilimumab and tremelimumab have two fully humanized monoclonal anti-CTLA-4 antibodies that have already received FDA approval for the treatment of melanoma and mesothelioma [36, 37]. A survey of tremelimumab has been completed in phase II clinical trials for treating advanced gastric and esophageal cancer (n = 18). Although only a 5% response rate was observed, four patients were controlled and one patient was observed with partial remission (25.4 Mo) after treatment and continued for several months [38]. The results of ongoing clinical trials are expected to further highlight the clinical value of monoclonal anti-CTLA-4 antibodies in esophageal cancer.

2.4. Vaccine regimens

Tumor vaccine treatment involves the administration of TAAs into patients thus triggering specific anti-tumor immune responses. Rosenberg et al. [39, 40] conducted a comprehensive review of 1306 cancer vaccine usage studies conducted before 2004 and found that the overall target response rate was only 3.3%. The explanation may be that these immune cells have low affinity or are inhibited by endogenous factors like the checkpoints mentioned above.

For the treatment of esophageal cancer, some vaccine-based clinical trial reports have been published. A Phase I clinical trial of 10 patients with refractory stage III or IV esophageal squamous cell carcinoma treated with peptide vaccine found that 9 patients developed antigen-specific T cell immune response. One of the patients with liver metastases showed complete remission for 7 months, another had partial remission within all metastatic lung lesions, and 3 patients had progression-free survival lasting 2.5 months. The peptide vaccine used was derived from three HLA-A24-restricted cancer testis antigens (TTK protein kinase, lymphocyte antigen 6 complex locus K, and insulin-like growth factor-II mRNA binding protein 3) [41]. The multicenter, phase II clinical trial of the vaccine evaluated the OS, PFS, and immune response after vaccinations in patients with HLA-A*2402 positive and negative esophageal squamous cell carcinoma, and immune response was observed in HLA-A*2402 positive patients (n = 35), but there was no statistical difference in OS compared to HLA-A*2402-negative patients (n = 25) (4.6 mo vs. 2.6 mo, P > 0.05), yet there is a significant difference in PFS (P = 0.032) [42]. In a tumor vaccine trial hosted by Saito et al. [43] (n = 20), 4 patients with high levels of MAGE-A4 or MHC class I antigen in autologous tumor cells not only showed MAGE-A4 specific immune responses after vaccination, but compared with patients without using antibodies, their OS was also significantly prolonged. Wada et al. [44] used NY-ESO-1 as a cancer vaccine in 8 patients with esophageal cancer. The results showed that 7 patients had an immune response. Of the 6 patients evaluated for efficacy, 1 patient experienced partial remission, 2 patients continued to maintain progression-free status, and 2 patients had mixed clinical responses. Given the preliminary results of these peptide vaccines in clinical trials, safety inspections and the related researches combined with radiotherapy and chemotherapy are also being carried out gradually in treating multiple cancer types including esophageal cancer.

2.5. Adoptive cell therapy regimens

The concept of ACT (adoptive cell therapy) was first proposed by Dietrich et al. [45]. It refers to the treatment of utilizing autologous or allogeneic immune cells by infusing them back into the patients after being amplified *in vitro* by certain means. Currently effector cells can be divided into two categories: the first type is non-specific immune cells, including autologous lymphokine-activated killer cells (LAK), cytokine-induced killer cells (CIK) and NK cells. Cells are isolated from peripheral blood cells and are stimulated by lymphokines or cytokines; another type of effector cells is antigen-specific T cells, including TILs, cytotoxic T cells (CTL) and genetically engineered T cells including T cell receptor transferred T-cells (TCR-T) and CAR-T [46].

The first ACT trial in human improved the survival of patients with metastatic cancer by reintroduction of CIK and recombinant IL-2 to their body, which has been successfully applied to the treatment of refractory metastatic melanoma, and for other types of cancer such as glioma, renal cell carcinoma, non-small cell lung cancer, etc. The objective response rate varies from 20 to 72% [47], encouraging its further usage in esophageal cancer, too.

So far, ACT treatment of esophageal cancer has been evaluated in several clinical trials. In the first published study by Besser et al. [48] and Toh et al. [49], mononuclear cells were isolated from peripheral blood of esophageal squamous cell carcinoma patients and were given autologous tumor cell stimulation *in vitro*. Latter results showed that half of the patients had an objective response, and 36% of the subjects achieved complete remission or partial remission. CTL and TIL cells are now hot spots for carrying out immunotherapy for solid tumors as the mechanism of killing tumor is rather clear.

TCR-T cells transduce the α and β chains of the antigen-specific high-affinity TCR into T cells and express them on the cell surface, thereby effectively identifying and killing the tumor cells expressing the antigen. Currently, the most common TAAs found in esophageal cancer are cancer testis MAGE-A3/4 and NY-ESO-1. Several studies [50, 51] showed that the expression ratio of MAGE-A3 in esophageal cancer was about 90%, and the expression rate of NYESO-1 in esophageal cancer was up to 40–90%. A preliminary phase 1 clinical trial of genetically engineered T cells was carried out by Kageyama et al. [52], TCR-T cells were readopted to patients with MAGE-A4-positive recurrent esophageal cancer, and administered the MAGE-A4 peptide vaccine subsequently, the level of TCR-T cells in the peripheral blood of 10 subjects was monitored for 5 months, and 5 of them were able to detect specific T cells continuously. Seven subjects appeared tumor progress after 2 months of treatment, but another 3 subjects survived more than 27 months.

CAR-T is another type of genetically engineered T cells. CAR-T was obtained by translocating chimeric antigen receptor such as CARs into T cells. Gross et al. [53] successfully constructed the structure of CARs into T cells for the first time to exert their specific killing function. Up to now, tens of clinical trial data of CAR-T treatment on malignant hematological malignancies have been published. The Novartis' tisagenlecleucel, a synthetic bioimmune product of anti-CD19 CAR-T cells has been approved by FDA on treating relapsed/refractory B-cell acute lymphoblastic leukemia (B-ALL) in 2017 [54]. The early generation of CAR-T therapy for solid tumors did not appear ideal outcomes during clinical use [55]. The reasonable explanation might be lack of unique TAAs in solid tumors, less efficiency and persistency of T cell homing to tumor sites, and the intratumoral immunosuppressive environment strongly inhibited CAR-T cell function. Clinical trials targeting solid tumors using second or third-generation CAR techniques had been limited, but some of the more significant clinical trials are carrying out good results. Patients with metastatic or recurrent HER2-positive medulloblastoma treated with HER2-CAR-T had came out with stable conditions [56]. Feng et al. [57] showed the results of a clinical trial of an EGFR-CAR-T treatment for EGFR-positive relapsed/refractory NSCLC patients revealed partial remission in 2 of the 11 patients involved in the evaluation and 5 patients had a stable condition ranging from 2 to 8 months. There were no obvious adverse reactions in the entire clinical trial. In the treatment of esophageal cancer, no CAR-T therapy-related studies have been conducted yet. However, anti-tumor targets are now erupting in esophageal cancer. Points such as HER2 can also provide references for future steps in the development of research.

3. Combined treatment

Currently, comprehensive therapy shed light on tumor treatment to a large degree. Clinical practice has proven that it is difficult to achieve the best results with any single treatment method. Therefore, the principle of treatment for most tumors depends on comprehensive treatment. Recent research results showed that the combined usage of immunotherapy and chemotherapy in a variety of cancer treatment achieved better results than a single therapy, it can not only reverse the immunosuppression effects caused by the late stage of the tumor, increase the cross-presentation of tumor antigens, promote the proliferation of killer T cells and make it more easy to kill tumor cells, but can also reduce the incidence of adverse reactions from chemotherapy and reduce drug resistance of tumor cells to some extent. Combination of chemotherapy and immunotherapy has been a common available method in some cancer types. Neoadjuvant chemotherapy regimens together with HER2-targeted therapy achieved pathologic complete response in relapse-free survival among patients with breast cancer [58].

New treatment targeting specific mutant genes illustrated clinical success in a phase II study of metastatic melanoma combined with interleukin-2 aldesleukin and BRAF inhibitor vemurafenib [59]. The effectiveness of combined therapy can even cover the metastatic areas, in melanoma brain metastases, complete intracranial response was observed after using dual checkpoint-inhibition of talimogene laherparepvec (T-Vec), pembrolizumab and whole brain radiotherapy. Additionally, immunotherapy also showed potential augmented effect plus cryotherapy [60], focused ultrasound therapy [61] and photothermal therapy [62], etc. Tumor vaccine also took another leap when combined with other immunotherapies, clinical results showed that nivolumab in combination with talimogene laherparepvec (T-Vec) in resected melanoma carried out better outcomes [63]. The clinical value of immunotherapy and radiotherapy showed even more outstanding clinical effects, anti-tumor immune response was enhanced by anti-PD-1 immunotherapy in recurrent nasopharyngeal carcinoma, showing a bright prospect of further combination [64]. In treating esophageal cancer, there are also many creative comprehensive treatment methods that are constantly developing. In patients with drug-resistant esophageal cancer, a phase Ib/II study of low-dose decitabine-primed chemoimmunotherapy showed undeniable safety and efficacy [65]. A combination therapy of multi-peptide vaccine with chemoradiation therapy performed satisfying safety thus can be an effective treatment for patients with unresectable ESCC [66]. Novel multitarget tyrosine kinase inhibitor anlotinib in a third-line treatment of refractory advanced non-small-cell lung cancer (RA-NSCLC) provided significant PFS benefits compared with placebo, and accompanied with acceptable toxicity [67]. Though has a guaranteed future, there need to be more rational and effective trials of combinations to be excavated in the field of treating esophageal cancer together with other solid tumors.

4. Conclusions and future directions

The success of immunotherapy in some tumors came from years of research deep into the immune system and tumor itself and brought hope of healing cancer. It is worth mentioning that several immune checkpoint blockers have been or are being approved by the FDA, and it is expected that the next step will be to accelerate the pace of application of single drug or other treatment modes in combination within clinical usage. However, opportunities and challenges coexist, and there are still some key questions that have not been answered in immunotherapy. First of all, many targeted cancer drugs that treat cancer need to be explored to determine the biological dose that achieves the greatest clinical benefit with minimal toxicity. Second, given that most of the current immunotherapy is mainly to activate anti-tumor effects by activating the immune system, this kind of treatment requires patient to have some degree of immunity before receiving the initial immunotherapy. Therefore, it is imperative to fully evaluate patient's immune status and find biomarkers that predict the effectiveness of immunotherapy. In addition, there is abundant evidence that exposure to radiation and chemotherapy drugs may affect the rate of DNA mutations in tumor cells, prompting the formation of some new antigens. As the current immunotherapy is always combined with radiotherapy and chemotherapy, determining the proper dose for each regimen is the prerequisite for maximum benefit of combined therapy.

Immunotherapy has a broad application prospect in the treatment of malignant tumors. The high frequency of esophageal cancer mutations and the effective results of immunotherapy highlighted in other gastrointestinal cancers provide strong evidence for the study of esophageal cancer immunotherapy. Treatment strategies combined with existing or new treatment modes will be the direction of future esophageal cancer treatment.

Author details

Tian Wang and Yi Zhang*

*Address all correspondence to: yizhang@zzu.edu.cn

Biotherapy Center, The First Affiliated Hospital of Zhengzhou University, Zhengzhou, Henan, China

References

[1] GBD 2015 Disease and Injury Incidence and Prevalence, Collaborators. Lancet. 2016; **388**(10053):1545-1602. DOI: 10.1016/S0140-6736(16)31678-6. PMC: 5055577 PMID: 277-33282

[2] GBD 2015 Mortality and Causes of Death, Collaborators. Lancet. 2016;**388**(10053): 1459-1544. DOI: 10.1016/s0140-6736(16)31012-1. PMC: 5388903 PMID: 27733281

[3] Chang S, Kohrt H, Maecker HT. Monitoring the immune competence of cancer patients to predict outcome. Cancer Immunology, Immunotherapy. 2014;**63**:713-719. DOI: 10. 1007/s00262-014-1521-3. PMID: 24487923

[4] Smyth E, Thuss-Patience PC. Immune checkpoint inhibition in gastro-oesophageal cancer. Oncology Research and Treatment. 2018;**41**(5):272-280. DOI: 10.1159/000489099. PMID: 29705787

[5] Li F, Zhang T, Cao L, Zhang Y. Chimeric antigen receptor T cell based immunotherapy for cancer. Current Stem Cell Research & Therapy. 2018 Apr 19. DOI: 10.2174/1574888X 13666180420110239. PMID: 29676233

[6] Kueberuwa G, Kalaitsidou M, Cheadle E, Hawkins RE, Gilham DE. CD19 CAR T cells expressing IL-12 eradicate lymphoma in fully lymphoreplete mice through induction of host immunity. Molecular Therapy—Oncolytics. 2017 Dec 19;**8**:41-51. DOI: 10.1016/j. omto.2017.12.003 eCollection 2018 Mar 30. PMID: 29367945

[7] Enzinger PC, Mayer RJ. Esophageal cancer. The New England Journal of Medicine. 2003;**349**:2241-2252. DOI: 10.1056/NEJMra035010 PMID: 14657432

[8] Rubenstein JH, Shaheen NJ. Epidemiology, diagnosis, and management of esophageal adenocarcinoma. Gastroenterology. 2015;**149**:302-17.e1. DOI: 10.1053/j.gastro.2015.04.053 PMID: 25957861

[9] Paget S. The distribution of secondary growths in cancer of the breast. 1889. Cancer Metastasis Reviews. 1989;**8**:98-101 PMID: 2673568

[10] Karakasheva TA, Dominguez GA, Hashimoto A, Lin EW, Chiu C, Sasser K, Lee JW, Beatty GL, Gabrilovich DI, Rustgi AK. CD38+ M-MDSC expansion characterizes a subset of advanced colorectal cancer patients. JCI Insight. 2018 Mar 22;**3**(6):pii-97022. DOI: 10.1172/jci.insight.97022 PMID: 29563330

[11] Whiteside TL. The tumor microenvironment and its role in promoting tumor growth. Oncogene. 2008;**27**:5904-5912. DOI: 10.1038/onc.2008.271 PMID: 18836471

[12] Zhu Y, Zhang L, Zha H, Yang F, Hu C, Chen L, Guo B, Zhu B. Stroma-derived fibrinogen-like protein 2 activates cancer-associated fibroblasts to promote tumor growth in lung cancer. International Journal of Biological Sciences. 2017 Jun 1;**13**(6):804-814. DOI: 10.7150/ijbs.19398 eCollection 2017. PMID: 28656005

[13] Okano S, Abu-Elmagd K, Kish DD, Keslar K, Baldwin WM 3rd, Fairchild RL, Fujiki M, Khanna A, Osman M, Costa G, Fung J, Miller C, Kayashima H, Hashimoto K. Myeloid-derived suppressor cells increase and inhibit donor-reactive T cell responses to graft intestinal epithelium in intestinal transplant patients. American Journal of Transplantation. 2018 Mar 6. DOI: 10.1111/ajt.14718. PMID: 29509288

[14] Parker KH, Beury DW, Ostrand-Rosenberg S. Myeloid-derived suppressor cells: Critical cells driving immune suppression in the tumor microenvironment. Advances in Cancer Research. 2015;**128**:95-139. DOI: 10.1016/bs.acr.2015.04.002

[15] Spallanzani RG1, Dalotto-Moreno T, Raffo Iraolagoitia XL, Ziblat A, Domaica CI, Avila DE, Rossi LE, Fuertes MB, Battistone MA, Rabinovich GA, Salatino M, Zwirner NW. Expansion of CD11b(+)Ly6G (+)Ly6C (int) cells driven by medroxyprogesterone acetate in mice bearing breast tumors restrains NK cell effector functions. Cancer Immunology, Immunotherapy. 2013 Dec;**62**(12):1781-1795. DOI: 10.1007/s00262-013-1483-x. PMID: 24114144

[16] Fleming V, Hu X, Weber R, Nagibin V, Groth C, Altevogt P, Utikal J, Umansky V. Targeting myeloid-derived suppressor cells to bypass tumor-induced Immunosuppression. Frontiers in Immunology. 2018 Mar 2;**9**:398. DOI: 10.3389/fimmu.2018.00398 eCollection 2018. PMID: 29552012

[17] Ahrends T, Borst J. The opposing roles of CD4+ T cells in anti-tumor immunity. Immunology. 2018 Apr 27. DOI: 10.1111/imm.12941. PMID: 29700809

[18] Yang G, Li H, Yao Y, Xu F, Bao Z, Zhou J. Treg/Th17 imbalance in malignant pleural effusion partially predicts poor prognosis. Oncology Reports. 2015 Jan;**33**(1):478-484. DOI: 10.3892/or.2014.3576

[19] Wang Y, Xu G, Wang J, Li XH, Sun P, Zhang W, Li JX, Wu CY. Relationship of Th17/Treg cells and radiation pneumonia in locally advanced esophageal carcinoma. Anticancer Research. 2017 Aug;**37**(8):4643-4647

[20] Qiao Y, Zhang C, Li A, Wang D, Luo Z, Ping Y, Zhou B, Liu S, Li H, Yue D, Zhang Z, Chen X, Shen Z, Lian J, Li Y, Wang S, Li F, Huang L, Wang L, Zhang B, Yu J, Qin Z, Zhang Y. IL6 derived from cancer-associated fibroblasts promotes chemoresistance via CXCR7 in esophageal squamous cell carcinoma. Oncogene. 2018 Feb 15;**37**(7):873-883. DOI: 10.1038/onc.2017.387

[21] Guo W, Wang P, Li N, Shao F, Zhang H, Yang Z, Li R, Gao Y, He J. Prognostic value of PD-L1 in esophageal squamous cell carcinoma: A meta-analysis. Oncotarget. 2017 Dec 27;**9**(17):13920-13933. DOI: 10.18632/oncotarget.23810. PMID: 29568405

[22] Freeman GJ, Long AJ, Iwai Y, Bourque K, Chernova T, Nishimura H, Fitz LJ, Malenkovich N, Okazaki T, Byrne MC, Horton HF, Fouser L, Carter L, Ling V, Bowman MR, Carreno BM, Collins M, Wood CR, Honjo T. Engagement of the PD-1 immunoinhibitory receptor by a novel B7 family member leads to negative regulation of lymphocyte activation. The Journal of Experimental Medicine. 2000;**192**:1027-1034. DOI: 10.1084/jem.192.7.1027. PMID: 11015443

[23] Walsh EM, Kelly RJ. Single agent anti PD-1 inhibitors in esophageal cancer—A first step in a new therapeutic direction. Journal of Thoracic Disease. 2018 Mar;**10**(3):1308-1313. DOI: 10.21037/jtd.2018.03.43

[24] Caja L, Dituri F, Mancarella S, Caballero-Diaz D, Moustakas A, Giannelli G, Fabregat I. TGF-β and the tissue microenvironment: Relevance in fibrosis and cancer. International Journal of Molecular Sciences. 2018 Apr 26;**19**(5). DOI: 10.3390/ijms19051294

[25] Song S, Maru DM, Ajani JA, Chan CH, Honjo S, Lin HK, Correa A, Hofstetter WL, Davila M, Stroehlein J, Mishra L. Loss of TGF-β adaptor 2SP activates notch signaling and SOX9 expression in esophageal adenocarcinoma. Cancer Research. 2013;**73**:2159-2169. DOI: 10.1158/0008-5472.CAN-12-1962

[26] Givel AM, Kieffer Y, Scholer-Dahirel A, Sirven P, Cardon M, Pelon F, Magagna I, Gentric G, Costa A, Bonneau C, Mieulet V, Vincent-Salomon A, Mechta-Grigoriou F. miR200-regulated CXCL12β promotes fibroblast heterogeneity and immunosuppression in ovarian cancers. Nature Communications. 2018 Mar 13;**9**(1):1056. DOI: 10.1038/s41467-018-03348-z

[27] Nazari A, Khorramdelazad H, Hassanshahi G. Biological/pathological functions of the CXCL12/CXCR4/CXCR7 axes in the pathogenesis of bladder cancer. International Journal of Clinical Oncology. 2017 Dec;**22**(6):991-1000. DOI: 10.1007/s10147-017-1187-x. PMID: 29022185

[28] Liu J, Li F, Ping Y, Wang L, Chen X, Wang D, Cao L, Zhao S, Li B, Kalinski P, Thorne SH, Zhang B, Zhang Y. Local production of the chemokines CCL5 and CXCL10 attracts CD8+ T lymphocytes into esophageal squamous cell carcinoma. Oncotarget. 2015;**6**: 24978-24989. DOI: 10.18632/oncotarget.4617

[29] Liu Z, McMichael EL, Shayan G, Li J, Chen K, Srivastava RM, Kane LP, Lu B, Ferris RL. Novel effector phenotype of Tim-3+ regulatory T cells leads to enhanced suppressive

function in head and neck cancer patients. Clinical Cancer Research. 2018 Apr 30. DOI: 10.1158/1078-0432.CCR-17-1350. PMID: 29712685

[30] Borghaei H, Paz-Ares L, Horn L, Spigel DR, Steins M, Ready NE, Chow LQ, Vokes EE, Felip E, Holgado E, Barlesi F, Kohlhäufl M, Arrieta O, Burgio MA, Fayette J, Lena H, Poddubskaya E, Gerber DE, Gettinger SN, Rudin CM, Rizvi N, Crinò L, Blumenschein GR, Antonia SJ, Dorange C, Harbison CT, Graf Finckenstein F, Brahmer JR. Nivolumab versus docetaxel in advanced nonsquamous non-small-cell lung cancer. The New England Journal of Medicine. 2015;**373**:1627-1639. DOI: 10.1056/NEJMoa1507643. PMID: 26412456

[31] Long GV, Atkinson V, Lo S, Sandhu S, Guminski AD, Brown MP, Wilmott JS, Edwards J, Gonzalez M, Scolyer RA, Menzies AM, McArthur GA. Combination nivolumab and ipilimumab or nivolumab alone in melanoma brain metastases: A multicentre randomised phase 2 study. The Lancet Oncology. 2018 Mar 27. DOI: 10.1016/S1470-2045(18)30139-6. PMID: 29602646

[32] Huang H, Zhang G, Li G, Ma H, Zhang X. Circulating CD14(+)HLA-DR(−/low) myeloid-derived suppressor cell is an indicator of poor prognosis in patients with ESCC. Tumour Biology. 2015;**36**:7987-7996. DOI: 10.1007/s13277-015-3426-y. PMID: 25967454

[33] Doi T, Piha-Paul SA, Jalal SI, Saraf S, Lunceford J, Koshiji M, Bennouna J. Safety and antitumor activity of the anti-programmed death-1 antibody pembrolizumab in patients with advanced esophageal carcinoma. Journal of Clinical Oncology. 2018 Jan 1;**36**(1): 61-67. DOI: 10.1200/JCO.2017.74.9846

[34] Santoni G, Amantini C, Morelli MB, Tomassoni D, Santoni M, Marinelli O, Nabissi M, Cardinali C, Paolucci V, Torniai M, Rinaldi S, Morgese F, Bernardini G, Berardi R. High CTLA-4 expression correlates with poor prognosis in thymoma patients. Oncotarget. 2018 Mar 30;**9**(24):16665-16677. DOI: 10.18632/oncotarget.24645. eCollection 2018 Mar 30

[35] Liu D, Badell IR, Ford ML. Selective CD28 blockade attenuates CTLA-4-dependent CD8+ memory T cell effector function and prolongs graft survival. JCI Insight. 2018 Jan 11;**3**(1). DOI: 10.1172/jci.insight.96378 PMID: 29321374

[36] Diao K, Bian SX, Routman DM, Yu C, Ye JC, Wagle NA, Wong MK, Zada G, Chang EL. Stereotactic radiosurgery and ipilimumab for patients with melanoma brain metastases: Clinical outcomes and toxicity. Journal of Neuro-Oncology. 2018 Apr 25. DOI: 10.1007/s11060-018-2880-y. PMID: 29696531

[37] Maio M, Scherpereel A, Calabrò L, Aerts J, Cedres Perez S, Bearz A, Nackaerts K, Fennell DA, Kowalski D, Tsao AS, Taylor P, Grosso F, Antonia SJ, Nowak AK, Taboada M, Puglisi M, Stockman PK, Kindler HL. Tremelimumab as second-line or third-line treatment in relapsed malignant mesothelioma (DETERMINE): A multicentre, international, randomised, double-blind, placebo-controlled phase 2b trial. The Lancet Oncology. 2017 Sep;**18**(9):1261-1273. DOI: 10.1016/S1470-2045(17)30446-1 Epub 2017 Jul 17. PMID: 28729154

[38] Ralph C, Elkord E, Burt DJ, O'Dwyer JF, Austin EB, Stern PL, Hawkins RE, Thistlethwaite FC. Modulation of lymphocyte regulation for cancer therapy: A phase II trial of tremelimumab in advanced gastric and esophageal adenocarcinoma. Clinical Cancer Research. 2010;**16**:1662-1672. DOI: 10.1158/1078-0432.CCR-09-2870. PMID: 20179239

[39] Rosenberg SA, Yang JC, Restifo NP. Cancer immunotherapy: Moving beyond current vaccines. Nature Medicine. 2004;**10**:909-915. DOI: 10.1038/nm1100. PMID: 15340416

[40] Rosenberg SA, Sherry RM, Morton KE, Scharfman WJ, Yang JC, Topalian SL, Royal RE, Kammula U, Restifo NP, Hughes MS, Schwartzentruber D, Berman DM, Schwarz SL, Ngo LT, Mavroukakis SA, White DE, Steinberg SM. Tumor progression can occur despite the induction of very high levels of self/tumor antigen-specific CD8+ T cells in patients with melanoma. Journal of Immunology. 2005;**175**:6169-6176. DOI: 10.4049/ jimmunol.175.9.6169. PMID: 16237114

[41] Kono K, Mizukami Y, Daigo Y, Takano A, Masuda K, Yoshida K, Tsunoda T, Kawaguchi Y, Nakamura Y, Fujii H. Vaccination with multiple peptides derived from novel cancer-testis antigens can induce specific T-cell responses and clinical responses in advanced esophageal cancer. Cancer Science. 2009;**100**:1502-1509. DOI: 10.1111/j.1349-7006.2009. 01200.x. PMID: 19459850

[42] Kono K, Iinuma H, Akutsu Y, Tanaka H, Hayashi N, Uchikado Y, Noguchi T, Fujii H, Okinaka K, Fukushima R, Matsubara H, Ohira M, Baba H, Natsugoe S, Kitano S, Takeda K, Yoshida K, Tsunoda T, Nakamura Y. Multicenter, phase II clinical trial of cancer vaccination for advanced esophageal cancer with three peptides derived from novel cancer-testis antigens. Journal of Translational Medicine. 2012;**10**:141. DOI: 10.1186/1479-5876-10-141. PMID: 22776426

[43] Saito T, Wada H, Yamasaki M, Miyata H, Nishikawa H, Sato E, Kageyama S, Shiku H, Mori M, Doki Y. High expression of MAGE-A4 and MHC class I antigens in tumor cells and inductionof MAGE-A4 immune responses are prognostic markers of CHP-MAGE-A4 cancer vaccine. Vaccine. 2014;**32**:5901-5907. DOI: 10.1016/j.vaccine.2014.09.002. PMID: 25218300

[44] Wada H, Sato E, Uenaka A, Isobe M, Kawabata R, Nakamura Y, Iwae S, Yonezawa K, Yamasaki M, Miyata H, Doki Y, Shiku H, Jungbluth AA, Ritter G, Murphy R, Hoffman EW, Old LJ, Monden M, Nakayama E. Analysis of peripheral and local anti-tumor immune response in esophageal cancer patients after NY-ESO-1 protein vaccination. International Journal of Cancer. 2008;**123**:2362-2369. DOI: 10.1002/ijc.23810. PMID: 18729190

[45] Dietrich A, Mitchison NA, Rajnavölgyi E, Schneider SC. Primed lymphocytes are boosted by type II collagen of their hosts after adoptive transfer. Journal of Autoimmunity. 1994;**7**:601-609. DOI: 10.1006/jaut.1994.1044. PMID: 7840853

[46] Alsina M, Moehler M, Lorenzen S. Immunotherapy of esophageal cancer: Current status, many trials and innovative strategies. Oncology Research and Treatment. 2018;**41**(5): 266-271. DOI: 10.1159/000488120. Epub 2018 Apr 20

[47] Rosenberg SA, Lotze MT, Muul LM, Leitman S, Chang AE, Ettinghausen SE, Matory YL, Skibber JM, Shiloni E, Vetto JT. Observations on the Systemic Administration of Autologous Lymphokine-Activated Killer Cells and Recombinant Interleukin-2 to Patients with Metastatic Cancer

[48] Besser MJ, Shapira-Frommer R, Schachter J. Tumor-infiltrating lymphocytes: Clinical experience. Cancer Journal. 2015;**21**:465-469 PMID: 26588677. DOI: 10.1097/PPO.0000000000000154

[49] Toh U, Yamana H, Sueyoshi S, Tanaka T, Niiya F, Katagiri K, Fujita H, Shirozou K, Itoh K. Locoregional cellular immunotherapy for patients with advanced esophageal cancer. Clinical Cancer Research. 2000;**6**:4663-4673. PMID: 11156218

[50] Chen X, Wang L, Yue D, Liu J, Huang L, Yang L, Cao L, Qin G, Li A, Wang D, Wang M, Qi Y, Zhang B, van der Bruggen P, Zhang Y. Correlation between the high expression levels of cancer-germline genes with clinical characteristics in esophageal squamous cell carcinoma. Histology and Histopathology. 2017 Aug;**32**(8):793-803. DOI: 10.14670/HH-11-847. Epub 2016 Nov 21

[51] Bujas T, Marusic Z, Peric Balja M, Mijic A, Kruslin B, Tomas D. MAGE-A3/4 and NY-ESO-1 antigens expression in metastatic esophageal squamous cell carcinoma. European Journal of Histochemistry. 2011;**55**:e7. DOI: 10.4081/ejh. 2011.e7. PMID: 21556122

[52] Kageyama S, Wada H, Muro K, Niwa Y, Ueda S, Miyata H, Takiguchi S, Sugino SH, Miyahara Y, Ikeda H, Imai N, Sato E, Yamada T, Osako M, Ohnishi M, Harada N, Hishida T, Doki Y, Shiku H. Dose-dependent effects of NY-ESO-1 protein vaccine complexed with cholesteryl pullulan (CHP-NY-ESO-1) on immune responses and survival benefits of esophageal cancer patients. Journal of Translational Medicine. 2013;**11**:246. DOI: 10.1186/1479-5876-11-246. PMID: 24093426

[53] Gross G, Waks T, Eshhar Z. Expression of immunoglobulin-T-cell receptor chimeric molecules as functional receptors with antibodytype specificity. Proceedings of the National Academy of Sciences of the United States of America. 1989;**86**:10024-10028. DOI: 10.1073/pnas.86.24.10024. PMID: 2513569

[54] Liu Y, Chen X, Han W, Zhang Y. Tisagenlecleucel, an approved anti-CD19 chimeric antigen receptor T-cell therapy for the treatment of leukemia. Drugs Today (Barc). 2017 Nov;**53**(11):597-608. DOI: 10.1358/dot.2017.53.11.2725754. PMID: 29451276

[55] Kershaw MH, Westwood JA, Parker LL, Wang G, Eshhar Z, Mavroukakis SA, White DE, Wunderlich JR, Canevari S, Rogers-Freezer L, Chen CC, Yang JC, Rosenberg SA, Hwu P. A phase I study on adoptive immunotherapy using gene-modified T cells for ovarian cancer. Clinical Cancer Research. 2006;**12**:6106-6115. DOI: 10.1158/1078-0432.CCR-06-1183. PMID: 17062687

[56] Nellan A, Rota C, Majzner R, Lester-McCully CM, Griesinger AM, Mulcahy Levy JM, Foreman NK, Warren KE, Lee DW. Durable regression of Medulloblastoma after regional

and intravenous delivery of anti-HER2 chimeric antigen receptor T cells. Journal for Immunotherapy of Cancer. 2018 Apr 30;**6**(1):30. DOI: 10.1186/s40425-018-0340-z

[57] Feng K, Guo Y, Dai H, Wang Y, Li X, Jia H, Han W. Chimeric antigen receptor-modified T cells for the immunotherapy of patients with EGFR expressing advanced relapsed/ refractory nonsmall cell lung cancer. Science China. Life Sciences. 2016;**59**:468-479. DOI: 10.1007/s11427-016-5023-8. PMID: 26968708

[58] Weiss A, Bashour SI, Hess K, Thompson AM, Ibrahim NK. Effect of neoadjuvant chemotherapy regimen on relapse-free survival among patients with breast cancer achieving a pathologic complete response: An early step in the de-escalation of neoadjuvant chemotherapy. Breast Cancer Research. 2018;**20**:27. DOI: 10.1186/s13058-018-0945-7

[59] Mooradian MJ, Reuben A, Prieto PA, Hazar-Rethinam M, Frederick DT, Nadres B, Piris A, Juneja V, Cooper ZA, Sharpe AH, Corcoran RB, Flaherty KT, Lawrence DP, Wargo JA, Sullivan RJ. A phase II study of combined therapy with a BRAF inhibitor (vemurafenib) and interleukin-2 (aldesleukin) in patients with metastatic melanoma. Oncoimmunology. 2018 Feb 1;**7**(5):e1423172. DOI: 10.1080/2162402X.2017.1423172. eCollection 2018

[60] Abdo J, Cornell DL, Mittal SK, Agrawal DK. Immunotherapy plus cryotherapy: Potential augmented abscopal effect for advanced cancers. Frontiers in Oncology. 2018 Mar 28;**8**:85. DOI: 10.3389/fonc.2018.00085. eCollection 2018

[61] Mauri G, Nicosia L, Xu Z, Di Pietro S, Monfardini L, Bonomo G, Varano GM, Prada F, Della Vigna P, Orsi F. Focused ultrasound: Tumour ablation and its potential to enhance immunological therapy to cancer. The British Journal of Radiology. 2018 Feb;**91**(1083):20170641. DOI: 10.1259/bjr.20170641

[62] Mi FL, Burnouf T, Lu SY, Lu YJ, Lu KY, Ho YC, Kuo CY, Chuang EY. Self-targeting, immune transparent plasma protein coated nanocomplex for noninvasive photothermal anticancer therapy. Advanced Healthcare Materials. 2017 Jul;**6**(14). DOI: 10.1002/ adhm.201700181

[63] Blake Z, Marks DK, Gartrell RD, Hart T, Horton P, Cheng SK, Taback B, Horst BA, Saenger YM. Complete intracranial response to talimogene laherparepvec (T-Vec), pembrolizumab and whole brain radiotherapy in a patient with melanoma brain metastases refractory to dual checkpoint-inhibition. Journal for Immunotherapy of Cancer. 2018 Apr 6;**6**(1):25. DOI: 10.1186/s40425-018-0338-6

[64] Finazzi T, Rordorf T, Ikenberg K, Huber GF, Guckenberger M, Schueler G, HI. Radiotherapy-induced anti-tumor immune response and immune-related adverse events in a case of recurrent nasopharyngeal carcinoma undergoing anti-PD-1 immunotherapy. BMC Cancer. 2018 Apr 6;**18**(1):395. DOI: 10.1186/s12885-018-4295-8

[65] Chen M, Nie J, Liu Y, Li X, Zhang Y, Brock MV, Feng K, Wu Z, Li X, Shi L, Li S, Guo M, Mei Q, Han W. Phase Ib/II study of safety and efficacy of low-dose decitabine-primed chemoimmunotherapy in patients with drug-resistant relapsed/refractory alimentary tract cancer. International Journal of Cancer. 2018 Apr 16. DOI: 10.1002/ijc.31531

[66] Iinuma H, Fukushima R, Inaba T, Tamura J, Inoue T, Ogawa E, Horikawa M, Ikeda Y, Matsutani N, Takeda K, Yoshida K, Tsunoda T, Ikeda T, Nakamura Y, Okinaga K. Phase I clinical study of multiple epitope peptide vaccine combined with chemoradiation therapy in esophageal cancer patients. Journal of Translational Medicine. 2014 Apr 3;**12**:84. DOI: 10.1186/1479-5876-12-84

[67] Han B, Li K, Zhao Y, Li B, Cheng Y, Zhou J, Lu Y, Shi Y, Wang Z, Jiang L, Luo Y, Zhang Y, Huang C, Li Q, Wu G. Anlotinib as a third-line therapy in patients with refractory advanced non-small-cell lung cancer: A multicentre, randomised phase II trial (ALTER0302). British Journal of Cancer. 2018 Mar 6;**118**(5):654-661. DOI: 10.1038/bjc.2017.478

4

Minimally Invasive Esophagectomy

Rafael Cholvi Calduch, Isabel Mora Oliver,
Fernando Lopez Mozos and Roberto Martí Obiol

Abstract

Minimally Invasive Surgery (MIS) for esophageal carcinoma has improved the outcome of patients. This approach has been shown to decrease the rate of respiratory complications, the intensive care unit (ICU) stay, and to allow a faster recovery of patients. Also, an improvement in perioperative care has contributed to better outcomes compared to the open approach. MIS has been shown to be as safe as open surgery in terms of resectability, harvested lymph nodes, and overall survival.

Keywords: esophageal carcinoma, anesthesia, minimally invasive esophagectomy, thoracoscopic esophagectomy, laparoscopic esophagectomy, surgical technique, prone position, postoperative care, postoperative prognosis

1. Introduction

Neoplasm of the esophagus is one of the most aggressive diseases with poor survival rate despite of the improvements in staging procedures, multimodality treatments, supportive care, and surgical techniques. It is the eighth most common cause of cancer and the sixth leading cause of cancer death worldwide [1]. Patients often are diagnosed at an advanced stage with metastatic disease in more than 50% at the time of presentation. Surgery is the gold standard for treatment both for early stage disease and for advanced disease after chemoradiotherapy neoadjuvant treatment. Surgery of esophageal cancer is probably one of the most demanding and challenging procedure for the surgeon and the patient alike—with a significant morbidity and mortality, particularly in inappropriately selected patients. Surgical treatment must consist on a radical R0 en-bloc esophagectomy associated with a two-field lymphadenectomy [2].

Traditionally, open approaches have been used to resect esophageal cancer, performed by transhiatal, transthoracic, or combined approach. Esophagectomy is a complex challenge for the surgeon, dealing with wide areas of the neck, mediastinum, and abdomen. Open esophagectomy is considered to be one of the most traumatic oncologic procedures performed in gastrointestinal surgery because of the extent of resection and dissection required [3]. It entails a significant risk of morbidity (at least a half of patients develop complications) and mortality, that ranges from 6–7% in high-volume centers to 20–28% in low-volume centers.

Orringer et al. [4] reported a large series of 1085 patients who underwent open esophagectomy by transhiatal approach, which has served as a standard to compare postoperative outcomes: hospital mortality rate of 4%; 53% of patients were discharged by 10th postoperative day; and an anastomotic leak rate of 13%. The most frequently reported complications of open approach have been pneumonia (21%), respiratory failure (16%), prolonged ventilatory support more than 48 h (22%), according to the report published by Bailey et al. [5].

In an attempt to avoid extensive tissue aggression and reduce the high morbidity and mortality, the minimal invasive approach has been introduced in the field of gastroesophageal surgery [6]. Cuschieri et al. [7] and DePaula et al. [8] were the first to apply a laparoscopic approach to patients with esophageal cancer. Cuschieri et al. performed six subtotal endoscopic esophagectomies through a right thoracoscopic approach with a mean duration of stay in the ICU of 19 h (range 16–26 h) and a median hospital stay of 11 days (8–18 days). DePaula et al. reported a small series of 12 patients who underwent transhiatal esophagectomy conducted by videolaparoscopy with no mortality and minimal blood loss.

Thanks to the improvements in technology and instrumentation, as well as the surgeons' training in advanced minimally invasive procedures, the practice of this technique has been extended since the 1990s. There are several single institution series reports [7–10] (retrospective and prospective) comparing Minimally Invasive Esophagectomy (MIE) versus open surgery [11, 12], and recent meta-analyses [13, 14] that have confirmed the safety and feasibility of the procedure and the advantages of minimally invasive surgery. These reports show that MIE can reduce the mortality and morbidity of open operations as well as allow a faster recovery. All these findings have been confirmed at the only available level I evidence study, the TIME-trial [15].

2. Patient selection

Tumor staging is essential for planning surgical treatment, and surgery should not be performed for patients without a chance of cure, such as those with distant metastases, or in those unable to survive the physiologic insult of the operation. The main objective of surgery must be to achieve a R0 resection. Nowadays, neoadjuvant chemoradiation plays a key role because it downstages the tumor and allows an adequate micro and macroscopic tumoral resection. From a surgical perspective, the drawback is that it may further complicate the procedure by distorting the peri-esophageal microanatomy and by causing a significant postradiation fibrosis. Tissue plane may be unclear and surgery will not be easy in this situation.

The difficult dissection as a result of neoadjuvant therapy and surgeons' fear to use a minimally invasive approach in advanced tumors, especially during their learning curve, cause an important discussion about MIE effectiveness in these situations. In a multicenter, open-label, randomized controlled trial published in 2012 by Biere et al. [15] that compares open surgery with MIE in advanced tumors, both with a similar number of patients, did not show significant differences between both in terms of margins resection. Thus, the minimally invasive approach would not be a contraindication in advanced stages. However, a previous history of abdominal or thoracic surgeries due to a significant underlying adhesion process could represent a real hindrance for minimally invasive technique.

3. Evaluation of physiological reserve

Predicting which patients are going to develop complications is not easy. Even so, we must know which indicators can increase postoperative morbidity and mortality. Many risk factors have been identified: Karnofsky score less than 80, liver cirrhosis, chronic obstructive pulmonary disease (COPD), ischemic heart disease, advanced age, locally advanced tumor, active smoking, alcoholism, and malnutrition [16–19] are some of them. Evaluating individual risk is important for patient selection and a proper preoperative management, regardless of the surgical approach to be performed (MIE or open surgery). However, there are physiological conditions of patients that cannot be improved.

The risk factors suggestive of preoperative optimization are the following:

- In cases of COPD, the use of long-acting β-agonists, combined with inhaled steroids [20, 21] and preoperative inspiratory muscle training, may reduce postoperative pulmonary complications [22].
- If significant coronary ischemia is discovered in perioperative time, coronary revascularization with angioplasty and stenting could be performed, although antiplatelet agents prescribed after this technique could delay esophagectomy.
- Alcoholism and smoking—The UK National Institute for Health and Clinical Excellence (NICE) recommends the use of nicotine as a replacement therapy for smokers to help stop smoking, because smoking is associated with higher risk of 30-day mortality and serious postoperative complications [23].
- Malnutrition is considered an independent risk factor that influences the development of postoperative infections, mortality, length of stay, and hospital costs in patients undergoing surgery [24]. We must bear in mind that most patients with esophageal neoplasia have difficulties for an adequate intake, which generates poor nutritional status and immunosuppression. Therefore, patients with nutritional risk screening (NRS) score ≥3 should have an optimized nutritional support that includes both enteral nutrition to maintain the intestinal barrier function and parenteral nutrition to avoid malnutrition and infection due to long-term insufficient feeding. These measures will help to improve clinical outcomes in these patients [25, 26].

- Patients who have a Forced Expiratory Volume in one second (FEV 1) < 70% of the predicted normal in the pulmonary function tests with normal arterial gas blood measurements are considered of moderate risk and those with FEV 1 < 50% or if the arterial gas bold analysis show hypoxemia or carbon dioxide retention must be considered of high risk.
- Patients with Child C stage cirrhosis must not be eligible for surgery.

4. Anesthetic challenges of MIE

The anesthetic challenges of MIE include prolonged surgery, difficulties of lung isolation, and one lung ventilation (OLV) when patient is positioned right up and complications related to extraperitoneal CO_2. Pain relief has been described as a protective factor to avoid postoperative respiratory complications, so it is highly recommended to use regional techniques for reducing postoperative pain. Also, the amount of fluids administered perioperatively can lead to the development of pulmonary complications and should be adequately evaluated to avoid fluid overload.

4.1. Prolonged surgery

MIE is a long procedure and may extend at least 5–6 h, depending on the experience of the surgeon. Such prolonged surgery increases the risk of hypothermia which can lead to reduce oxygen delivery and increase myocardial work, stress response, and postoperative infection. Our main objective is to maintain normothermia. If at the end of the surgery the patient is normothermic, extubation will be possible and postoperative ventilation will not be necessary [27].

Balanced anesthesia, by an inhalation approach (sevoflurane and desflurane) or by propofol target-controlled infusion with remifentanil, may help promote early recovery after MIE. There is evidence that both sevoflurane and desflurane, when compared with propofol, produce a beneficial local immunomodulatory effect in patients undergoing OLV for thoracic surgery, significantly reducing inflammatory mediators, adverse postoperative events, and improving clinical outcomes [28, 29].

4.2. One lung ventilation

MIE with a patient in right up position requires a period of one lung ventilation during the mobilization of thoracic esophagus. Inadequately managed lung isolation contributes to mortality and morbidity [30].

When surgery is performed thoracoscopically, retraction of an inadequately collapsed lung or lobe results more difficult than in open surgery, and this is important when choosing the method used to achieve lung isolation. The options described to reach an adequate lung isolation are a left or right double lumen tube or a single lumen tracheal tube and a bronchial blocker. A retrospective study has not found differences in intraoperative hypoxemia, hypercapnia, and high airway pressures whether a left- or right-sided tube was placed for OLV [31].

As a consequence most MIE techniques involve access to the right thorax; a left double-lumen tube perhaps would be preferable, especially when the thoracic approach is done in lateral decubitus. If we used the prone position (PP), a single-lumen endotraqueal tube is a valid alternative. Whichever method of lung isolation is selected, a fiberoptic bronchoscope should be used to check correct positioning both after intubation and after moving the patient before surgery [32].

The combination of OLV and esophageal surgery results in an inflammatory response that will increase alveolar injury, leading to the development of acute lung injury (ALI) [33]. During and after OLV, the alveolar concentrations of IL-6 and IL-8 are increased. The lung protective ventilatory strategy can reduce airway pressure and airway resistance. It can decrease the release of IL-6 and IL-8 and inhibit lung inflammatory response during OLV and postoperatively [34]. Some of the consequences that may cause ventilator-induced lung injury are volutrauma (high tidal volume), barotrauma (excessive transpulmonary pressure), atelectrauma (repeated opening and closing of alveoli resulting), and biotrauma (caused by inflammatory mediators) [35].

Thus, it is essential for the implementation of protective ventilatory strategies to reduce the severity of lung injuries during mechanical ventilation. These strategies include restrict tidal volume to 5–6 ml/kg during OLV, optimizing positive expiratory end pressure (PEEP), and limiting plateau and peak inspiratory pressures to less than 25 cm H_2O and less than 35 cm H_2O, respectively [36]. In addition to reduce lung injury, these actions promote early extubation [37].

4.3. Complications of extra-peritoneal carbon dioxide

MIE may require a large period of capnoperitoneum, while laparoscopic dissection and mobilization of the stomach are being performed. As a consequence of surgical communication between the chest and abdomen, carbon dioxide may pass into the right chest, where drain tube has been placed in thoracic step, and this gas can be vented by this drain. In this situation, laparoscopic abdominal dissection could be difficult. Moreover, carbon dioxide may diffuse into the mediastinum (capnomediastinum), into the left chest, and it can cause subcutaneous emphysema around the chest, axilla, and neck. We can realize that gas is spreading to these spaces if we object a rapid increase in end-tidal CO_2. If CO_2 is accumulated inside thorax cavity, an increase of airway pressures and lung compression might occur, leading to oxygen desaturation. This fact could negatively affect cardiac output.

We can solve all these problems by reducing the pressure at which the capnoperitoneum is maintained, and this will reduce the diffusion of gas to thoracic cavity without impairing abdominal dissection. Anyway, if extra-abdominal CO_2 compromises cardiac or respiratory function, the capnoperitoneum should be evacuated. We should not extubate patients with significant emphysema until we achieve normocarbia [27].

4.4. Fluid management—goal directed therapy (GDT)

Maintaining adequate fluid balance is essential in both open surgery and MIE. While excessive fluid administration may be associated with increased postoperative pulmonary complication, tissue edema, and compromised perfusion, an inadequate intravascular volume can predispose to ischemia, end-organ dysfunction, and risk of anastomotic failure and leak.

In esophagectomy patients, an accurate fluid balance is essential to achieve adequate perfusion pressure and oxygen delivery to vital organs. The form of fluid replacement therapy, which is currently recommended, seems to be based on the principles of goal-directed therapy (GDT) with the aim to increase cardiac output in high-risk surgical patients. Various studies have found that GDT-based fluid administration improves intraoperative hemodynamic stability and reduces intensive care unit admissions, the incidence of complications, and mortality [38].

Some authors have suggested that restrictive fluid therapy is preferable to fluid overload because it leads to improved gastrointestinal recovery time, reduced overall morbidity [39], improved respiratory parameters, decreased incidence of postoperative pulmonary complications and shorter recovery periods [40]. On the other hand, fluid overload causes lung injury and has negatively impact to intestinal anastomoses [41].

4.5. Thoracic epidural analgesia (TEA) versus paravertebral analgesia

Even with reduction in trauma access, MIE may still result in an important postoperative pain, and optimal multimodal analgesia is required. Effective analgesia accelerates extubation, recovery, and early mobilization. Despite the importance of regular postoperative simple analgesia, a regional technique is essential.

Thoracic epidural analgesia (TEA) offers many benefits in esophagectomy, reducing respiratory complications, such us pneumonia [42–44] and postoperative pain. TEA has also been associated with decreased incidence of anastomotic leakage [37], possibly as a consequence of improving microcirculation in the gastric conduit [45]. Moreover, epidural analgesia also decreases the risk of prolonged ventilation or reintubation and improves some lung function parameters and blood oxygenation [46]. However, TEA also has some disadvantages: the incidence of failure may reach 12%, there are risks in the application technique, and it does not only promote urinary retention but also cause hypotension which makes necessary additional fluid administration [47–49]. Contraindications to an epidural access include sepsis or bacteraemia, infection at the insertion site, hypovolemia or shock, coagulopathy or thrombocytopenia and increased intracranial pressure [50].

Paravertebral blockade has recently been shown to provide analgesia comparable with TEA after thoracic step of esophagectomy. It is associated with less incidence of failed block and reduces hypotension and urinary retention when it is compared with TEA. Several recent reviews and meta-analyses defend its benefits [51–53], and it is a standard practice in some UK hospitals for minimally invasive esophagectomy. Local data also show shorter stays in the intensive therapy unit comparing with TEA.

4.6. Conclusion

MIE supposes many anesthetic challenges, some of them unique for this type of procedure and requires an accurate knowledge of the different surgical steps performed. Moreover, it is essential to know and treat complications of one lung anesthesia and extra-peritoneal spread of CO_2. Paravertebral blockade might have more benefits than TEA to improve postoperative pain in patients undergoing for MIE.

5. Operative technique

Minimally invasive esophageal resection for cancer involves a three-stage operation that includes a thoracosopy and laparoscopy, either with a cervical or intrathoracic anastomosis. It has been described as different combinations of laparotomy, thoracotomy, thoracoscopy, and laparoscopy approaches called hybrid techniques. These techniques have 1 step of the procedure completed via an open approach.

5.1. Thoracoscopy phase

The operation starts with thoracoscopic mobilization of the esophagus and thoracic lymphadenectomy. The thoracic phase can be performed through a lateral right thoracic approach by blocking the right tracheal bronchus, or in prone position without selecting any blocking.

In the first case, the patient is positioned in the left lateral decubitus position (LDP) and a right lung blocking is achieved employing a double-lumen tube. The surgeon stands on the left side of the patient and the assistant on the right. Three to four thoracoscopic ports are used in this approach and placed as follows:

- 10-mm camera port is placed at the 7th to 8th intercostal space, just anterior to the midaxillary line.
- A 5-mm port is placed at the 8th or 9th intercostal space, posterior to the posterior axillary line.
- A 10-mm port is placed at the 4th intercostal space in the anterior axillary line.
- The last 5-mm port is placed just posterior to the scapula tip.

When thoracoscopy is performed in a prone position (**Figure 1**), the mobilization of the esophagus takes place with a right prone posterior approach. Patients are intubated with a single-lumen endotracheal tube and the right lung remains partially collapsed because of the positive pressure of pneumothorax created and due to the gravity. The right upper limb is abducted 80–100°. The surgeon stands on the right side of the patient, the first assistant (camera) to the left of the surgeon, and the second assistant stands on the left side of the patient. Three ports are used and placed as follow:

- 10-mm camera port is placed at the 7th intercostal space below the inferior angle of the scapula.
- 5–10 mm port for right-hand working is placed at the 5th intercostal space right lateral from the spinous process.
- 5 mm for left-hand working is placed at the 9th intercostal space right lateral from the spinous process.

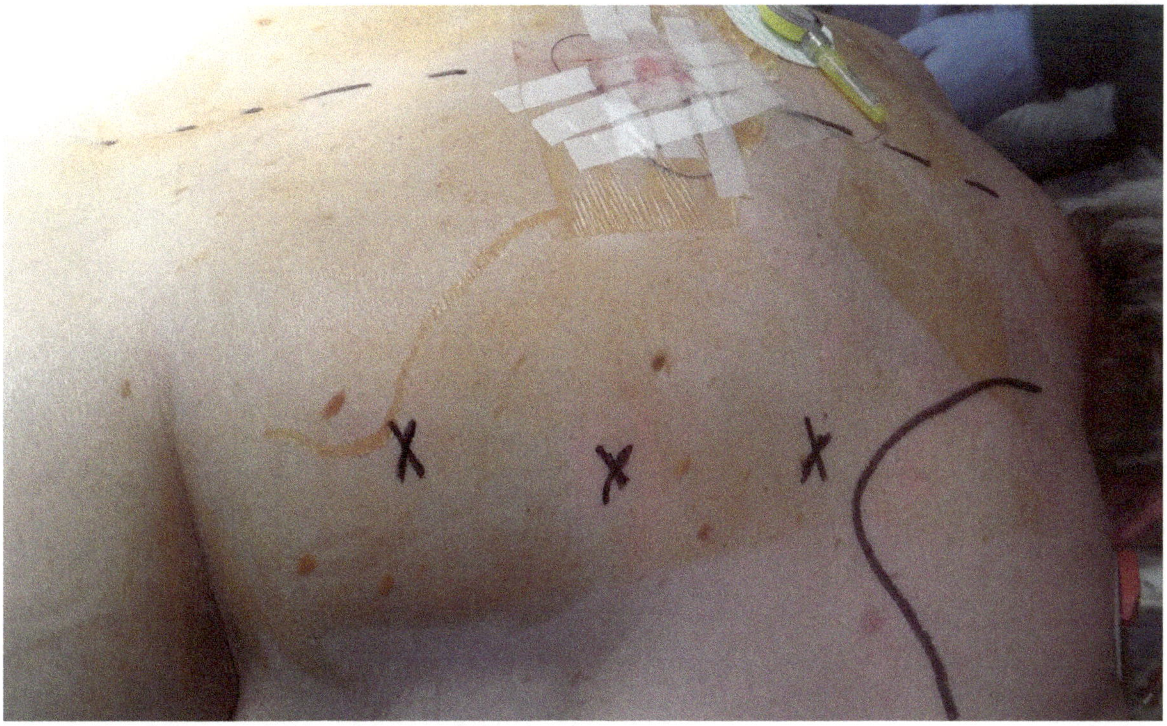

Figure 1. Thoracic trocar position on the right chest for thoracoscopic esophagectomy.

Pneumothorax is created and the insufflation pressure must be maintained at 6–8 mmHg. A single retracting suture in the diaphragm could be used to provide downward traction allowing good exposure of the distal esophagus, although in most occasions this is not necessary.

After a general survey of the tumor area and pleura, the inferior pulmonary ligament and the mediastinal pleura over the esophagus are divided up to the level of the azygos vein (**Figure 2**), which is sectioned with an endoscopic vascular stapler. The proximal esophagus is exposed and dissected circumferentially up to the level of 1–2 cm above the carina, using 5-mm harmonic shears, from the pericardium, chest wall, descending thoracic aorta, and superior cava vein, including all surrounding lymph nodes (**Figure 3**), periesophageal tissue, and fat. A tape is used for retraction of the esophagus to facilitate the dissection around it. Any aortoesophageal vessel and any lymphatic branches must be clipped. The thoracic duct has to be protected. The vagal trunks are identified and divided.

The dissection should be performed near the esophagus to avoid trauma to the posterior membranous trachea and the recurrent laryngeal nerves, which is the most difficult step. Laterally, dissection is carried down to the left pleura and continues to the thoracic inlet. A careful lymph nodal clearance must be achieved in the supracarinal space. Mobilization of the distal esophagus poses no problem, and it is important to limit it in order to avoid difficulty in maintaining pneumoperitoneum during the abdominal phase.

After the placement of a chest tube, the right lung is allowed to expand fully (or inflated in left lateral decubitus approach). Some surgeons infiltrate intercostal spaces with local anesthetic. Trocars are removed, and ports are closed.

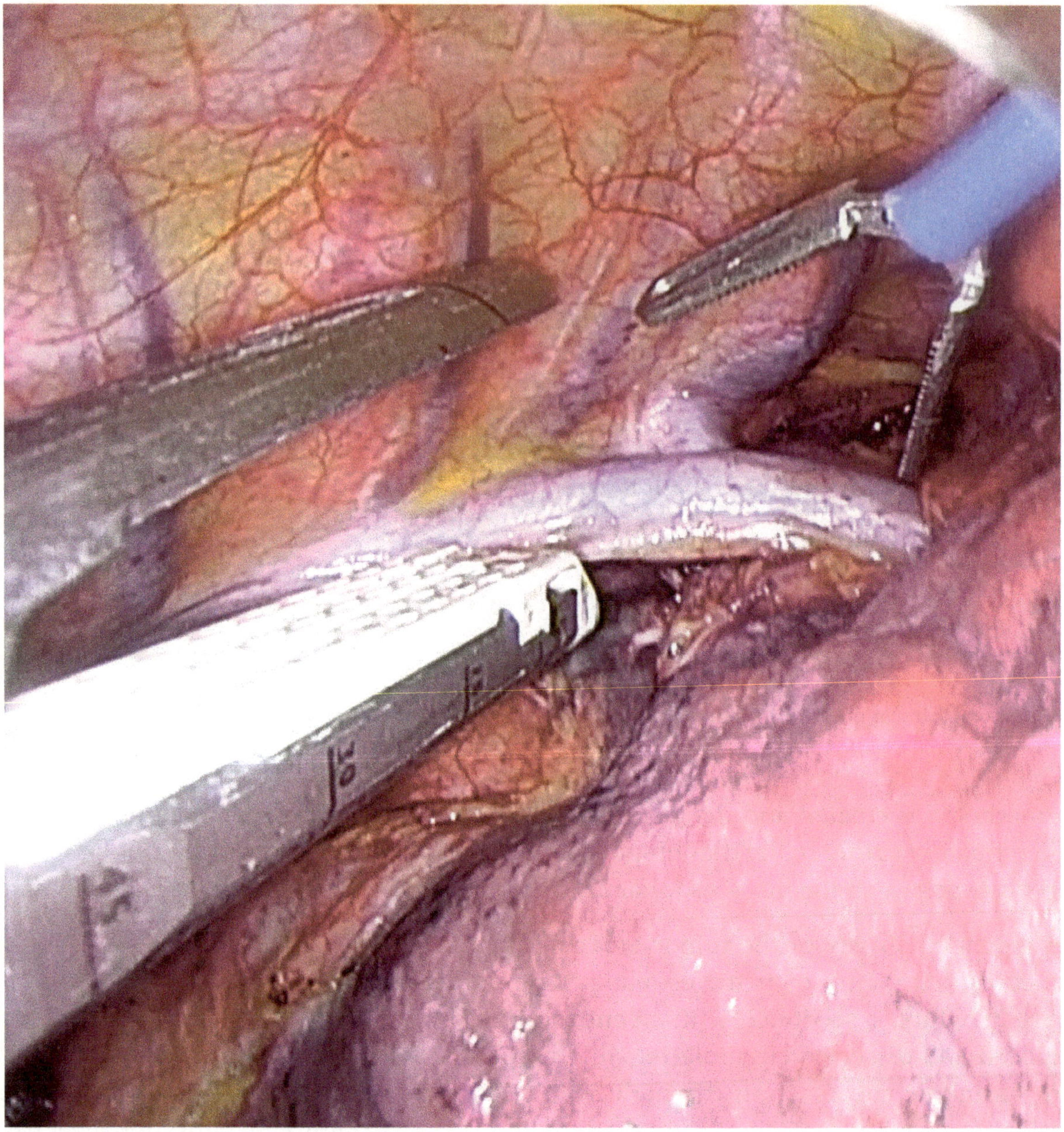

Figure 2. Division of the azygos vein using a stappler.

5.2. Laparoscopy and cervical phase

The second stage starts turning the patient to a modified Lloyd-Davis position with reverse Trendelemburg and neck exposing the left cervical area. The surgeon remains between the legs of the patient. The first and second assistants stand to the right and to the left of the patient, respectively. Five abdominal ports are used for the dissection: 10-mm supraumbilical port for camera; 5 mm epigastric port for retraction of left lobe of the liver, 5–10 mm right midclavicular port for left-hand working; 5–10 mm left midclavicular port for right-hand working; and 5–10 mm left anterior axillary port for gastric retraction. It is advisable to use trocars of a diameter of 10 mm for the possibility of using staplers from any port.

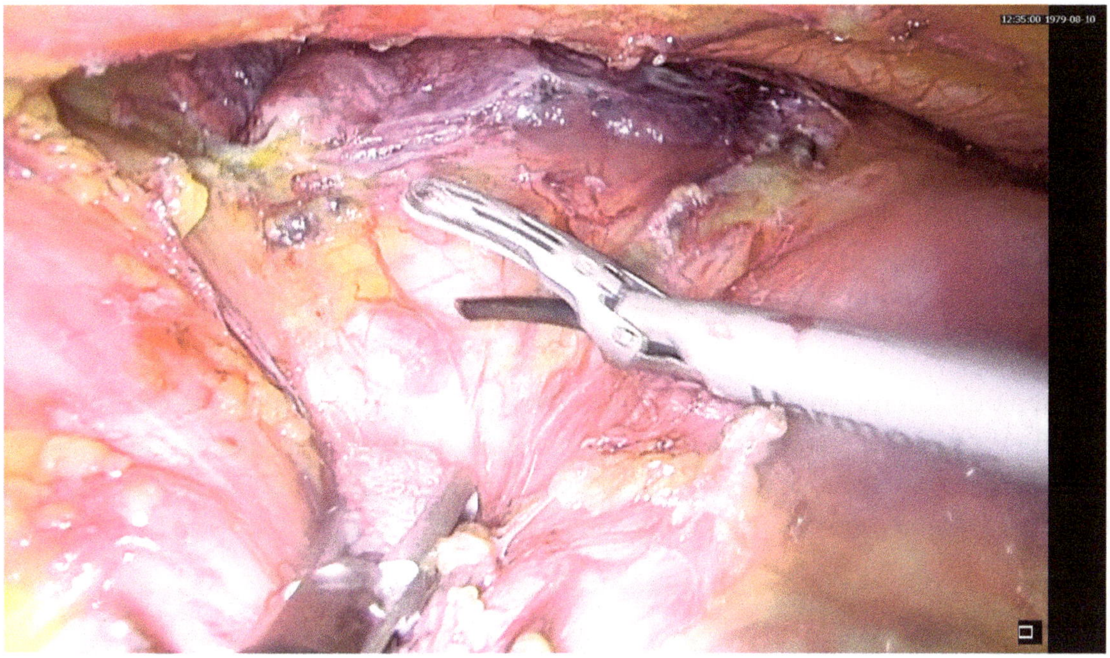

Figure 3. Mediastinal periesophageal lymph node.

After placement of the ports, an abdominal general survey must be performed. The gastrohepatic omentum is divided; the right and left crura of the diaphragm are dissected to allow easy passage of the gastric tube through the hiatus (preventing later gastric outlet obstruction). Left gastric artery and vein are dissected and divided using an endoscopic stapler with vascular load and a careful lymph node clearance over the left gastric pedicle, celiac axis, common hepatic, and splenic artery must be achieved. The stomach is mobilized by dividing the short gastric vessels in the gastrocolic omentum, using ultrasonic coagulating shears taking care of preserving the right gastroepiploic arcade. The fundus is dissected from the superior pole of the spleen and the pancreaticogastric ligaments are divided. Authors do not recommend pyloroplasty since it has been widely demonstrated that this does not improve gastric emptying.

Then the gastric tube is constructed with the stapler by dividing the stomach starting at the lesser curve. The construction of the gastric tube may vary depending on the characteristics of the tumor (if the tumor is located in the gastroesophageal junction or it has gastric extension, it may be necessary to resect some of the proximal stomach and to make an intrathoracic anastomosis). It is preferably a gastric tube with 5–6 cm in diameter. Most of the groups place a feeding jejunostomy laparoscopically. Authors prefer to leave a nasojejunal feeding tube to avoid complications derived from a jejunostomy.

The phrenoesophageal membrane is dissected, and gastric conduit is pulled through posterior mediastinum and brought up to the neck. Torsion is avoided by ensuring that the greater curvature always lies toward the left crus.

The last stage consists of a careful dissection of the cervical esophagus. A 4–6 cm left skin crease cervical incision is made. The tape looped around the esophagus left during the thoracic dissection allows the surgeon to pull it out through the neck to facilitate the dissection. The esophagogastric specimen is pulled out of the neck incision and the esophagus is transected 2–3 cm distal to the upper esophageal sphincter. A very high anastomosis is performed between the cervical esophagus and gastric tube in an end-to-end manner using an End-to-end anastomosis stapler (EEA sta-pler) or something similar. Some groups suture the gastric conduit to the prevertebral fascia. Neck wound is closed and a cervical drain could be placed. To prevent hiatal herniation, laparoscopic tacking sutures between the gastric tube and the diaphragm should be placed. If the anastomosis is performed intrathoracicaly, cervical stage is not performed.

Some groups pull out the specimen through a minilaparotomy incision incorporating camera port, and they construct the gastric tube in an extracorporeal way. This is recommended in cases of bulky tumors because it facilitates extraction of the specimen and allows to achieve a longer gastroplasty in case of performing the anastomosis in the neck.

One tube-drain is placed close to the hiatus. Trocars are removed, and ports are closed.

6. Minimally invasive surgery versus open approaches

Minimally invasive esophagectomy emerges as an attempt to reduce the significant morbidity and mortality of classic open techniques and allows a faster recovery of the patient.

Different groups have reported their experience in implementation of minimally invasive surgery in esophageal cancer in order to assess the potential advantages and disadvantages. One of the largest series was published by Luketich et al. [9]. They showed their outcomes in 222 patients after MIE: 30-day operative mortality of 1.4%, median intensive care unit stay of 1 day (range 1–3), hospital stay of 7 days (range 3–75), lower incidence of pneumonia, and adult respiratory distress syndrome (ARDS) (7.6 and 5%, respectively); anastomotic leak rate of 11.7%; and excellent health-related quality of life (HRQL) scores at a mean follow-up of 19 months, showing that MIE is a safety procedure and have potential advantages over open approach. Palanivelu et al. [10] reported their experience in 130 patients who underwent MIE with prone thoracoscopy: median ICU stay of 1 day (range 1–32 days), median hospital stay of 8 days (range 4–68 days), postoperative morbidity of 20.76%, perioperative mortality of 1.54%, anastomotic leak rate of 2.31%, lower incidence of pneumonia, and ARDS (1.54 and 0.77%, respectively), minimum blood loss. Both series showed a stage-specific survival similar to an open approach.

These findings have been confirmed in a recent meta-analysis [13] of 57 studies containing 15,790 patients with resectable esophageal cancer. Less intraoperative blood loss, short hospital stay, reduction of the incidence of total and pulmonary complications (OR: 0.700, 95% CI 0.626–0.781 and OR: 0.527, 95% CI: 0.431–0.645, $p < 0.05$, respectively), and high operative time than Open esophagectomy were found. However, ICU stay, the number of harvested lymph nodes, and anastomotic leak had no significant differences.

As we have mentioned previously in this chapter, traditional open esophagectomy carries a significant risk of postoperative complications that involves a profound detrimental impact on patient's quality of life. Quality of life typically returns to baseline after 1 year [54]. Minimally invasive techniques avoid thoracoabdominal incisions and reduce the levels of tissue trauma. The recovery rate after minimally invasive esophagectomy seems to be faster than after open approach. Parameswaran et al. [11] assessed this question in a prospective longitudinal nonrandomized study in 62 patients, measuring health-related quality of life (HRQL) after MIE. Their study noticed that although patients reported marked deterioration in most aspects of HRQL 6 weeks after the operation, they started to recover by 3 months and returned to baseline levels by 6 months, except reflux and diarrhea.

There is concern about if oncologic outcomes are equivalent to that of the open approach. When minimally invasive surgery was introduced in the management of colorectal cancer, there was also a concern about safety and oncological quality of resections. However, several randomized prospective trials demonstrated that the laparoscopic approach was not only safe but also oncologically sound [12].

While the advantages over short-term postoperative outcomes have been widely published by different institutions, there is a lack on the available data about oncologic efficacy and survival after MIE compared with the open approach. Different groups have tried to demonstrate that the adequacy of surgical margins and lymphadenectomy can be maintained or even improved with a MIE approach [55]. Berger and colleagues [12] found in their retrospective review that there were no differences between the groups in the R0 resection rates and a significant increase in nodal harvest in the MIE group (median 20 versus 9; $p < 0.0001$). Because of the known impact of neoadjuvant treatments on lymph node yields, they also examined lymph node harvest by the presence or absence of neoadjuvant chemoradiation, and they did not find differences in both groups. However, patients in the open group had a more advanced stage disease, and most of them had received neoadjuvant treatments.

The same group published a later work, Palazzo et al. [56], that compares survival of patients undergoing MIE and open or hybrid esophagectomy (OHE) in a retrospective analysis. They found on Kaplan-Meyer univariate analysis, a significantly improved 5-year survival with MIE (MIE 64%, OHE 35%, $p < 0.001$) and after adjusting for potential confounding factors (lymph nodes harvested, neoadjuvant treatments, stage, etc.) in a multivariate analysis demonstrated that patients undergoing OHE had a significantly worse survival. They made the same selection bias as in their previous study.

Nevertheless, these results are based on nonrandomized small series with heterogeneous data and could be affected by patient selection bias (frequently MIE group include a higher number of patients who have early disease stages and thus, less patients who received neoadjuvant chemoradioteraphy). Advanced tumors and the use of neoadjuvant therapy have been considered to be contraindications to MIE by many surgeons and limited its use, especially in patients with advanced disease.

All these studies have culminated in TIME-trial published in *The Lancet* in 2012 by Biere et al. [15, 57]. It is the first randomized trial to investigate the potential advantages of minimally invasive esophagectomy. They undertook a multicenter, open-label, randomized controlled trial at five study centers in three different countries. They compared open with minimally invasive esophagectomy with a right thoracoscopy in the prone position in a total of 115 patients with resectable esophageal cancer, excluding cervical allocation. The results showed that significantly fewer patients had postoperatory pulmonary infections, shorter hospital stay, and less blood loss in the minimally invasive group than in the open group. No difference was found in ICU stay. Also, short-term postoperative quality of life measured by SF 36, EORTC C30, and esophageal-specific OES18 questionnaire were significantly better for patients in the minimally invasive group, and they had less pain according to the Visual Analogue Scale (VAS) pain score. However, pathological parameters of the resected specimen and 30-day and in-hospital mortality did not differ between groups. They concluded that patients undergoing the minimally invasive approach have short-term benefits in pulmonary infections, hospital stay, and quality of life outcomes with no compromise in the quality of the resected specimen.

More randomized clinical trials are needed in order to assess the long-term advantages of minimally invasive surgery.

7. Prone position versus lateral decubitus position for thoracic step

To minimize morbidity and mortality after an esophagectomy, a thoracoscopic approach was introduced as a minimally invasive option [58, 59]. This procedure is most commonly performed with the patient in the left lateral decubitus position, but prone position is a valid alternative. Cuschieri et al. [60] first explained the prone position (PP) for thoracoscopic esophageal mobilization in 1994. They described this technique in 6 patients and compared the results with those of left lateral position in 20 patients. They suggested that PP had technical advantages and reduced postoperative complications. However, this technique was not widely used at that time, and more than 10 years have passed by to find publications that talk about PP again. In 2006, Palanivelu et al. [10] reported their experience with 130 patients treated by thoracoscopic esophagectomy in PP raising new interest in this procedure. Many reports about that have been published so far.

The primary benefit of the PP is derived from the anatomical exposure: the lung falls away as a consequence of gravity and the esophagus is better visualized. This permits performance of the operation without the need for collapsing the right lung using a double-lumen endotracheal tube. If we use a single-lumen endotracheal tube, the partial or intermittent ventilation of the right lung reduces the venous shunt effect and results in opening up a great percentage of the alveoli helping in prevention atelectasis. Moreover, this type of ventilation does not make difficult the surgical procedure or prolong its duration. In a prone position, we have better functional residual capacity than in a supine position. Furthermore, ventilation perfusion ratio is well maintained, and hypoxia and hypercarbia are avoided. All of this, aided by gravity, reduces lung injury. All that was mentioned previously could explain why Cuschieri et al. [60] described a decrease in respiratory complications in PP. Luketich group [9] performed the thoracoscopic surgery in LDP and reported the incidence of pneumonia in 7.6% and adult respiratory distress syndrome (ARDS) in 5% of the patients. Palanivelu et al. [10] talks about pneumonia in 1.54% of the patients and ARDS in 0.77% with PP approach.

As we have described already, gravity and artificial pneumothorax may improve mediastinal organs and structures exposure without any help of an assistant: this is another benefit of the PP. It makes possible the use of only three trocars, while four of them are needed in lateral decubitus approach. Prone position also promotes blood and other fluids from accumulating in the right anterior thorax, instead of posterior mediastinum that takes part of operative field. Thus, intermittent suction of accumulated fluids is not required during surgery. In the lateral position, the esophagus is in a dependent place and any pooling of blood obscures the surgical field.

Recently, Javed et al. [61] have published a comparative study between MIE in prone versus lateral decubitus position (LDP). They described the surgery in LDP using an additional trocar (four in total) for the assistant to retract the lung and to suction out the blood, whereas they only need three for PP technique. In this study, authors report low blood loss intraoperative, which was significantly less in PP group. Kubo et al. [62] also describe significantly lower blood loss with this approach. This fact could be explained due to a better exposure in PP that allows a more meticulous dissection avoiding damage to vessels and other thoracic structures and decreasing bleeding.

Noshiro et al. [63] have published a study to describe whether lymphadenectomy along the left recurrent laryngeal nerve is facilitated in the PP. Lymph nodes along this nerve are frequently involved by carcinoma cells, and their complete dissection is required [58]. They conclude that when PP is compared with LDP, lower blood loss and better exposure of the surgical field around the left recurrent laryngeal nerve occurs in first group. Although they describe slightly higher number of the resected lymph nodes in the PP, they do not find significant differences. On the other hand, Javed et al. [61] show a significantly higher lymph node yield in PP and the number of patients with affected lymph nodes is also significantly higher.

Most of the reports [10, 61] describe a shorter operative time for a thoracoscopic esophagectomy in PP than in LDP. As we have said before, the best exposure of the surgical field allows for faster and better quality surgery.

Fabian et al. [64] suggested that the learning curve for the prone position approach appears to be relatively short, within the first five cases. This author also says that prone approach may result in better dissection into the neck explained by pneumatic dissection from the thoracic cavity cranially along the esophagus. This maneuver simplifies the neck surgery that could lead to less morbidity in cervical step.

The incidence of complications, such as anastomosis leak, gastric tip necrosis, chylothorax, tracheal, or vocal cord injury is comparable between PP and LDP according to many reports. Other clinical outcomes seem to be similar between both: median length of stay, discharged within 10 days, and in-hospital mortality [63, 64]. As we have commented at the beginning, it might be possible to reduce respiratory morbidity using PP approach.

In addition, in PP the surgeon's wrist and shoulder joins are in a neutral position in relation to the forearms and upper arms, minimizing fatigue and maximizing ergonomic function. The view of the monitor stands parallel to operative field and ergonomic position of the surgeon makes easier hand-eye coordination. In contrast in LDP, the surgeon's view of the monitor must be turned upside down to avoid the counterimage when two monitors are set on each side. In this situation, hand-eye coordination cannot be obtained smoothly if a scope-holding assistant does not work correctly.

One disadvantage with the prone technique could be the need for conversion to open required electively when many adhesions preclude a minimally invasive approach or emergently as a consequence of uncontrollable bleeding. Although a posterior thoracotomy can be performed in this position, it is a less familiar approach that hinders dissection. Moreover, if we have performed the thoracic step without the use of a double-lumen endotracheal tube, we have to know that if a conversion is required, isolated lung ventilation would be invaluable. Thus, there are authors that continue using double-lumen intubation in the prone approach [64].

In conclusion, the PP may be performed with comparable outcomes to the LDP. The technique improves exposure of the operative field and reduces surgical times without compromising patient's safety or oncological results. Moreover, PP brings on an ergonomic position for the surgeon that makes easy the dissection.

8. Fast-track surgery (FTS) protocol on patient undergoing MIE

The concept of fast-track surgery (FTS) was first introduced by Kehlet and Mogensen [65], and the objective of his study was to show less postoperative stress, reduce morbidity associated with complications, accelerate recovery, and reduce postoperative cost in patients submitted for colon surgery after a rehabilitation programme [66]. It is essentially a multidisciplinary team to perform a fast-track approach during perioperative period for reaching an optimal outcome [67]. To date, the fast-track protocol has been applied in many surgical fields such as colon, rectum, or liver, but there is limited literature talking about the safety of using this protocol in esophageal surgery, especially in those cases where a minimally invasive technique is going to be performed.

Patients must receive health instructions and adequate information about FTS in the preoperative period. As we have explained previously, it is essential to optimize nutritional support with enteral and parenteral nutrition in those patients with long-term insufficient feeding and nutritional deficiencies. Recall that this measure has not been carried out in conventional care [68].

Many anesthesiologists have always been wary of allowing an esophageal cancer patient to ingest liquids 3 h before induction of anesthesia, defending the risk of aspiration pneumonia with this maneuver. But National and European Anesthesia Societies now recommend intake of clear fluids until 2 h before the induction of anesthesia as well as a 6 h fast for solid food [69]. Following these guidelines, Pan and his group, who have recently published a FTS protocol for MIE [70], instructed patients to drink fluid meals until 6 h before surgery and a carbohydrate drink until 3 h before surgery. They do not notice more pulmonary complications in FTS group than in conventional management group.

The use of the nasogastric tube (NGT) during the postoperative period is still controversial, although data describes disturbance of water, electrolyte, and acid base, and more digestive fluid reflux using nasogastric tube, which can increase pulmonary morbidity [71]. Some studies also show that NGT can delay normal gastrointestinal function [72]. Removal of NGT in the immediate postoperative period promotes early oral diet introduction that has some physiological advantages: decreases bacterial translocation, ensures function of intestinal mucosal cells, activates digestive secretory system, reduces postoperative infection, and accelerates organ recovery [73]. Oral feeding can be initiated during the first 48 h, following a stepwise programme from water to fluid meals, and finally to semifluid meals and normal food. Pan et al. [70] do not report gastroenterological complications, including anastomosis leak, without using NGT in postoperative period, and they suggest that an early oral diet in patients with MIE is safe and feasible. Enteral nutrition through jejunostomy may be initiated on the first postoperative day, even before oral intake. Both, oral and enteral nutrition, promote faster recovery of gastrointestinal function. Lewis et al. [74] concluded in their meta-analysis that early enteral nutrition can reduce anastomosis leakage and mortality. Jejunostomy can be removed when patients are able to ingest normal food.

The evidence about restrictive fluid administration intraoperatively and postoperatively, as we have reported in section called "anesthetic challenges of MIE," show less cardiopulmonary complications with this therapy. Earlier oral and enteral nutrition promotes that postoperative intravenous fluids can be reduced to as little as possible and removed during the first 24–48 h.

Abdominal and chest tube are also points of discussion in the FTS programme:

- Abdominal cavity drainage allows monitoring active bleeding and anastomosis leak, but it also can lead to abdominal infection and intestinal obstruction. While conventional care prefers to maintain drainage a few days, supporters of the fast-track protocol suggest that we should not leave drainage if there is no evidence of intraoperative complications. Jesus et al. [75] do not report more mortality or morbidity without using abdominal drainage.
- Chest tube causes pain and limits patient's mobility, so it has to be removed as soon as possible. A recent study has showed that it is safe to remove thoracic drainage when its volume is between 250 and 450, and there is no air leak.

The fast-track protocol also includes early perambulation after surgery for preventing venous thromboembolism that can be facilitated if patients are not carrying any type of drainage. Adequate analgesia can also accelerate perambulation and promote the recovery of intestinal function. Moreover, chest physiotherapy and incentive spirometry should be instituted. In their study, Pan et al. [70] reported that hospital stay and the days until intestinal activity are significantly shortened in the FTS group without an increase in morbidity and mortality. Patients undergoing MIE and fast-track protocol can be discharged earlier, even in the first week.

In summary, FTS program can be used safely in patients undergoing MIE because it promotes early recovery without increasing morbidity and mortality. We must offer the patient adequate preoperative information about the fast-track protocol to facilitate its implementation in the immediate postoperative period.

9. Conclusion

The minimally invasive approach to esophageal cancer is a safe and feasible procedure with favorable outcomes when compared to open esophagectomy. The data available reported by the different studies describe fewer respiratory complications, a reduction of hospital stay and faster patient recovery without compromising the oncologic efficacy related with harvested lymph nodes and R0 margin resection. The thoracoscopic approach in prone position is an alternative that offers more benefits than the lateral decubitus technique. Moreover, the implementation of a fast-track protocol allows an early recovery without increasing morbidity and mortality.

Acknowledgements

Thanks to Mrs. Noelia Tomás Marín-Baldo for her contribution in correcting English.

Author details

Rafael Cholvi Calduch, Isabel Mora Oliver, Fernando Lopez Mozos* and Roberto Martí Obiol

*Address all correspondence to: ferlomo@gmail.com

Division of Oesophageal and Upper Gastrointestinal Surgery, Department of Surgery, Hospital Clínico Universitario de Valencia, Valencia, Spain

References

[1] Zhang Y. Epidemiology of esophageal cancer. World Journal of Gastroenterology. 2013; **19**(34):5598-5606

[2] Griffin SM, Raimes SA. Oesophagogastric Surgery: A companion to Specialist Surgical Practice. 4th ed. Philadelphia: Saunders, Elsevier, 2009

[3] D'Journo XB, Thomas PA. Current management of esophageal cáncer. Journal of Thoracic Disease. 2014;**6**(S2):S253-S264

[4] Orringer MB, Marshall B, Lannettoni MD. Transhiatal esophagectomy: Clinical experience and refinements. Annals of Surgery. 1999;**230**:392-403

[5] Bailey SH, Bull DA, Harpole DH, et al. Outcomes after esophagectomy: A ten-year prospective cohort. Annals of Thoracic Surgery. 2003;**75**(1):217-222

[6] T. Kim, S. N. Hochwald, G. A. Sarosi, A. et al. Review of Minimally Invasive Esophagectomy and Current Controversies. Gastroenterology Research and Practice, vol. 2012, Article ID 683213, 7 pages, 2012.

[7] Cuschieri A, Shimi S, Banting S. Endoscopic oesophagectomy through a right thoracoscopic approach. Journal of the Royal College of Surgeons of Edinburgh. 1992;**37**(1):7-11

[8] DePaula AL, Hashiba K, Ferreira EA, et al. Laparoscopic transhiatal esophagectomy with esophagogastroplasty. Surgical Laparoscopy and Endoscopy. 1995;**5**(1):1-5

[9] Luketich JD, Alvelo-Rivera M, Percival O, et al. Minimally invasive esophagectomy. Outcomes in 222 patients. Annals of Thoracic Surgery. 2003;**238**:486-495

[10] Palanivelu C, Prakash A, Senthilkumar R, et al. Minimally invasive esophagectomy: thoracoscopic mobilization of the esophagus and mediastinal lymphadenectomy in prone position experience of 130 patients. Journal of American College of Surgeons. 2006;**203**:7-16

[11] Parameswaran E, Blazeby JM, Hughes R, et al. Health-related quality of life after minimally invasive oesophagectomy. British Journal of Surgery. 2010;**97**:525-531

[12] Berger AC, Bloomenthal A, Weksler B, et al. Oncologic e cacy is not compromised and may be improved with minimally invasive esophagectomy. J Am Coll Surg. 2011;**212**: 560-566 (discussion 566-568)

[13] Yibulayin W, Abulizi S, Hongbo LV, et al. Minimally invasive oesophagectomy versus open esophagectomy for resectable esophageal cancer: A meta-analysis. World Journal of Surgical Oncology. 2016;**14**:304

[14] Lv L, Hu W, Ren Y, et al. Minimally invasive esophagectomy versus open esophagectomy for esophageal cancer: A meta-analysis. OncoTargets and Therapy. 2016;**9**:6751-6762

[15] Biere SS, Berge Henegouwen MI, Maas KW, et al. Minimally invasive versus open oesophagectomy for patients with oesophageal cancer: A multicentre, open-label, randomised controlled trial. The Lancet. 2012;**379**:1887-1892

[16] 17.Bartels H, Stein HJ, Siewert JR. Preoperative risk analysis and postoperative mortality of oesophagectomy for resectable oesophageal cancer. British Journal of Surgery. 1998;**85**:840-844

[17] Fekete FBJ. Nutrition Factors and Oesophageal Resection. Edinburgh: Churchill Livingstone; 1988

[18] Law S, Wong KH, Kwok KF, et al. Predictive factors for postoperative pulmonary complications and mortality after esophagectomy for cancer. Annals of Surgery. 2004; **240**:791-800

[19] Bollschweiler E, Schroder W, Holscher AH, et al. Preoperative risk analysis in patients with adenocarcinoma or squamous cell carcinoma of the oesophagus. British Journal of Surgery. 2000;**87**:1106-1110

[20] Ueda K, Tanaka T, Hayashi M, et al. Role of inhaled tiotropium on the perioperative outcomes of patients with lung cancer and chronic obstructive pulmonary disease. Journal of Thoracic and Cardiovascular Surgery. 2010;**58**:38-42

[21] Bolukbas S, Eberlein M, Eckhoff J, et al. Short-term effects of inhalative tiotropium/formoterol/budenoside versus tiotropium/formoterol in patients with newly diagnosed chronic obstructive pulmonary disease requiring surgery for lung cancer: A prospective randomized trial. European Journal of Cardio-Thoracic Surgery. 2011;**39**:995-1000

[22] Hulzebos EH, Helders PJ, Favié NJ, et al. Preoperative intensive inspiratory muscle training to prevent postoperative pulmonary complications in high-risk patients undergoing CABG surgery: A randomized clinical trial. JAMA. 2006;**296**:1851-1857

[23] Turan A, Mascha EJ, Roberman D, et al. Smoking and perioperative outcomes. Anesthesiology. 2011;**114**:837-846

[24] Correia MI, Caiaffa WT, Da Silva AL, et al. Risk factors for malnutrition in patients undergoing gastroenterological and hernia surgery: an analysis of 374 patients. Nutrición Hospitalaria. 2001;**16**:59-64

[25] Jie B, Jiang ZM, Nolan MT, et al. Impact of preoperative nutritional support on clinical outcome in abdominal surgical patients at nutritional risk. Nutrition. 2012;**8**:1022-1027

[26] Kuppinger D, Hartl WH, Bertok M, et al. Nutritional screening for risk prediction in patients scheduled for extra-abdominal surgery. Nutrition. 2013;**29**:399-404

[27] Rucklige M, Sanders D, Alastair M. Anaesthesia for minimally invasive oesophagectomy. Continuing Education in Anaesthesia, Critical Care & Pain. 2010;**10**:43-47

[28] De Conno E, Steurer MP, Wittlinger M, et al. Anaesthetic-induced improvement of the inflammatory response to one-lung ventilation. Anesthesiology. 2009;**110**:1316-1326

[29] Schilling T, Kozian A, Kretzschmar M, et al. Effects of propofol and desflurane anaesthesia on the alveolar inflammatory response to one-lung ventilation. British Journal of Anaesthesia. 2007;**99**:368-375

[30] Sherry K. Management of patients undergoing oesophagectomy. In: Gray AJG, Hoile RW, Ingram GS, Sherry KM, editors. The Report of the National Confidential Enquiry into Perioperative Deaths 1996/1997. London: NCEPOD; 1998. pp. 57-61

[31] Ehrenfeld JM, Walsh JL, Sandberg WS. Right and left-sided Mallinckrodt double-lumen tubes have identical clinical performance. Anesthesia and Analgesia. 2008;**106**:1847-1852

[32] Pennefather SH, Russel GN. Placement of double lumen tubes—Time to shed light on an old problem. British Journal of Anaesthesia. 2000;**84**:308-310

[33] Kooguchi K, Kobayashi A, Kitamura Y, et al. Elevated expression of induciblenitric oxide synthase and inflammatory cytokines in the alveolar macrophages after esophagectomy. Critical Care Medicine. 2002;**30**:71-76

[34] Lin WQ, Lu XY, Cao LH, et al. Effects of the lung protective ventilatory strategy on proinflammatory cytokine release during one-lung ventilation. Ai Zheng. 2008;**27**:870-873

[35] Badenes R, Belda FJ, Aguilar G. Mechanical ventilation in cardiac surgery. Current Anaesthesia & Critical Care. 2010;**21**:250-254

[36] Slinger P. Pro: Low tidal volume is indicated during one-lung ventilation. Anesthesia and Analgesia. 2006;**103**:268-270

[37] Michelet P, D'Journo XB, Roch A, et al. Protective ventilation influences systemic inflammation after esophagectomy: A randomized controlled study. Anesthesiology. 2006;**105**:911-919

[38] Mayer J, Boldt J, Mengistu AM, et al. Goal-directed intraoperative therapy based on autocalibrated arterial pressure waveform analysis reduces hospital stay in high-risk surgical patients: A randomized, controlled trial. Critical Care. 2010;**14**:R18

[39] Nisanevich V, Felsenstein I, Almogy G, et al. Effect of intraoperative fluid management on outcome after intra-abdominal surgery. Anesthesiology. 2005;**103**:25-32

[40] Kita T, Mammoto T, Kishi Y. Fluid management and postoperative respiratory disturbances in patients with transthoracic esophagectomy for carcinoma. Journal of Clinical Anesthesia. 2002;**144**:252-256

[41] Licker M, de Perrot M, Spiliopoulos A, et al. Risk factors for acute lung injury after thoracic surgery for lung cancer. Anesthesia and Analgesia. 2003;**97**:1558-1565

[42] Ballantyne JC, Carr DB, deFerranti S, et al. The comparative effects of postoperative analgesic therapies on pulmonary outcome: cumulative meta-analyses of randomized, controlled trials. Anesthesia and Analgesia. 1998;**86**:598-612

[43] Watson A, Allen PR. Influence of thoracic epidural analgesia on outcome after resection for esophageal cancer. Surgery. 1994;**115**:429-432

[44] Whooley BP, Law S, Murthy SC, et al. Analysis of reduced death and complication rates after esophageal resection. Annals of Surgery. 2001;**233**:338-344

[45] Lázár G, Kaszaki J, Abraham S, et al. Thoracic epidural anesthesia improves the gastric microcirculation during experimental gastric tube formation. Surgery. 2003;**134**:799-805

[46] Cense HA, Lagarde SM, de Jong K, et al. Association of no epidural analgesia with postoperative morbidity and mortality after transthoracic esophageal cancer resection. Journal of American College of Surgeons. 2006;**202**:395-400

[47] Pathak D, Pennefather SH, Russell GN, et al. Phenylephrine infusion improves blood flow to the stomach during oesophagectomy in the presence of a thoracic epidural analgesia. European Journal of Cardio-Thoracic Surgery. 2013;**44**:130-133

[48] Al-Rawi OY, Pennefather SH, Page RD, et al. The effect of thoracic epidural bupivacaine and an intravenous adrenaline infusion on gastric tube blood flow during esophagectomy. Anesthesia and Analgesia. 2008;**106**:884-887

[49] Richards ER, Kabir SI, McNaught CE, et al. Effect of thoracic epidural anaesthesia on splanchnic blood flow. British Journal of Surgery. 2013;**100**:316-321

[50] Joshi GP, Bonnet F, Shah R, et al. A systematic review of randomized trials evaluating regional techniques for postthoracotomy analgesia. Anesthesia and Analgesia. 2008;**107**:1026-1040

[51] Davies RG, Myles PS, Graham JM. A comparison of the analgesic efficacy and side-effects of paravertebral vs. epidural blockade for thoracotomy—A systematic review and meta-analysis of randomized trials. British Journal of Anaesthesia. 2006;**96**:418-426

[52] Baidya DK, Khanna P, Maitra S. Analgesic efficacy and safety of thoracic para-vertebral and epidural analgesia for thoracic surgery: A systematic review and meta-analysis. Interactive Cardiovascular and Thoracic Surgery. 2014;**18**:626-635

[53] Ding X, Jin S, Niu X, et al. A comparison of the analgesia efficacy and side effects of para-vertebral compared with epidural blockade for thoracotomy: An updated meta-analysis. PLoS One. 2014;**9**:e96233

[54] Zieren HU, Jacobi CA, Zieren J, et al. Quality of life following resection of oesophageal carcinoma. British Journal of Surgery. 1996;**83**:1772-1775

[55] Burdall OC, Boddy AP, Fullick J, et al. A comparative study of survival after minimally invasive and open oesophagectomy. Surgical Endoscopy. 2015;**29**:431-437

[56] Palazzo F, Rosato EL, Chaudhary A, et al. Minimally invasive esophagectomy provides significant survival advantage compared with open or hybrid esophagectomy for patients with cancer of the esophagus and gastroesophageal junction. Journal of American College of Surgeons. 2014

[57] Biere SS, Maas KW, Bonavina L, et al. Tradicional invasive vs. minimally invasive esophagectomy: A multi-center, randomized trial (TIME-trial). Study Protocol. BMC Surgery. 2011;**11**:2

[58] Akiyama H, Tsurumaru M, Udagawa H, et al. Radical lymph node dissection for cancer of the thoracic esophagus. Annals of Surgery. 1994;**220**(3):364-372

[59] Fujita H, Kakegawa T, Yamana H, et al. Mortality and morbidity rates, postoperative course, quality of life, and prognosis after extended radical lymphadenectomy for esophageal cancer. Comparison of three-field lymphadenectomy with two-field lymphadenectomy. Annals of Surgery. 1995;**222**(5):654-662

[60] Cuschieri A. Thoracoscopic subtotal oesophagectomy. Endoscopic Surgery and Allied Technologies. 1994;**2**(1):21-25

[61] Javed A, Manipadam JM, Jain A, et al. Minimally invasive oesophaguectomy in prone position versus lateral decubitus position: A comparative study. Journal of Minimal Access Surgery. 2016;**12**(1):10-15

[62] Kubo N, Ohira M, Yamashita Y, Sakurai K, Lee T, Tokokawa T, et al. Thoracoscopic esophaguectomy in the prone position versus in the lateral position for patients with esophagueal cancer: A comparison of short- term surgical results. Surgical Laparoscopy, Endoscopy & Percutaneous Techniques. 2014;**24**:158-163

[63] Noshiro H, Iwasaki H, Kabayashi K, et al. Lymphadenectomy along the left recurrent laryngeal nerve by minimally invasive esophaguectomy in the prone position for thoracic esophageal cancer. Surgical Endoscopy. 2010;**24**:2965-2973

[64] Fabian T, Martin J, Katigbak M, et al. Thoracoscopic esophageal mobilization during minimally invasive esophagectomy: A head-to-head comparison of prone versus decubitus positions. Surgical Endoscopy. 2008;**22**(11):2485-2491

[65] Kehlet H, Mogensen T. Hospital stay of 2 days after open sigmoidectomy with a multimodal rehabilitation programme. British Journal of Surgery. 1999;**86**:227-230

[66] Kehlet H. Multimodal approach to control postoperative pathophysiology and rehabilitation. British Journal of Anaesthesia. 1997;**78**:606-617

[67] Hubner M, Muller S, Bonnard L, et al. Fast track surgery. Revue Médicale Suisse. 2008; **4**:2001-2004

[68] Jin-Yi W, Xuan H, Guo-Han C, et al. Clinical application of the fast track surgery model based on preoperative nutritional risk screening in patients with esophageal cancer. Asia Pacific Journal of Clinical Nutrition. 2015;**24**:206-211

[69] Cerfolio RJ, Bryant AS, Bass CS, Alexander JR, Bartolucci AA. Fast tracking after Ivor Lewis esophagogastrectomy. Chest. 2004;**126**:1187-1194

[70] Pan H, Hu X, Yu Z, et al. Use of a fast-track surgery protocol on patients undergoing minimally invasive oesophagectomy: Preliminary results. Interactive Cardiovascular and Thoracic Surgery. 2014;**19**:441-447

[71] Nguyen NT, Slone J, Wooldridge J, et al. Minimally invasive esophagectomy without the use of postoperative nasogastric tube decompression. American Surgeon. 2009;**75**:929-931

[72] Koukouras D, Mastronikolis NS, Tzoracoleftherakis E, et al. The role of nasogastric tube after elective abdominal surgery. Clinical Therapeutics. 2001;**152**:241-244

[73] Henriksen MG, Jensen MB, Hansen HV, et al. Enforced mobilization, early oral feeding, and balanced analgesia improve convalescence after colorectal surgery. Nutrition. 2002;**18**:147-152

[74] Lewis SJ, Andersen HK, Thomas S. Early enteral nutrition within 24 h of intestinal surgery versus later commencement of feeding: A systematic review and meta-analysis. Journal of Gastrointestinal Surgery. 2009;**13**:569-755

[75] Jesus EC, Karliczek A, Matos D, et al. Prophylactic anastomotic drainage for colorectal surgery. Cochrane Database of Systematic Reviews. 2004;CD002100.

5

Tissue Engineering of Esophagus

Yabin Zhu, Mi Zhou and Ruixia Hou

Abstract

The incidences of esophageal diseases like atresia, tracheoesophageal fistula, esophagitis, and even carcinoma rise rapidly worldwide. Traditional therapies such as surgery, chemotherapy, or/and radiotherapy, etc. always meet problems, leading to deterioration of the patients' life quality and sometimes the reduced survival rate. Tissue-engineered esophagus, a novel biologic substitute with tissue architecture and bio-functions, has been believed to be a promising replacement in the future. However, the research of esophageal tissue engineering is still at the early stage. Considerable research has been focused on the issues of developing ideal scaffolds with optimal materials and fabrication methods. The *in vivo* tests and clinic attempts are being progressed.

Keywords: materials, scaffolds, fabrication technology, tissue engineering, regeneration

1. Introduction

The incidences of esophageal diseases like atresia, tracheoesophageal fistula, esophagitis, and even carcinoma rise rapidly worldwide. For example, Barrett's esophagus, a complication of chronic gastroesophageal reflux disease (GERD), is a metaplasia of epithelial cells and often causes adenocarcinomas at a rate of approximately 1%. Among them, only 5–10% patients had chance to survive for 5 years if they do not receive treatment at the earliest stage [1]. The atresia of esophagus is a relatively common malformation occurred with a frequency of one in 2500 births [2]. Recently, more than 500,000 individuals are diagnosed with esophageal cancer each year with possibility of 850,000 by 2030 [3]. Esophageal cancer (EC) is a destructive disease. The treatment is usually tough and protracted, so as to inevitably reduce the patients' life quality, and may indirectly contribute to the mortality rate. Badly, the rate of esophageal cancer is 10–100 times higher in Iran, India, Northern China, and Southern Africa than the people in other place of the world [4]. The traditional therapies like surgery, radiotherapy, or/and chemotherapy, and surgically replacing with stomach, colon, small intestine, etc. did not improve greatly the survival rate. In addition, esophagus donor is too rare to get autologous/allogeneic replacement from human body. A tissue-engineered substitute with integrated structure and function is thought to be a promising and effective alternative for treating esophageal disease, which will eliminate the need to harvest replacement tissues from the patients' own body or other human body.

The esophagus is a muscular canal extending from pharynx to stomach and has functions to transport food and water from mouth to stomach. There are three types of cells, i.e., stratified squamous epithelial cells, fibroblasts, and smooth/skeletal muscle cells, which constitute four layers of this tissue, namely the mucosa, submucosa, muscularis externa, and adventitia. **Figure 1** shows the sketch and histological structure of human esophagus, in which a folding lumen is observed in a resting state (**Figure 1a**). The stratified squamous epithelial cells (E) compose the lumen epithelium that serves as a barrier or protective layer against mechanical stresses produced by food bolus. The epithelial cells are supported by the underlying basement membrane (**Figure 1b**, arrows). The topography of the basement membrane is a rugged and uneven stripe that consists of interwoven fibers. The diameters of these fibers were measured to be from 28 to 165 nm with an average of 66 ± 24 nm. The pores displayed between fibers with unequal size (**Figure 1**c). The molecular components of the basement membrane

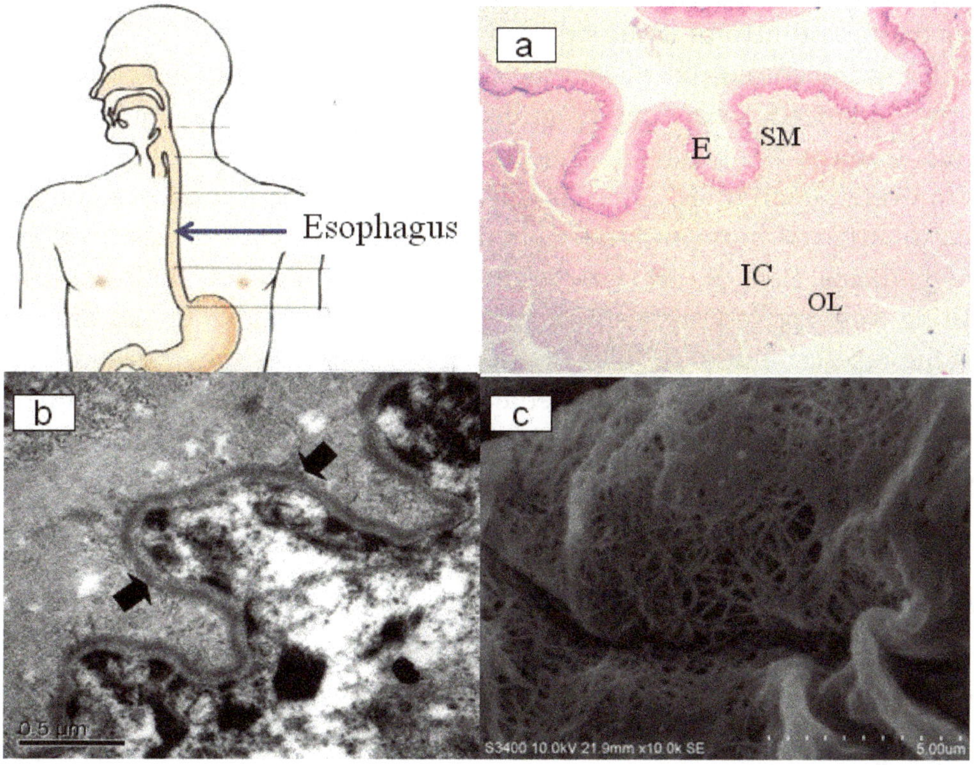

Figure 1. Overview and histological structure of esophagus (a). There are four tissue layers, i.e., mucosa containing epithelium (E), lamina propria and muscularis mucosae, submucosa (SM), muscularis externa consisting of two sublayers of inner circular (IC) and outer longitudinal (OL) muscle, and adventitia in esophagus organ. The stratified squamous epithelial cells (E) lined the esophagus lumen (H&E staining). Cross-section and topography of basement membrane were observed under transmission electron microscope (TEM) (b, c).

were detected to be collagen IV, laminin, entactin, and proteoglycans, mainly; among them collagen IV is slightly less than that of laminin but ~50 times more than that of entactin, but the quantity of proteoglycans was ~5 times more than that of entactin [5].

The muscle component in esophagus is responsible for motor function via peristalsis longitudinally and circumferentially. It consists of striated skeletal muscle in upper third, mixture of skeletal and smooth muscle in the middle third, and pure smooth muscle in the lower third. The muscle exhibits a bilaminar arrangement. The endo-circular and exo-longitudinal myofibrils (**Figure 1a**, IC and OL) are packed bilaminarly in order to propel the swallowing food and water into stomach through sequential contraction of the circular muscles via occluding the esophagus lumen, and longitudinal muscle by shortening the duct and enlarging the lumen, or enhancing the fibril density of the circular muscle, which in turn improves the contracting efficiency of the circular muscle [6–8].

Tissue engineering is an interdisciplinary field that applies the principles of engineering and life sciences toward the development of biological substitutes that restore, maintain, or improve tissue function, proposed by Langer and Vacanti. Scaffolds, cells, and their combination are the main three topics of tissue engineering research. Material is the necessary substratum in scaffold fabrication. There are various types of materials that have been developed as scaffold matrices to constitute esophagus tissue, for example, resorbable substances, decellularized matrices, acellular patches, and the composites from natural and/or synthesized polymers. Among them, a number of tissue-derived extracellular matrix (ECM) like decellularized urinary bladder submucosa, gastric acellular matrix, aortal acellular matrix, acellular dermal grafts, and decellularized esophagus have been much investigated for the applications as esophagus replacement. Some have also been tested for healing injury of esophagus in animal models or even human trials. Alternatively, synthesized and/or natural materials or their composites also attracted more and more attentions in researches of tissue engineering and regenerative medicine. Refs. [9, 10] reported that poly(glycolic acid) (PGA) and silicone with collagen coating were applied to constitute tubular scaffold. Small intestinal submucosa (SIS) was used as the replacement of tubular organs, for example, esophagus and large-diameter vascular grafts, as literature reports. Nonetheless, the complications or postoperative problems like inflammation, leakage, stenosis, and extrusion in long-term implantation are still presented when the materials or scaffolds are implanted into bodies.

2. Materials for scaffold constitution

Since the ancient times, some allogeneic materials have been adopted for medicinal purposes. In the past decades, after the concept of tissue engineering was submitted, many natural and artificial materials were adopted to produce scaffolds. Some achievements have been obtained toward improving tissue regeneration in laboratory scaffold, serving as a temporary platform to support or promote the growth of cells or/and tissues, which is one of the key issues in the research of tissue engineering. For esophagus, a variety of natural or/and artificially synthesized materials have been investigated as scaffold substrate.

2.1. Natural biomaterials

Natural biomaterials, for example, collagen, chitosan, gelatin, decellularized extracellular matrix (ECM), etc., all of which are derived from animal sources, have been widely studied in scaffold constitution, since all these materials possesses good biocompatibility and have biospecific signals cued from the molecules secreted by the resident cells. Thus, they are believed to be able to direct the *in vivo* remodeling process. These natural materials also have been used in a variety of tissue engineering applications, such as the grafts of heart, heart valve, skeletal muscle, skin, cardiovascular grafts, etc. For the research of esophageal tissue engineering, some ECMs like acellular dermal grafts, gastric acellular matrix, aortal acellular matrix grafts, and decellularized esophagus and urinary bladder submucosa had once been tested to repair esophagus in animal models [11–14]. For example, Marzaro et al. seeded porcine esophageal smooth muscle cells (SMC) on the acellular esophagus aiming at healing the defected porcine esophagus. They got results that SMCs grew on the ECM without obvious inflammation and rejection after implantation for 3 weeks [14].

The research team led by Professor Badylak pioneers the scaffold fabrication using decellularized ECM like porcine urinary bladder matrix (UBM) and small intestinal submucosa (SIS) toward *in vitro* and *in vivo* repairing of esophagus organ [15–17]. For example, they implanted the acellular UBM at the esophagus defects of female mongrel dogs, where the circumferential endo-mucosa/submucosa had been resected. The results showed that complete epithelialization took place on the scaffold surface at day 35, neovascularization and formation of muscle bundles took place at day 50, and the immature nerves and Schwann cells were observed at day 91. After implantation for 230 days, neonatal esophagus with the formation of well-organized tissue laminar and tissue motility had grown [12]. Another important application is skeletal muscle ECM. They decellularized skeletal muscle with enzymes and chemicals to obtain acellular ECM. This ECM was verified to contain the growth factors, glycosaminoglycans, and basement membrane structural proteins. Expectedly, these components greatly promoted myogenic cells' growth and proliferation *in vitro,* and also promoted the myogenesis when the ECM was implanted into a rat abdominal wall. The ECM scaffold was found to degrade gradually at the implant site [16]. The xenogeneic ECM derived from porcine SIS combined with endoscopic technique was adopted to repair dysfunctional esophagus of five male patients who had esophageal adenocarcinoma, Barrett's or/and high-grade dysplasia (HGD). After 24 months, patients restored the mature squamous epithelium and returned a normal diet without significant dysphagia. Unfortunately, among these five patients, some recurred Barrett's esophagus, mainly at the gastroesophageal junction [17]. It was the first and very important report about clinical application of tissue-engineered esophagus in human body. A model of the human esophageal mucosa was reported recently by the MacNeil laboratory [18]. Unlike conventional 2D cell culture systems, they seeded primary human esophageal fibroblasts and epithelial cells in a porcine-derived acellular esophageal scaffold and discovered an esophageal mucosa recapitulation after 20 days. It provided a biologic-relevant experiment model of human esophageal mucosa.

Some literatures reported that three-dimensional biological scaffolds made from nonautologous extracellular matrix (ECM) can act as an inductive template for tissue and organ reconstruction after the ECM was recellularized with autologous stem cells or differentiated cells. This kind of ECM/cells was tried to repair and reconstruct some complex tissues like esophagus, trachea, and skeletal muscle in animal models. Porcine SIS was once attempted to be used as the scaffold by Wei et al., on which the canine oral epithelial cells were preseeded before transplantation into animal body followed by suturing across an esophageal gap in the cervical portion (~5 cm). Not only reepithelization but also muscle formation was discovered in the cell-seeded SIS after implantation in animal body for 8 weeks [19]. Urita et al. used the decellularized stomach tissue to evaluate the esophageal mucosa regeneration [13]. Isch et al. implanted a commercial decellularized product, AlloDerm® (LifeCell™), for the esophagoplasty of canine cervical esophagus. Complete epithelialization on the membrane surface was achieved after 2 weeks, without obvious anastomotic fistula or stenosis [20]. Bhrany compared the growth of rat epithelial cells on esophageal ECMs decellularized by deoxycholic acid and Triton X-100. The results indicated that treatment with deoxycholic acid was better than Triton X-100 treatment in epithelium regeneration [11]. Koch et al. decellularized a porcine esophagus and implanted subcutaneously into Sprague-Dawley rats. The decellularized esophagus was shown to maintain its native matrix morphology and extracellular matrix composition [21]. Considering the findings in these literatures, we believed that the decellularized ECM is a good scaffold candidate in esophageal tissue engineering.

Proteins or/and proteoglycans derived from animal ECM are also the important materials that have been actively researched previously. Saxena et al. seeded rat esophageal epithelial cells on the collagen-based scaffolds (OptiMaix-3D001315). After cultured *in vitro*, cells were tested to display positive pan cytokeratin PCK-26 which broadly recognizes the epitopes present in most human epithelial tissues [22]. Qin et al. fabricated a cross-linked collagen-chitosan sponge and implanted into the latissimus dorsi of nude mice after it was preseeded with fetal canine esophageal epithelial cells. Ten layers of mature epithelial cells formed after 2 weeks and the collagen-chitosan implant degraded totally after 4 weeks [23]. Saito et al. implored the feasibility of collagen that used to be the substrate of tissue-engineered esophagus [24]. They constituted an artificial esophagus using collagen sponge together with a latissimus dorsi muscle flap and split-thickness skin and replaced the esophagus of rabbits. Five in 12 total experimental rabbits survived without anastomotic leakage or stenosis. The longest survival period in these rabbits was 16 days.

Although many interesting achievements about natural biomaterials have been obtained in some *in vitro* or *in vivo* experiments, problems like weak mechanical strength, fast degradation, and source limitation of these natural biomaterials are still to be worked out.

2.2. Polymeric materials

Artificial polymers have been much investigated as scaffold substrates in tissue engineering because these materials possess many attracting features, for example, good availability, low cost, and high possibility of designing and production. Polyethylene (PE) tube was the earliest example to be an artificial conduit for esophageal replacement in a dog model in 1952 [25]. However, 6 in 20 experimental dogs died after the PE tube was replaced. Leakage and stricture in some dogs were discovered at the site of the PE junction. A fibrous sheath around this plastic tube was developed in all dogs, likely because of the nonbiodegradability of PE materials. Despite the failures, this study is the pioneering experiment of tissue engineering research of esophagus.

Since the concept of tissue engineering was put forward, the interests in using biocompatible and biodegradable polymers, such as polyglycolic acid (PGA), polycaprolactone (PCL), poly-L-lactic acid (PLLA), and their copolymers, has been increasing greatly, particularly after the regulatory approval from the U.S. Food and Drug Administration (FDA). Various kinds of biodegradable polymers have been investigated specifically for the tissue engineering of esophagus. For example, vicryl, made from PGA and collagen coating, is one type of biodegradable and absorbable scaffold with good biocompatibility. It has been tested as a porcine thoracic esophageal replacement in 1991 [26]. No matter what, it failed when the material was implanted into animal body. It was because the reflux gastric fluid dissolved the grafted tube, resulting in severe mediastinitis, leakage, and stenosis. In 1998, Shinhar used vicryl mesh to repair the porcine cervical esophagus. Here, stenosis still took place, though the stump fistula disappeared [27]. Miki et al. fabricated a tube using PGA mesh as a frame, and collagen containing esophageal fibroblasts and epithelial cells as the outer and inner layer, respectively. The fibroblasts were found to be able to accelerate the proliferation and differentiation of epithelial cells due to the keratinocyte growth factor secreted by fibroblasts. After the tube was implanted into muscle flaps of athymic rats for 14 days, nonstenosis was observed in the tube's lumen, but also 20 layers of stratified epithelium were developed from histological examination [28].

One key issue of those synthetic materials used as scaffold matrices is the materials' hydrophobic and biologically inert surface, which will inevitably lead to the inferior reactions between material and cells when the host cells come into contact with the scaffold surface upon implantation. Zhu et al. developed some methods to modify the surface chemistry aiming at enhancing cell-polymer interactions. In order to graft proteins or other biomolecules onto polymer surface, a reaction of ester groups from the substrate polyesters (e.g., PLLA, PU, PCL, and their copolymers) and amino groups (-NH_2) of hexanediamine was firstly introduced to produce pendent amino groups on polyester surfaces through formation of amide bonds. This reaction was called as aminolysis. The density of amino group produced from the aminolysis reaction was quantified using ninhydrin method and fluorescein labeling. Second, this pendent -NH_2 reacted with one aldehyde group (-CHO) from glutaraldehyde (GA). Third, the other aldehyde of GA was used in covalently bond proteins or other biomolecules. Collagen, gelatin, chitosan, fibronectin, polypeptides, growth factors, etc. were thus grafted on the polymeric scaffold surface. Finally, the protein or other biomolecule-grafted surfaces were produced. The water soluble carbodiimide (WSC) can also induce the reaction between the pendent -NH_2 on the aminolyzed surface and –COOH of target proteins, so that the proteins were covalently bonded to the material surface as the **Scheme 1** demonstrated [29–31].The introduction of the amino groups also allows layer-by-layer (LBL) assembly on the polymer surface, because the aminolyzed polyester can be used as a polycationic substratum, on which polyanions can be assembled by means of electrostatic attraction. For example, LBL assemblies of poly(styrene sulfonate, sodium salt) (PSS)/chitosan and chondroitin sulfate (CS)/collagen were performed on the aminolyzed poly-L-lactide (PLLA-NH_2) surface (**Scheme 1**) [32, 33].

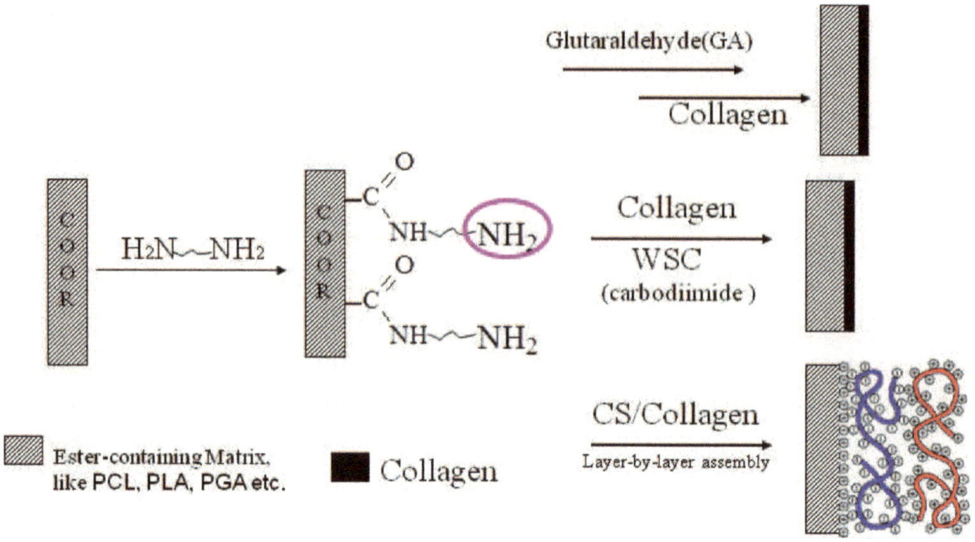

Scheme 1. Diagram of reactions between ester groups from synthesized polyesters and amino groups from diamine, aiming at introducing pendent amino groups onto substrate surface, through which many biomolecules containing amino or/and carboxylic groups can be bonded via crosslinking reagents or layer-by-layer assembly technology.

We tried another method, photo-oxidation plus copolymerization, to modify the material surface chemistry. This method was processed under UV initiation to introduce carboxylic groups (-COOH) onto material surface. Through these carboxylic groups, molecules like protein or other bio-molecules (containing COOH) will be bonded onto the surface under the catalysis of 1-ethyl-3-(3-dimethylamino propyl) carbodiimide hydrochloride (EDAC). As a result, covalent immobilization of proteins onto the material surface took place [34]. The optimal conditions for each method with respect to cell functions have been elucidated by *in vitro* evaluation of endothelial cells or esophagus cells including epithelial cell, fibroblast, and smooth muscle cell [30, 35–39].

Another important issue regarding polymers is the catalyst used during synthesis. Those ester-containing polymers are usually synthesized under catalyzing of stannum compounds [40, 41]. However, this kind of catalyst covalently links to the molecular chain of the ultimate products. We know, these stannum-containing materials are harmful to human body when it is implanted *in vivo* as a scaffold substrate, because the bonded stannum will release and accumulate in body as the material gradually degrades. Thus, it is necessary to develop new methods to catalyze efficient polymerizations but no toxicity giving off. Stolt et al. explored the reaction of L-lactide ring-opening polymerization using catalysts generated from iron and acetic acid, isobutyric acid, butyric acid, trifluoroacetic acid, dichloroacetic acid, etc. They discovered that the iron acetate, iron isobutyrate, and iron trifluoroacetate were the efficient catalysts for ring-opening reaction to yield poly(l-lactide) (PLLA) with a molar mass (weight average molecular weight, Mw) of 150 kDa. The monomers' conversion was up to over 85% under the optimum reaction conditions [42]. After this, they produced lactic acid-based poly(ester-urethane) (PEU) using iron monocarboxylates as the initiators, which were prepared from the reaction between iron powder and acetic acid, trifluoroacetic acid, or isobutyric acid. These iron monocarboxylates were considered as catalysts in reactions of hydroxyl-terminated prepolymers and further linking with hexamethylene diisocyanate. The final product, PEU with high Mw, was achieved under the catalyst of fluorinated iron acetate [43]. Zhu group investigated the polymerizing of ester-containing monomers like lactide, caprolactone, glycolic acid, etc. using ferric chloride ($FeCl_3$), ethanol iron ($Fe(OC_2H_5)_3$), iron (III) acetylacetonate ($Fe(acac)_3$), or iron (II) acetylacetonate $Fe(acac)_2$, as the catalyst. The result was that $Fe(acac)_3$ was the most efficient catalyst among them to yield products with high monomer conversion and number average molecular weight [44]. Based on these studies, an oligomer, poly(ethylene glycol-co-lactide) dimethacrylate (PLEGDMA) was further synthesized via ring-opening polymerization of L-LA and polyethylene glycol (PEG) under $Fe(acac)_3$ initiation. After cross-linking with PEG diacrylate and NIPAAm, or with linear prepolyurethane in the homemade mold, biodegradable tubular scaffolds with good mechanical properties were fabricated (**Figure 2**). These scaffolds were verified to be good enough to support the growth of porcine esophageal cells like epithelial, fibroblast, and muscle cell.

3. Fabrication of 3D scaffold for esophageal tissue engineering

Biodegradable 3D scaffolds serve as analogues of extracellular matrix (ECM) in the engineered tissue or organ. Therefore, the scaffold's chemistry and macro and/or microscale architecture must be helpful to maintain cell's functions including cell-matrix adhesion, cell-cell adhesion, cell migration, proliferation, differentiation, etc. On the other hand, 3D scaffold should provide spatial cues for cell infiltration, so that cells are capable of integrating with the underlining substrate. People are always seeking techniques to fabricate spatial scaffolds. Some technologies like foaming, porogen leaching, electrospinning, or other fiber processing, phase separation, 3D microprinting, etc. were developed to construct 3D porous scaffolds. In particular, electrospinning technology and thermally induced phase separation (TIPS) method have been extensively studied to constitute 3D scaffolds in tissue engineering of esophagus.

3.1. Phase separation

Phase separation of polymeric materials is often induced by thermal alteration. That is called thermally induced phase separation, shortened as TIPS. TIPS is one of the most practical

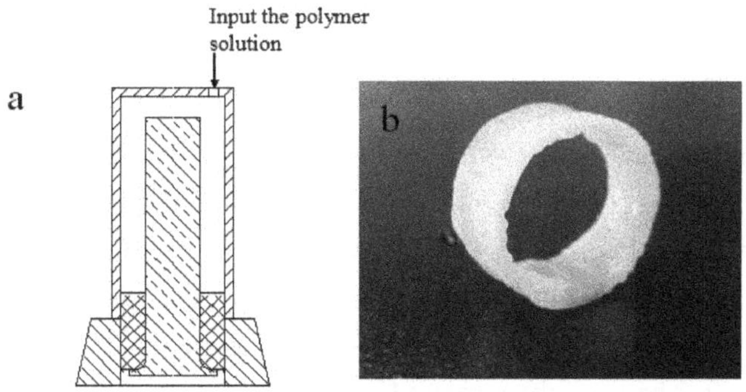

Figure 2. (a) A tubular mold; (b) overview of the tubular scaffold made from crosslinking of PLEGDMA, PEG diacrylate and NIPAAm.

techniques to prepare 3D scaffolds with optimal pore profiles by modulation of process parameters. It was firstly proposed by Castro as early as in 1981 [45] and extended to scaffold making after commencing of tissue engineering [36, 46–48]. The TIPS procedure usually involves four steps: (1) polymer dissolution in some solvent, (2) occurrence of phase separation, (3) polymer gelation, and (4) solvent extraction [49]. There are many advantages of TIPS over other traditional methods such as porogen leaching and foaming. For example, TIPS has the abilities to create a variety of pore structures by employing different parameters, and abroad applications for substrate sources because of its universality for various materials like crystal or noncrystal synthesized polymers [50, 51].

Zhu et al. prepared porous scaffolds with ≥100 μm pore size and good pore interconnectivity using TIPS technique [52, 53]. In order to simulate the ECM architecture, the original TIPS was modified, and thus a scaffold with an asymmetrical pore structure in a hierarchical order was created (**Figure 3**). The pore size on the scaffold surface was small, 1–10 μm, while that of the scaffold bulk was large, ≥100 μm (**Figure 3b**). Primary porcine epithelial cell was cultured on this asymmetrical scaffold lumen surface and primary fibroblast was cultured in the scaffold bulk. The coculture results verified that the bulk with large pores allowed fibroblast migration and infiltration while the lumen superficies with micropores supported the growth of epithelial cells and served as a barrier against fibroblast penetration. The immuno-fluorescent staining (nuclei displayed as blue and keratin as green) of epithelial cells exhibited that several layers of epithelial cells had formed after *in vitro* culture for 14 days on the scaffold lumen (**Figure 3**, **a2** and **b2**). The *in vivo* test showed that a complete layer of epithelium was regenerated on porcine esophagus lumen while the scaffold was being degraded after implantation for 5 months [53].

Beckstead et al. prepared porous sheets with salt-leaching/gas foaming method. The ammonium bicarbonate salt with size from 38–75 to 150–250 μm was used as the porogen reagent. A mixture of 10% chloroform and 90% ethanol was adopted as the polymer solvent. After dissolved in the solvent completely, the polymer solution was evaporated while 50% aqueous citric acid solution was used to initiate gas foaming accompanying with salt leaching [54]. They evaluated the cell (rat esophageal epithelial cell) behaviors on the scaffolds derived from natural material (exemplified AlloDerm), and synthetic materials like poly(lactic-co-glycolic acid) (PLGA) and PCL/PLLA. The results exhibited that AlloDerm scaffold had superior epithelial organization and stratification over other artificial scaffolds. Further modification to the artificial scaffolds would be a necessary way to polish their chemistry and to improve the cell behaviors.

3.2. Electrospinning

The technique of electrospinning was first proposed by Formhals in 1934 [55]. After that, it was gradually applied in diverse regions, for example, filtration industry, wound dressings, controlled drug releasing, and scaffold making in tissue engineering, and so on. In particular, this technique has gained popularity in tissue engineering fields, as a means of making scaffold. The fiber sheets obtained from electrospinning process possesses many features similar to natural ECM, for example, fibers were loosely connected with nano to microscale diameters; the sheet has high porosity and high surface area to volume ratio. Therefore, this technology became an interesting and valuable way to constitute scaffolds for esophageal tissue engineering.

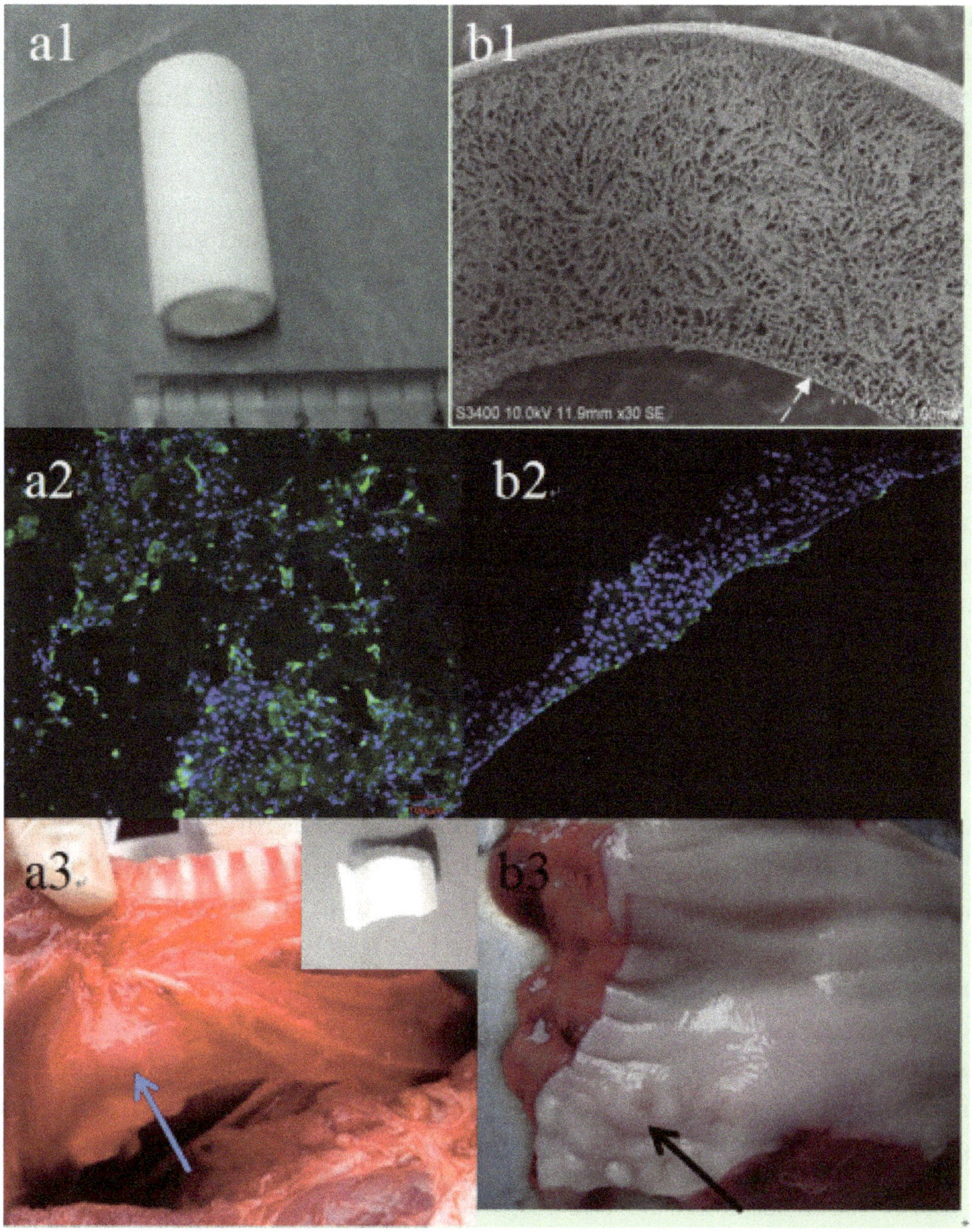

Figure 3. Overview of tubular scaffold (a1) and cross-section structure (b1). The scaffold was prepared with TIPS technique using biodegradable poly(l-lactide-co-caprolactone) as the substrate material. Primary epithelial cells were cultured on the scaffold lumen for 14 days and the immunofluorescence staining (nuclei displayed as blue and keratin as green), a2 is surface scanning and b2 is cross-section observation. The scaffold was surface grafted with fibronectin and implanted in porcine esophagus for 5 months (a3 and b3). Arrows in b1 indicate scaffold lumen, and in a3 and b3 referred the nude esophagus and scaffold-implanted site.

A typical electrospinning setup includes a syringe pump, a metallic collector, and a high-voltage generator. The parameters of this electrospinning system, including process parameters (e.g., electric potential, solution flow rate, distance between the spray nozzle and collector, etc.), polymer solution properties (e.g., solvents, solution viscosity, and concentration), and ambient parameters (e.g., temperature and humidity) influence the fiber features and internal construction.

Leong et al. yielded poly(D,L-lactide) fibers with the diameter of ~1 μm and nanoscale pores on each fiber through the method of electrospinning combined with phase separation. Large pores between the fibers in the whole sheet were also formed. Such multiporous structure greatly enhanced the cell-matrix interactions and thus promoted the adhesion of porcine esophageal epithelial cells onto the fibers [56].

We have set up a programmable electrospinning system (China Patent ZL 200810062323.8) to upgrade the apparatus's versatility. Besides the basic components, i.e., high-voltage generator and syringe pump, an electronic controller that allows manipulating the nozzle and metallic collector was automatically incorporated into the system. Two nozzles were applied in this system. They can be connected independently to two syringe pumps via silicone tube and operated under programmable monitor to spray polymer fibers individually, sequentially, or simultaneously. Using this upgrade system, a uniform composite fiber sheet consisting of polymers and natural biomaterials with the diameter ranging from 1 to 600 nm was created. These composite sheets derived from proteins and polymers showed good biocompatibility and good mechanical properties. Furthermore, a PCL fiber mesh with macroscopically alignment was electrospun on this setup. The interesting discovery is that this aligned fiber was able to switch smooth muscle cells from synthetic to contractile phenotype and hopefully to maintain the biological function of the cultured muscle tissue [57].

Grafting with ECM molecules is a good way for synthetic scaffolds to improve their bioactivity. For example, poly(L-lactide-co-caprolactone) (PLLC) was electrospun to form fibers. After then, they were grafted with fibronectin in order to promote epithelial cell growth [58]. According to the findings about the topographic features and protein quantifications of the basement membrane of porcine esophagus [4], an electrospun scaffold was fabricated using fibroin (extracted from pregnant silkworm originated in Zhejiang province, China) and polymer as the materials. In order to simulate the architecture of the basement membrane, proteins including collagen IV, laminin, entactin, proteoglycans (PG) extracted from porcine esophagus were coated on the above fibers, aiming at enhancing epithelium regeneration

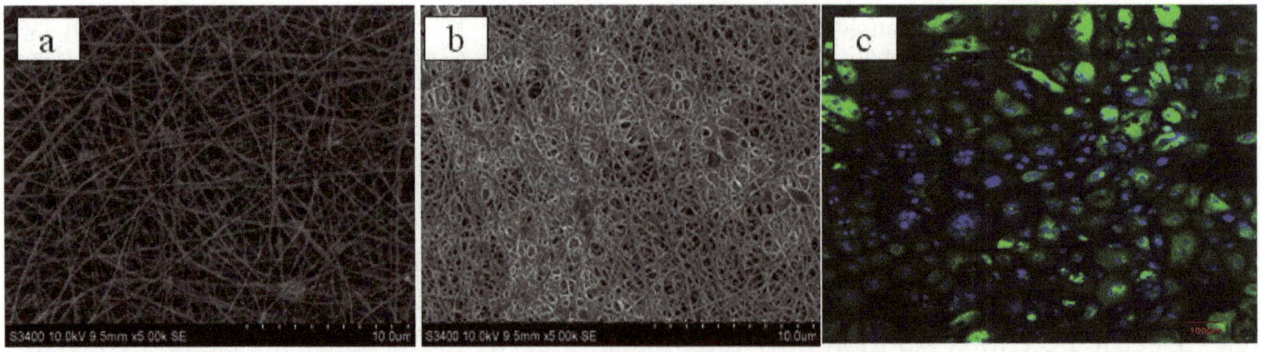

Figure 4. Scaffold morphology of PCL/SF (a), scaffold coated with basement membrane proteins that were extracted from porcine esophagus (b), and cell phenotype immune-histochemically stained with CK14 antibody (green) and nuclei with DAPI (blue) (c).

(**Figure 4**). Silk fibroin is known to have good physical and mechanical properties, and also good biocompatibility. Electrospun fibroin scaffolds together with optimal pore parameters and protein coating extracted from animal esophagus could be great candidates in esophageal tissue engineering [59].

4. Constitution of muscularis propria of the esophagus

The muscle tissue of esophagus consists of striated muscle (skeletal) in the upper third, mixture of skeletal and smooth muscle in the middle third, and pure smooth muscle in the lower third. These muscle contents arrange into endo-circular and exo-longitudinal sub-bilayers to play an important role in propelling the swallowed food or fluid into the stomach via muscle peristalsis. Generating an oriented muscle architecture to mimic the tissue of muscularis externa is an important issue to restore the functions of tissue-engineered esophagus. Many researchers studied the relationship between scaffold's chemistry and microstructure and muscle cells' phenotype. Stegemann once verified that the behaviors of smooth muscle cell (SMC) were positively correlated to the scaffold geometry (2D and 3D) [60]. Li et al. believed that the scaffold geometry played an important role in modulating SMC phenotype. They cultured SMCs and discovered that cells in 3D collagen (type I) gels had lower proliferation and higher collagen synthesis than the cells in 2D collagen substrate [61]. Chan-Park verified that smooth muscle α-actin of SMCs cultured in microchannels upregulated greatly, suggesting a phenotype shift from synthetic to contractile state of cells [62]. They thus believed that 3D microchannels could encourage cells to reorganize into orientation patterns because SMC have a natural self-arrangement propensity. Moreover, the narrow space of channels around 100 μm or less helped cells to achieve more uniform orientation. We also fabricated scaffolds with circular and longitudinal microchannel patterns (**Figure 5**). Further, the scaffold surface was grafted with silk fibroin using our method of diamine aminolysis and GA crosslinking. The primary esophageal SMC was cultured in these 3D protein-grafted channels in order to achieve SMC phenotype regulation and *in situ* muscle formation [63]. The results confirmed that primary esophageal smooth muscle cells exhibited fine alignment in all types of microchannels while SMCs in the interval channels communicated well through the gaps (**Figure 5**).

Some researchers had considered and investigated that mechanical stimulation might be an effective way to regulate SMC phenotype. Ritchie et al. designed a system to exert mechanical forces on esophageal smooth muscle cells. They discovered that cells on the flexile polyurethane membrane displayed alignment parallel to the force direction when low cyclic strains (2%) was used, but alignment perpendicular to the force direction when high strains (5 and 10%) used [64]. Cha et al. reported that muscle cells would orient according to the optimal movement of the tissue. They adopted cyclic mechanical strain (a homemade stretching chamber) on primary myofibroblasts, and promoted the cell differentiation, and further modulated the orientation and proliferation of the differentiated smooth muscle cell. Their conclusion was that myofibroblast/scaffold hybrids with cyclic strain could be applied to organize smooth muscle cells with muscle tissue functions [65].

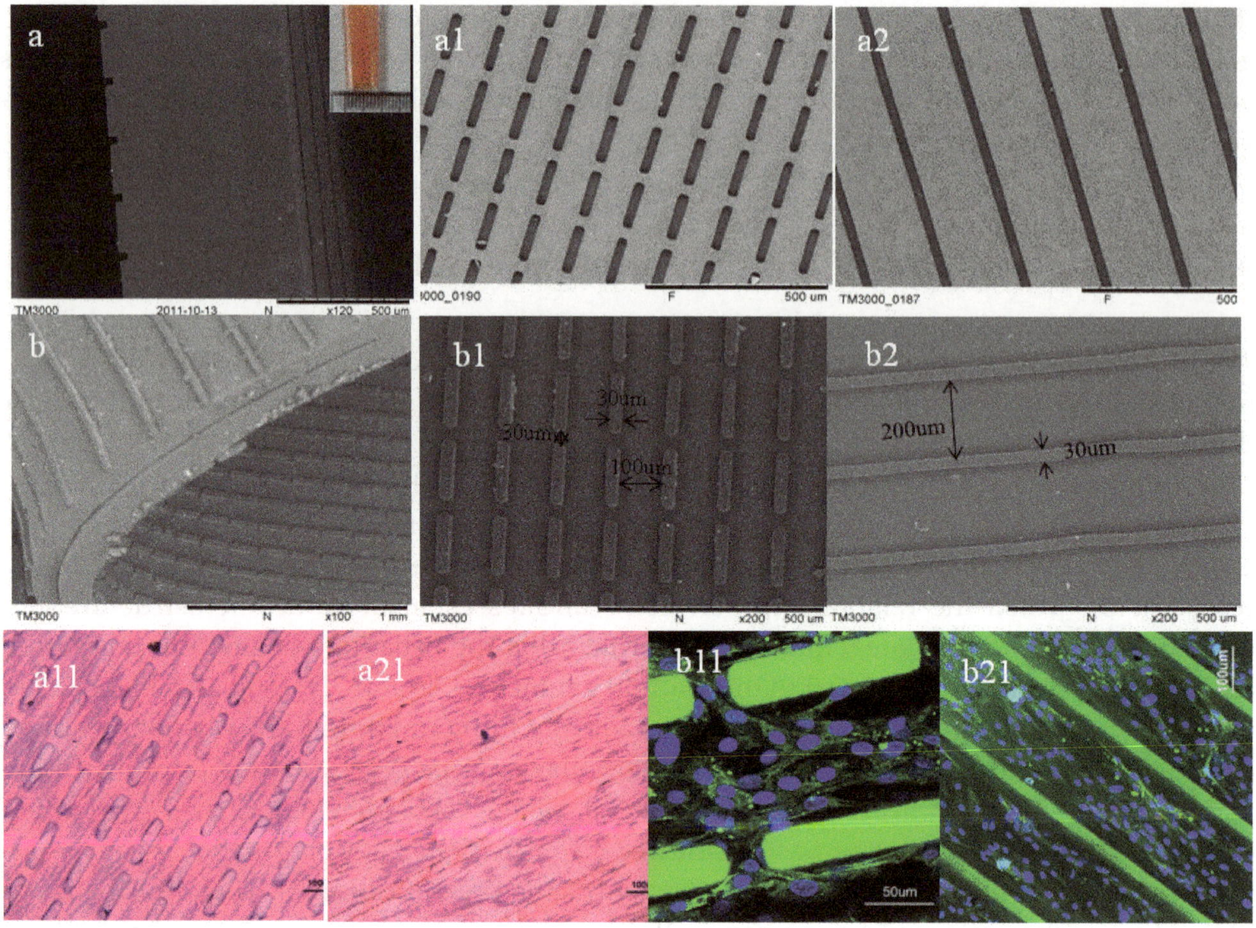

Figure 5. Overview of tubular scaffold (a, inserted) and tube wall's cross-section structure observed under SEM (a). (a1) Scaffold's morphologies of tube lumen and outer face, containing microchannels of 100 μm width with discontinuous channel walls intermitted by 30 μm gap, and both the wall thickness and depth are 30 μm; (a2) microchannels of 200 μm width with noninterval slits. (b) SEM picture of tubular scaffold with bulge wall (b1 and b2). The height of wall and gap between wall intervals is 30 μm. Esophageal smooth muscle cells were seeded and aligned in all scaffolds' channels while cells in the interval channels communicated through the wall gaps (a11, a21 and b11, b21). The scaffold was constructed through silica mold with predetermined patterns using biodegradable poly(ester-urethane) as the substrate material. The surface was grafted with silk fibroin via the method of diamine aminolysis and GA crosslinking. Cells of a11 and a21 were stained by H&E and cells of b11 and b21 were immuno-fluorescently stained with anti-α-smooth muscle as the primary antibody.

5. Clinical potential and future perspectives

With the development of stem cell technology, some kinds of stem cells, for example, embryonic stem cell, mesenchymal stem cell, progenitor stem cell, induced pluripotent stem cell, etc., are adopted to be the seeded cells in tissue reconstruct. In case of esophagus, bone mesenchymal stem cell (bMSC) is more often used to seed on scaffolds than other kinds of stem cells to regenerate or remodel the engineered esophagus. Taylor and Macchiarin reported that allogeneic mesenchymal stromal cells were seeded on the decellularized rat esophagi to orthotopically replace the entire cervical esophagus. After 14 days, the explanted grafts showed regeneration of all the major cell and tissue components of the esophagus including functional epithelium, muscle fibers, nerves, and vasculature. Thus, this tissue-engineered esophageal scaffold was considered as a significant step toward the clinical application of bioengineered esophagi [66].

In summary, the research of substrate materials and scaffold fabrications in esophageal tissue engineering has made great progress in past decades. Esophagus repairs in animal models and even clinical tests are being attempted and the techniques are being improved. Materials with appropriate physical and chemical properties are still being developed. Optimizing scaffolds and cells for epithelium regeneration or/and muscle constitution, and their combination have been in progress. Some crucial problems, such as complications from stricture to dilation, angiogenesis and innervation consideration, little or no muscle regeneration in the implants, etc., need to be issued before the tissue-engineered esophagus can be a viable conduit for surgical replacement in clinic. And, graft-to-host integration and remodeling of the organ functions like peristalsis and nerve guide would be the important gauge for the success in tissue engineering of esophagus. With the development of material science and engineering, stem cell biology, and other related theories and technologies, tissue-engineered esophagus is able to foresee the promising employment in clinic in near future.

Acknowledgements

Financial supports by the National Science Foundation (30870645, 81171476, 81471797) and Scientific Innovation Team Project of Ningbo (2015B11050), China, are gratefully acknowledged.

Author details

Yabin Zhu*, Mi Zhou and Ruixia Hou

*Address all correspondence to: zhuyabin@nbu.edu.cn

The Medical School of Ningbo University, Ningbo, China

References

[1] Powell J, McConkey CC, Gillison EW, Spychal RT. Continuing rising trend in oesophageal adenocarcinoma. International Journal of Cancer. 2002;**102**:422-427. DOI: 10.1002/ijc.10721

[2] Spitz L. Oesophageal atresia. Orphanet Journal of Rare Diseases. 2007;**2**:24-37. DOI: 10.1186/1750-1172-2-24

[3] Bloom D, Cafiero E, Jané-Llopis E, Abrahams-Gessel S, Bloom LR, et al. The Global Economic Burden of Noncommunicable Diseases. Available from: http://www.hsph.harvard.edu/pgda/WorkingPapers/2012/PGDA_WP_87.pdf

[4] Lambert R, Hainaut P. The multidisciplinary management of gastro-intestinal cancer. Epidemiology of oesophagogastric cancer. Best Practice & Research. 2007;**21**:921-945. DOI: 10.1016/j.bpg.2007.10.001

[5] Li YY, Zhu YB, Yu HW, Chen L, Liu YX. Topographic characterization and protein quantification of esophageal basement membrane for scaffold design reference in tissue engineering. Journal of Biomedical Materials Research Part B: Applied Biomaterials. 2012;**100B**:265-273. DOI: 10.1002/jbm.b.31949

[6] Goyal RK, Paterson WG. Handbook of Physiology: The Gastrointestinal System. Washington, DC: American Physiological Society; 1989. p. 865

[7] Wood JD. Physiology of the Gastrointestinal Tract. 2nd ed. New York: Raven Press; 1987. p. 67

[8] Schunke M, Schulte E, Schumacher U, Ross L, Lamperti E. Neck and Internal Organs (THIEME Atlas of Anatomy). Texas: Terry Telger; 2010

[9] Takimoto Y, Nakamura T, Teramachi M, Kiyotani T, Shimizu Y. Replacement of long segments of the esophagus with a collagen-silicone composite tube. ASAIO Journal. 1995;**41**:M605-M608. DOI: 10.1097/00002480-199507000-00082

[10] Sato M, Ando N, Ozawa S, Miki H, Hayashi K, Kitajima M. Artificial esophagus. Materials Science Forum. 1997;**250**:105-114

[11] Bhrany AD, Beckstead BL, Lang TC, Farwell DG, Giachelli CM, Ratner BD. Development of an esophagus acellular matrix tissue scaffold. Tissue Engineering. 2006;**12**:319-330. DOI: 10.1089/ten.2006.12.319

[12] Agrawal V, Brown BN, Beattie AJ. Evidence of innervation following extracellular matrix scaffold-mediated remodelling of muscular tissues. Journal of Tissue Engineering and Regenerative Medicine. 2009;**3**:590-600. DOI: 10.1002/term.200

[13] Urita Y, Komuro H, Chen G, Shinya M, Kaneko S, Kaneko M, Ushida T. Regeneration of the esophagus using gastric acellular matrix: An experimental study in a rat model. Pediatric Surgery International. 2007;**23**:21-26. DOI: 10.1007/s00383-006-1799-0

[14] Marzaro M, Vigolo S, Oselladore B, Conconi MT, Ribatti D, Giuliani S, Nico B, Perrino G, Nussdorfer GG, Parnigotto PP. In vitro anWd in vivo proposal of an artificial esophagus. Journal of Biomedical Materials Research. 2006;**77**:795-801. DOI: 10.1002/jbm.a.30666

[15] Badylak SF, Weiss DJ, Caplan A, Macchiarini P. Engineered whole organs and complex tissues. Lancet. 2012;**379**:943-952. PMID: 22405797. DOI: http://dx.doi.org/10.1016/S0140-6736(12)60073-7

[16] Wolf MT, Daly KA, Reing JE, Badylak SF. Biologic scaffold composed of skeletal muscle extracellular matrix. Biomaterials. 2012;**33**:2916-2925. PMID: 22264525

[17] Badylak SF, Hoppo T, Nieponice A, Gilbert TW, Davison JM, Jobe BA. Esophageal preservation in five male patients after endoscopic inner-layer circumferential resection in the setting of superficial cancer: A regenerative medicine approach with a biologic scaffold. Tissue Engineering. 2011;**17**:1643-50. DOI: 10.1089/ten.tea.2010.0739

[18] Green NH, Corfe BM, Bury JP, MacNeil S. Production, characterization and potential uses of a 3D tissue-engineered human esophageal mucosal model. JoVE—Journal of Visualized Experiments. 2015;**99**:e52693

[19] Wei RQ, Tan B, Tan MY. Grafts of porcine small intestinal submucosa with cultured autologous oral mucosal epithelial cells for esophageal repair in a canine model. Experimental Biology and Medicine (Maywood). 2009;**234**:453-461. DOI: 10.3181/0901-RM-5

[20] Isch JA, Engum SA, Ruble CA. Patch esophagoplasty using AlloDerm as a tissue scaffold. Journal of Pediatric Surgery. 2001;**36**:266-268. DOI: 10.1053/jpsu.2001.20685

[21] Koch H, Graneist C, Emmrich F, Till H, Metzger R, Aupperle H, Schierle K, Sack U, Boldt A. Xenogenic esophagus scaffolds fixed with several agents: Comparative in vivo study of rejection and inflammation. International Journal of Biomedicine and Biotechnology. 2012;**2012**:948320. DOI: 10.1155/2012/948320

[22] Saxena AK, Kofler K, Ainödhofer H. Esophagus tissue engineering: Hybrid approach with esophageal epithelium and unidirectional smooth muscle tissue component generation in vitro. Journal of Gastrointestinal Surgery. 2009;**13**:1037-1043. DOI: 10.1007/s11605-009-0836-4

[23] Qin X, Xu ZF, Shi HC. Artificial esophagus with cultured esophageal epithelial cells seeded on collagen-chitosan membrane. Academic Journal of Second Military Medical University. 2002;**23**:1134-1137

[24] Saito M, Sakamoto T, Fujimaki M. Experimental study of an artificial esophagus using a collagen sponge, a latissimus dorsi muscle flap, and split- thickness skin. Surgery Today. 2000;**30**:606-661

[25] Berman EF. The experimental replacement of portions of the esophagus by a plastic tube. Annals of Surgery. 1952;**135**:337-343

[26] Purushotham AD, Carachi R, Gorham SD. Use of a collagen coated vicryl tube in reconstruction of the porcine esophagus. European Journal of Pediatric Surgery. 1991;**1**(2):80-84. DOI: 10.1055/s-2008-1042464

[27] Shinhar D, Finaly R, Niska A. The use of collagen-coated vicryl mesh for reconstruction of the canine cervical esophagus. Pediatric Surgery International. 1998;**13**(2-3):84-87. DOI: 10.1007/s003830050254

[28] Miki H, Ando N, Ozawa S, Sato M, Hayashi K, Kitajima M. An artificial esophagus constructed of cultured human esophageal epithelial cells, fibroblasts, polyglycolic acid mesh, and collagen. ASAIO Journal. 1999;**45**:502-508. DOI: 10.1097/00002480-199909000-00025

[29] Zhu YB, Gao CY, Liu XY, Shen JC. Surface modification of polycaprolactone membrane via aminolysis and biomacromolecule immobilization for promoting cytocompatibility of human endothelial cells. Biomacromolecules. 2002;**3**:1312-1319. DOI: 10.1021/bm020074y

[30] Zhu YB, Gao CY, Liu XY, He T, Shen JC. Immobilization of biomacromolecules onto aminolyzed poly(L-lactic acid) towards acceleration of endothelium regeneration. Tissue Engineering. 2004;**10**:53-61. DOI: 10.1089/107632704322791691

[31] Zhu YB, Chan-Park M. Density quantification of collagen grafted on biodegradable polyester: Its application to esophageal smooth muscle cell. Analytical Biochemistry. 2007;**363**:119-127. DOI: 10.1016/j.ab.2007.01.007

[32] Zhu YB, Gao CY, He T, Liu XY, Shen JC. Layer-by-layer assembly to modify poly(L-lactic acid) surface toward improving its cytocompatibility to human endothelial cells. Biomacromolecules. 2003;**4**:446-452. DOI: 10.1021/bm025723k

[33] Gong YH, Zhu YB, Liu YX, Ma ZW, Gao CY, Shen JC. Layer-by-layer assembly of chondroitin sulfate and collagen on aminolyzed poly(L-lactic acid) porous scaffolds to enhance their chondrogenesis. Acta Biomaterialia. 2007;**3**:677-685. DOI: 10.1016/j.actbio.2007.04.007

[34] Zhu YB, Gao CY, Guan JJ, Shen JC. Promoting the cytocompatibility of polyurethane scaffolds via surface photo-grafting polymerization of acrylamide. Journal of Materials Science: Materials in Medicine. 2004;**15**:283-289. DOI: 10.1023/B:JMSM.0000015489.27261.f0

[35] Zhu YB, Chian KS, Chan-Park M, Mhaisalkar PS, Ratner BD. Protein bonding on biodegradable poly(l-lactide-co-caprolactone) membrane for esophageal tissue engineering. Biomaterials. 2006;**27**:68-78. DOI: 10.1016/j.biomaterials.2005.05.069

[36] Zhu YB, Chan-Park M, Chian KS. The growth improvement of porcine esophageal smooth muscle cells on collagen-grafted poly(DL-lactide-co-glycolide) membrane. Journal of Biomedical Materials Research: Applied Biomaterials. 2005;**75**:193-199. DOI: 10.1002/jbm.b.30305

[37] Zhu YB, Chan-Park M, Chian KS. Surface modification of poly(DL-lactide-co-glycolide) copolymer with covalently immobilized collagen for esophageal tissue engineering. Materials Forum. 2005;**29**:478

[38] Zhu YB, Gao CY, Shen JC. Surface modification of polycaprolactone with poly(methacrylic acid) and gelatin covalent immobilization for promoting its cytocompatibility. Biomaterials. 2002;**23**(24):4889-4895. DOI: 10.1016/S0142-9612(02)00247-8

[39] Zhu YB, Gao CY, Liu YX Shen JC. Endothelial cell functions in vitro cultured on poly(L-lactic acid) membranes modified with different methods. Journal of Biomedical Materials Research. 2004;**69A**(3):436-444. DOI: 10.1002/jbm.a.30007

[40] Kowalski A, Libiszowski J, Biela T, Cypryk M, Duda A, Penczek S. Kinetics and mechanism of cyclic esters polymerization initiated with tin(II) octoate. Polymerization of epsilon-caprolactone and L,L-lactide co-initiated with primary amines. Macromolecules. 2005;**38**:8170-8176. DOI: 10.1021/ma050752j

[41] Kricheldorf HR, Kreiser-Saunders I, Stricker A. Polylactones 48. Polylactones 48. SnOct2-initiated polymerizations of lactide: A mechanistic study. Macromolecules. 2000;**33**:702-709. DOI: 10.1021/ma991181w

[42] Stolt M, Södergård A. Use of Monocarboxylic iron derivatives in the ring-opening polymerization of l-lactide. Macromolecules. 1999;**32**:6412-6417. DOI: 10.1021/ma9902753

[43] Stolt M, Hiltunen K, Södergård A. Use of iron monocarboxylates in the two-step preparation of poly(ester-urethane)s. Biomacromolecules. 2001;**2**:1243-1248

[44] Lei YN, Zhu YB, Chen L, Hou LX. Polymerization of aliphatic cyclic ester using iron compounds as catalysts. Chinese Journal of Functional Polymers. 2011;**24**:297-302

[45] Castro AJ. Methods for making microporous products. US Patent 4247498, 1981-01-27

[46] Nam YS, Park TG. Porous biodegradable polymeric scaffolds prepared by thermally induced phase separation. Journal of Biomedical Materials Research. 1999;**47**:8-17. DOI: 10.1002/(SICI)1097-4636(199910)47:1<8::AID-JBM2>3.0.CO;2-L

[47] Zhu YB, Gao CY, Guan JJ, Shen JC. Engineering porous polyurethane scaffolds via photo-grafting polymerization of methacrylic acid for promotion of cytocompatibility to human endothelial cells. Journal of Biomedical Materials Research. 2003;**67A**:1367-1373

[48] Guan JJ, Fujimoto KL, Wagner WR. Preparation and characterization of highly porous, biodegradable polyurethane scaffolds for soft tissue applications. Biomaterials. 2005;**26**:3961-3971. DOI: 10.1016/j.biomaterials.2004.10.018

[49] Vasita R, Katti D. Nanofibers and their applications in tissue engineering. International Journal of Nanomedicine. 2006;**1**:15-30. DOI: 10.2147/nano.2006.1.1.15

[50] Li DM, Krantz WB, Greenberg AR, Sani RL. Membrane formation via thermally induced phase separation (TIPS): Model development and validation. Journal of Membrane Science. 2006;**279**:50-60. DOI: 10.1016/j.memsci.2005.11.036

[51] Gong YH, Ma ZW, Gao CY, Wang W, Shen JC. Specially elaborated thermally induced phase separation to fabricate poly(L-lactic acid) scaffolds with ultra large pores and good interconnectivity. Journal of Applied Polymer Science. 2006;**101**:3336-3342. DOI: 10.1002/app.23931

[52] Zhu YB, Ong WF, Chan WY, Li YY, Liu YX. Construct of asymmetrical scaffold and primary cells for tissue engineered esophagus. Materials Science and Engineering: C. 2010;**30**:400-406. DOI: 10.1016/j.msec.2009.12.009

[53] Hou L, Jin JC, Lv JJ, Chen L, Zhu YB, Liu XY. Constitution and in vivo test of microporoustubular scaffold for esophageal tissueengineering. Journal of Biomaterials Applications. 2015;**30**(5):568-578. DOI: 10.1177/0885328215596285

[54] Becksteada BL, Pan S, Bhrany AD, Bratt-Leal AM, Ratner BD, Giachelli CM. Esophageal epithelial cell interaction with synthetic and natural scaffolds for tissue engineering. Biomaterials. 2005;**26**:6217-6228. DOI: 10.1016/j.biomaterials.2005.04.010

[55] Formhals A. Process and apparatus for preparing artificial threads. US Patent: 1975504, 1934-10-02

[56] Leong MF, Chian KS, Mhaisalkar PS, Ratner BD. Effect of electrospun poly(D,L-lactide) fibrous scaffold with nanoporous surface on attachment of porcine esophageal epithelial cells and protein absorption. Journal of Biomedical Materials Research. 2009;**89A**:1040-1048. DOI: 10.1002/jbm.a.32061

[57] Zhu YB, Cao Y, Pan J, Liu YX. Macro-alignment of electrospun fibers for vascular tissue engineering. Journal of Biomedical Materials Research. 2010;**92B**:508-516. DOI: 10.1002/jbm.b.31544

[58] Zhu YB, Leong MF, Ong WF, Chan-Park M, Chian KS. Esophageal epithelium regeneration on fibronectin grafted poly(L-lactic acid-co-caprolactone) (PLLC) nanofiber scaffold. Biomaterials. 2007;**28**:861-868. DOI: 10.1016/j.biomaterials.2006.09.051

[59] Lv JJ, Chen L, Zhu YB, Hou L, Liu YX. Promoting epithelium regeneration for esophageal tissue engineering through basement membrane reconstitution. ACS Applied Materials & Interfaces. 2014;**6**:4954-4964. DOI:10.1021/am4059809

[60] Stegemann JP, Nerem RM. Altered response of vascular smooth muscle cells to exogenous biochemical stimulation in two- and three-dimensional culture. Experimental Cell Research. 2003;**283**:146-155

[61] Li S, Lao J, Chen BP, et al. Genomic analysis of smooth muscle cells in 3-dimensional collagen matrix. FASEB Journal. 2003;**17**:97-99 S

[62] Shen JY, Chan-Park M, He B, et al. Three-dimensional microchannels in biodegradable polymeric films for control orientation and phenotype of vascular smooth muscle cells. Tissue Engineering. 2006;**12**:2229-2240. DOI: 10.1089/ten.2006.12.2229

[63] Hou L, Gong CF, Zhu YB. In vitro construction and in vivo regeneration of esophageal bilamellar muscle tissue. Journal of Biomaterials Applications, 2016;**31**:1-12. DOI: 10.1177/0885328215627585

[64] Ritchie AC, Wijaya S, Ong WF, Zhong SP, Chian KS. Dependence of alignment direction on magnitude of strain in esophageal smooth muscle cells. Biotechnology and Bioengineering. 2009;**102**:1703-1711. DOI: 10.1002/bit.22190

[65] Cha JM, Park SN, Noh SH, Suh H. Time-dependent modulation of alignment and differentiation of smooth muscle cells seeded on a porous substrate undergoing cyclic mechanical strain. Artificial Organs. 2006;**30**:250-258. DOI: 10.1111/j.1525-1594.2006.00212.x

[66] Sjöqvist S, Jungebluth P, Lim ML, Haag J, Gustafsson Y, et al. Experimental orthotopic transplantation of a tissue-engineered oesophagus in rats. Nature Communications. 2014;**5**:1-51. DOI: 10.1038/ncomms4562

6

Eco-Epidemiology of Chagas Disease in Chile

Mauricio Canals Lambarri, Andrea Canals Cifuentes, Salvador Ayala, Valentina Tapia-Garay and Dante Cáceres Lillo

Abstract

There are four vector species of Chagas disease in Chile: *Triatoma infestans*, responsible for the domestic cycle; *Mepraia spinolai*, the main wild vector; and *M. gajardoi* and *M. parapatrica*, two coastal wild species whose importance as vectors is not well known. They are species of dry environments of the central-north region of Chile, whose best predictors of distribution are warm average temperatures and low rainfall. They are found in rock quarries, nests of birds, and small mammals, and *T. infestans* has sylvatic foci associated with a Bromeliaceae species. While human blood represents 70% of the diet of *T. infestans*, in *M. spinolai* this value is 7%, which means that a large part of Chagas disease in Chile is due to *T. infestans*. However, all species have high percentages of *T. cruzi* infection. Chagas disease in Chile follows the distribution of *T. infestans*, and although the cycle of domestic transmission by this vector is interrupted, there is still a constant prevalence and mortality and ascending incidences. Models predict that although climate change will not vary greatly the north-south distribution of vectors, it could increase the reproductive number of the disease, increasing risk areas of Chagas disease.

Keywords: Chagas disease, ecology, vectors, epidemiology, Chile

1. Introduction

American trypanosomiasis or Chagas disease is caused by the flagellated protozoan *Trypanosoma cruzi*, transmitted by several hematophagous insect species (Hemiptera, Reduviidae, and Triatominae) which in Chile are known as vinchucas. This protozoan species undergoes part of its development cycle (epimastigotes and trypomastigotes) in the insect vector, and when it ingests blood of a vertebrate host, the infectious trypomastigotes are eliminated with the dejections on the host; these are able to enter the bloodstream through the small wound or scratch lesions. Inside the *T. cruzi* continues its development with intracellular forms (amastigotes) and extracellular forms (trypomastigotes), producing damage which may be manifested in an acute form, although it generally does so after many years as a chronic form that compromises the digestive tract (megacolon or megaesophagus) and/or heart disease.

Two cycles of vector transmission in Chagas disease are described: (1) the domestic cycle maintained by domestic vectors, in Chile *Triatoma infestans*, which includes a man and an animal reservoir constituted by domestic and peridomestic animals such as cats, dogs, cows, horses, and others, and (2) the wild cycle maintained by wild vectors (such as *Mepraia spinolai*) and the wild animal reservoir composed of rodents, small marsupials, rabbits, etc. These cycles are not completely separated, since there are species that transit between the peridomestic and wild environments such as dogs, cats, goats, and other farm animals (**Figure 1**) [1–3]. In addition, wild vectors can penetrate into domestic environments and feed on humans [4], and domestic vectors can form wild colonies [5–7].

Its discovery is due to the Brazilian doctor Dr. Carlos R. J. Chagas, who in 1907 was the director of the Oswaldo Cruz Institute and director of the National Malaria Control Program. Dr. Chagas examined huts, finding a large number of insects that he named *Conorrhinus sanguessuga* (now *Panstrongylus megistus*) that contained "*Crithidia*." After experiments of inoculation

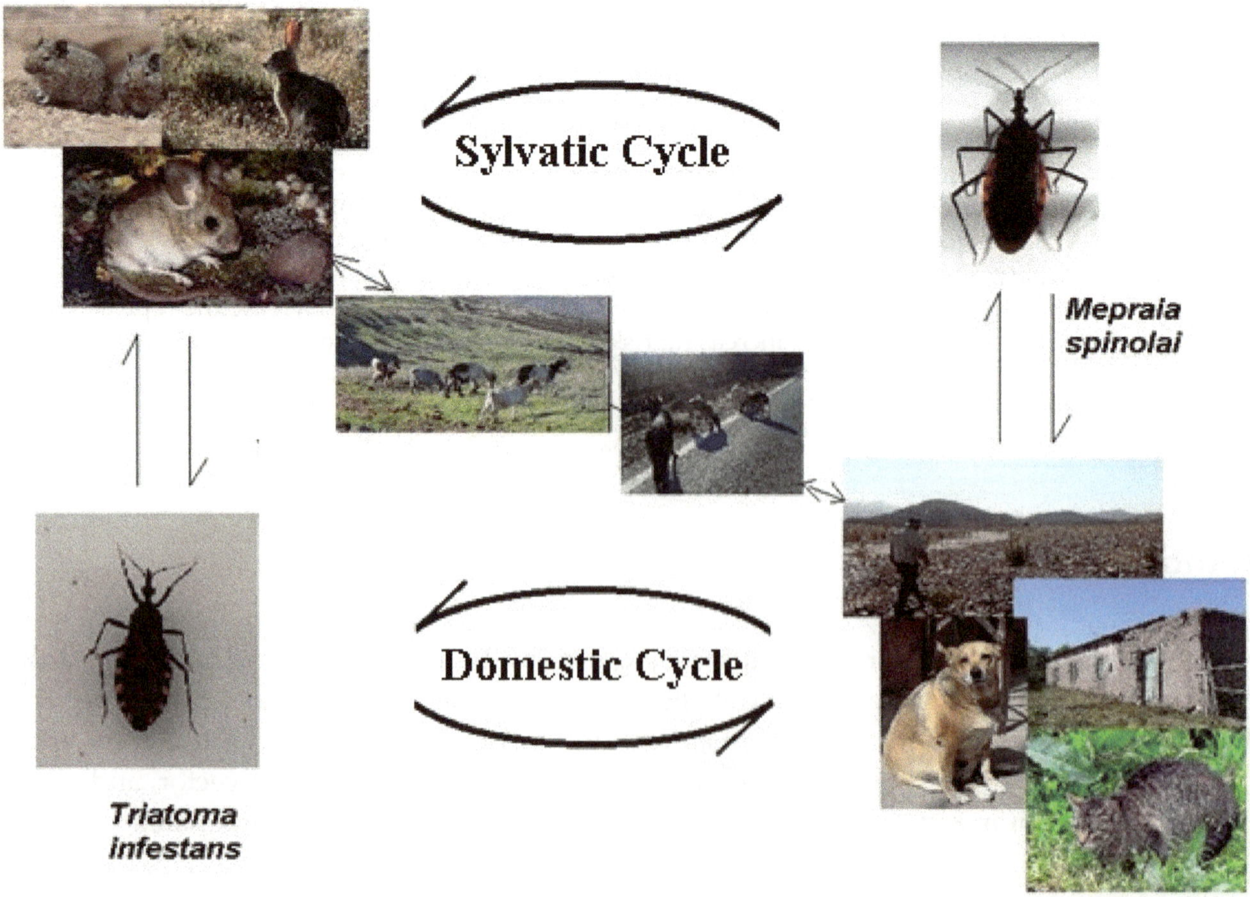

Figure 1. Domestic and wild cycles of Chagas disease.

in monkeys, he found a great quantity of flagellates, calling the new species *Shyzotrypanum cruzi* (today *Trypanosoma cruzi*) in honor of Dr. Oswaldo Cruz. Later, in 1909 he found a naturally infected cat and on April 14 found in the village of Santa Rita a 2-year-old girl named Berenice who lived in a house infested with *P. megistus* with a feverish condition and found in her blood the protozoan *T. cruzi*, describing the disease in 1909 [8]. Later, Carlos Chagas wrote about acute and chronic forms of the disease (1911) and the life cycle of *T. cruzi* (1931) [9], among other topics.

The first studies of Chagas disease in Chile were carried out by Dr. Juan Noé in 1921, with appreciation of *T. cruzi* in the vector *Triatoma infestans* around Santiago. Subsequently, the Argentine Dr. Salvador Massa, led by Noé, demonstrated the specificity of *T. cruzi* in cardiac fibers in experimental animals. With the creation of the Department of Parasitology of the State Health Office in 1937, systematic investigations led to the demonstration of the first case in Chile [10].

Knowledge of this disease has been progressively increasing in Chile thanks to the contribution of numerous researchers. Schenone, in 1980, [11] recognized three stages in the investigation of this disease. In the first stage, from 1937 to 1943, research focused on detecting the disease and tried to determine the endemic areas, detecting vector species and reservoirs. Important studies in this stage included those of Drs. G. Gasic, V. Bertín, *S. Massa*, and R. Gajardo Tobar. In the second stage, from 1944 to 1952, there was a more systematic study, determining the magnitude of the problem and conducting systematic surveys to determine the epidemiology better. The remarkable work of Dr. Amador Neghme was published in this period. The third stage can be established from 1953 to 1994 where there was a fruitful work of many researchers who have helped to clarify clinical aspects, congenital transmission, blood banks, epidemiology, distribution of endemic areas, the reservoir, natural history, ecology, physiology, and behavior of vectors. In this stage, the contributions of Drs. H. Schenone, W. Apt, and A. Atías and their teams stand out in epidemiological and clinical aspects. The fourth stage subsequent to 1995 had been added in which the investigation has focused more on specifying aspects not revealed in the previous periods and that has been marked by the acknowledgment of the interruption of the home transmission chain by *Triatoma infestans* which occurred in 1999. Research was focused mainly on laboratory and diagnostic improvement, on congenital and transfusion treatment and transmission, and on the study of the ecology of Chagas disease vectors and *T. cruzi*. There were important improvements in the detection of the disease, the control of blood banks and the success of domiciliary disinfestation carried out by the vector control area of the Ministry of Health. A negative effect of the declaration of the interruption of the vector transmission chain has been less interesting and resources for the study and control of this disease contributes to perpetuate it as an unattended disease.

2. Eco-epidemiology of vectors

Four species of insect vectors of Chagas disease have been described in Chile. The species responsible for the domestic cycle is *Triatoma infestans*, and the species involved in the wild cycle are *Mepraia spinolai* (**Figure 2**), *M. gajardoi*, and *M. parapatrica*.

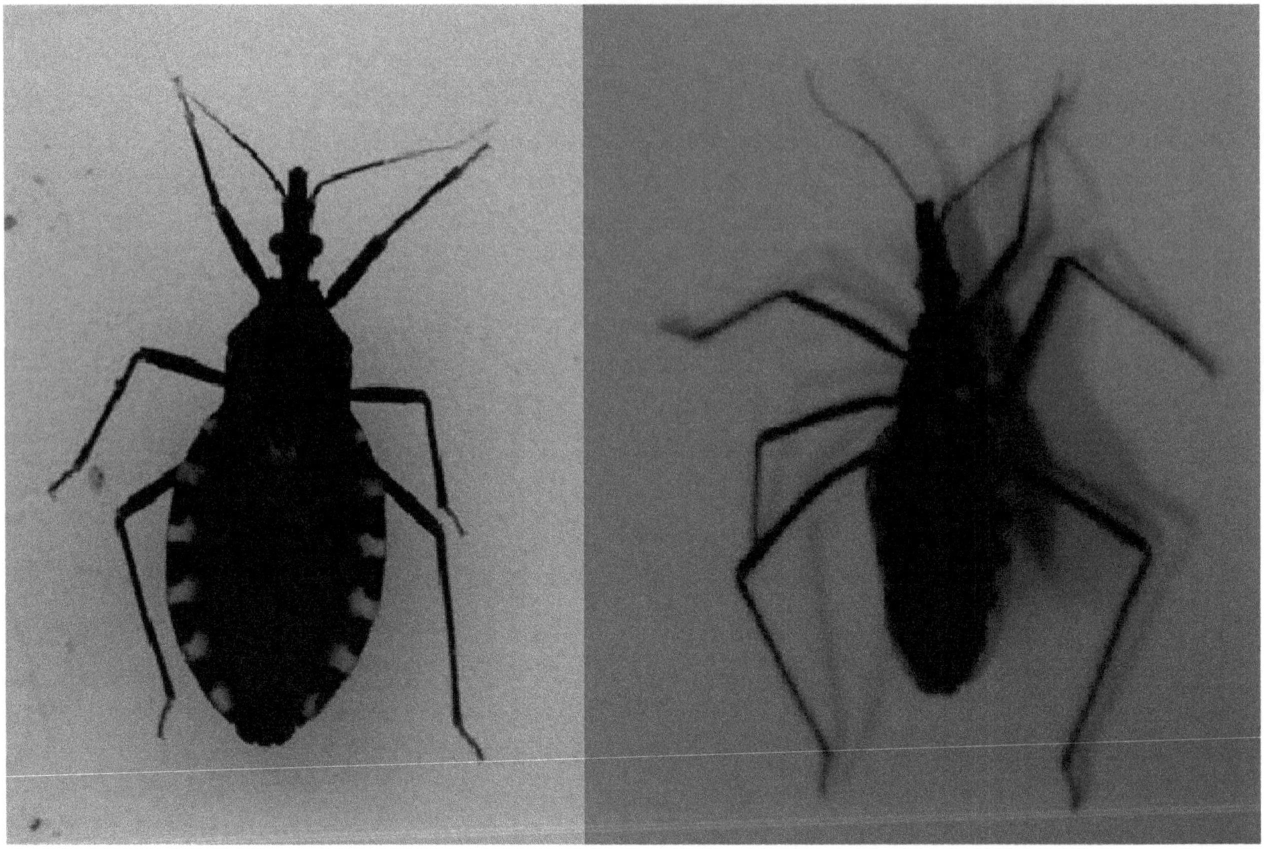

Figure 2. *Triatoma infestans* and *Mepraia spinolai,* the main vectors of Chagas disease in Chile.

2.1. Distribution and niche

The vector *T. infestans*, a bug with characteristic yellow spots in the connexivum, has the widest distribution in Chile, between 18 and 34°S (**Figure 3**). It is found in domestic habitats, but foci of reproductive populations have also been detected in wild habitats [5–7]. In the domestic habitats, it is found in cracks of adobe walls or in "quincha" (wooden branches covered with mud), roofs of branches, and dwellings and chicken coops of the peridomiciliary zone. In sylvatic habitats it has been found forming colonies associated with plants of *Puya chilensis* (Bromeliaceae).

Mepraia spinolai is a wild species endemic to Chile with high polymorphism, with apterous females, and apterous, winged, and brachypterous males with red spots in the connexivum [12–14]. It is found between 26 and 34°S, from the sea level to 3000 m (**Figure 3**) [11]. Their habitat is made up of rocky areas such as quarries and cracks, bird nests, and animal caves [15] and sometimes peridomiciliary pens and walls and in human dwellings [16, 17].

Mepraia gajardoi is a coastal, wild species that lives between latitudes 18 and 26°S, feeding on small reptiles and mammals in the area. The males have generally blackish coloration with small reddish lateral spots in the dorsal part of connexivum. Male brachypterous and female micropterous.

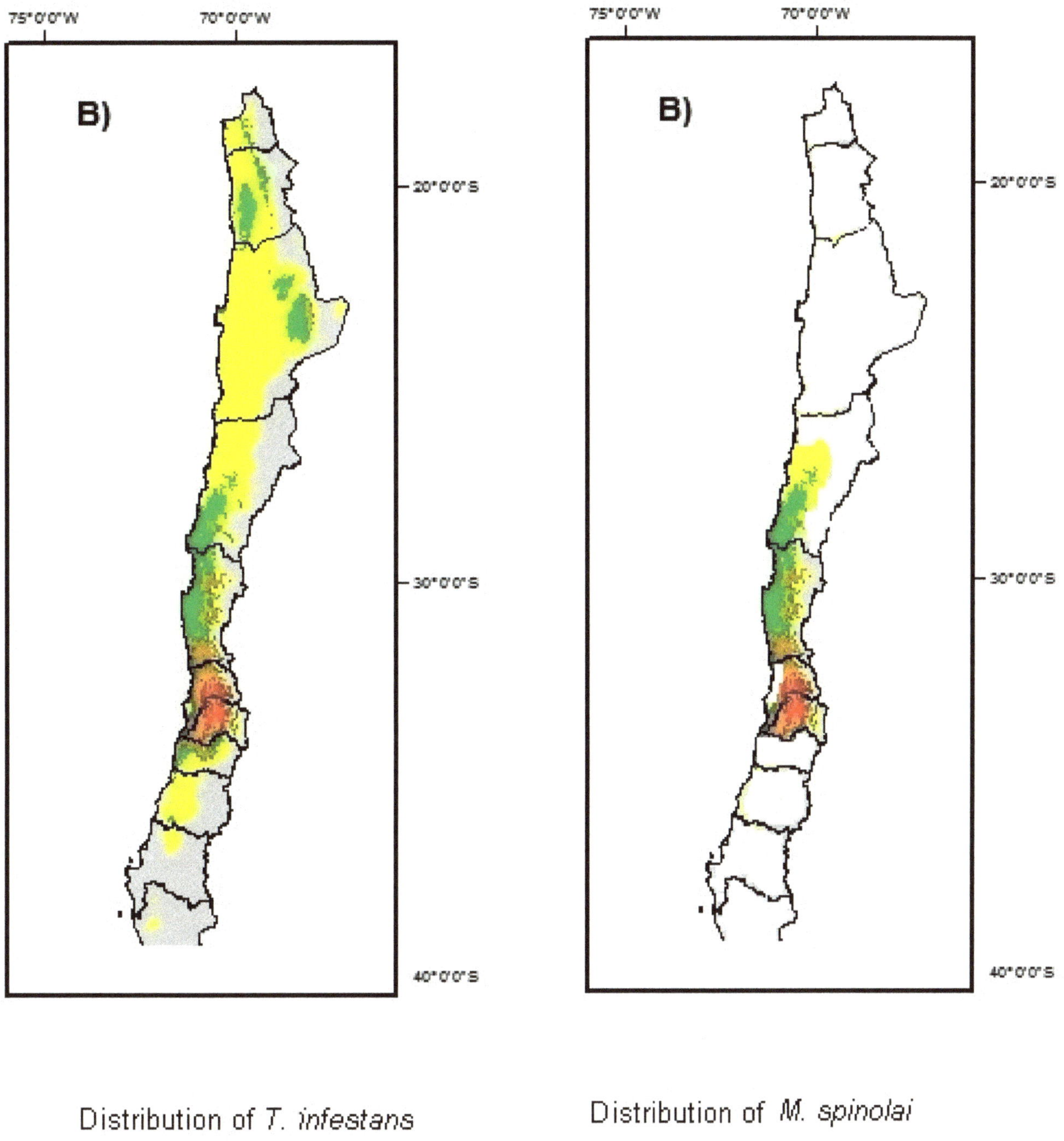

Figure 3. Approximate distribution of the two main vectors of Chagas disease (modified from [18] and [19]).

Mepraia parapatrica is a blackish species with red-orange spots in the connexivum, which only lives at 25°S. The females are micropterous, while the males are brachypterous and macropterous. It also lives on the coast, feeding on rodents and reptiles in the area.

Climate change predictions in Chile include an increase in temperature, with a gradient of higher to lower temperatures from north to south and from the Andes to the Pacific Ocean. During the 2011–2030 period, the temperature increase would be about 0.5°C in the southern zone and 1.5°C for the north and the Chilean altiplano. A decrease in precipitation of 5–15% is expected during the same period. The distribution of *T. infestans* and Chagas disease is associated with maximum temperature and the precipitation during the driest month [18]; thus, the distribution of *T. infestans* would be little affected by climate change. This is consistent with the decrease in suitable areas proposed for *M. spinolai* in the same area and is in contrast to the high impact on the distribution of *M. gajardoi*, a species with a small distribution on the coast of northern Chile [19]. Under the assumption of niche conservatism, the latter species would suffer disappearance of its habitat, while *M. spinolai*, a species with distribution similar to *T. infestans* from 25°S southward and with similar preferred environmental conditions, would decrease its distribution area in the interior valleys while increasing its distribution on the coast [19]. Since *T. infestans* is a species residing in arid and semiarid habitats, its distribution area would not be affected significantly. However, the transmission risk of Chagas disease in this zone could be increased because of changes in metabolism, survival, reproduction, biting rates, or densities of the insects.

2.2. Ecology and population dynamics

There are very few attempts to estimate the population density of vectors. A useful measure is the so-called triatomine index used for domestic vectors such as *T. infestans*, which is defined as the number of insects captured by a person in a house in 1 hour. Schenone estimated in these species indices of 54.5 for the Antofagasta Region in 1980, 19.8 for the Atacama Region, 26.7 for the Coquimbo Region, 37.0 for Valparaíso Region, 50.5 for the Metropolitan Region, and 17.2 for the O'Higgins Region. Later, Canals et al. [20] estimated the densities of vinchucas per human in high endemic rural areas, calculating for these zones an average of 25.3 individuals/humans, with a maximum in the Coquimbo Region of 39.1 individuals/human. For the case of *M. spinolai*, the maximum triatomine index in peridomiciliary zones was 64 vinchucas/person/hour, and the estimated maximum density was 4.59 vinchucas/human [21]. The density per square meter has been estimated in this species between 15 and 364 vinchucas/m^2, with an average of 79 vinchucas/m^2 in areas of rock walls in Colina [22]. This species can be found in high densities [22–26], even in mixed colonies with *T. infestans*, and has been found in human habitations [14, 17, 27, 28]. For example, Schenone et al. [27] reported the presence of 288 specimens in 50 rural dwellings in regions III, IV, V, and Metropolitan. In this sense *M. spinolai* is a potentially dangerous species, especially in areas where the usual contact with humans occurs, as in quarry areas, and in some areas around Santiago where it is currently being urbanized, such as Colina, Lampa, and Til-Til. Also, from the perspective of its food sources, *M. spinolai* is in the phase of domiciliation [4, 29, 30], with 7.4% human blood in its diet [29, 31].

Another approximation to get an idea of the density can be obtained from the number of specimens referred to the Institute of Public Health of Chile; these come in greater proportion from the regions of Antofagasta, Atacama, Coquimbo, Valparaiso, and Metropolitan (Santiago). A recent study [32] reported that 8331 triatomines have been received between 2005 and 2016. A 73.7% correspond to *T. infestans*, 24.0% to *M. spinolai*, and 2.3% to *M. gajardoi*. Their numbers increased over this period. This high proportion of *T. infestans* could be explained because this species, once eliminated from human habitations, has been able to recolonize wild habitats with several foci whose magnitude has not been completely clarified. From the first description of a wild focus in Chile in 2006 [5] in Calera de Tango, and in Til-Til, the new outbreaks in Sahondé, Putaendo [6] to the reports of wild foci in the cities of Valparaiso 2009, Atacama 2014, and Coquimbo 2015 [7].

The data reported by the Ministry of Health show the proportion of infested dwellings (home infestation) in 1999 and annual data since 2010 and divide the information into the percentage of colonized houses, that is, colonies with evidence of active reproduction, the individual visits to houses that receive adult individuals but without colonization, and the total (the sum of both). Household infestation has clearly decreased in this period, but the proportion of houses with individual visitors has increased. Currently, domiciliary infestation is estimated at 0.05% [32].

The vinchucas in Chile are long-lived species, surviving around 18 months in the laboratory [12, 13, 24, 33]. Their development is strongly affected by temperature and relative humidity like all triatomines [34]. The development of *T. infestans* completely ceases at temperatures below 16°C, and temperatures above 40°C are lethal [35]. The effect of relative humidity (RH) and its importance in molt periods has been discussed [36]. Combinations of variable ranges of low temperature and RH affect the maturation of *T. infestans* and *M. spinolai* (**Table 1**). While at constant temperature and humidity, the pre-imago period consisting of five nymph states (N1–N5) is 6.1 months in *T. infestans* [37]; this increases to 14.3 months in variable

	T. infestans	EC	*M. spinolai*	EC
Fecundity (eggs/female/week)	1.9	(15–32/40–90)	0.25	(28/70)
	1.0	(25/75)		
	5.4	(26/60)		
Egg viability (%)	74.6	(17/70)	27.7	(24/73)
	93.7	(24/73)		
Mortality rate (death/individual/day)	0.0083	(25/75)	0.0055	(24/73)
	0.0070	(15–32/40–90)		
Reproductive number (Ro)	1.36	(15–32/40–90)	22.9	(28/70)
	25.04	(26/60)		
Generation time (months)	14.7	(15–32/40–90)	13.2	(28/70)
	7.1	(26/60)		
Intrinsic rate of growth (r)	0.021	(15–32/40–90)	0.24	(28/70)
	0.45	(26/60)		

(EC: Temperature (°C)/Relative humidity (%)). References. Canals et al. [20].

Table 1. Some population parameters of *T. infestans* and *M. spinolai* in different environmental conditions.

environments [24, 38, 39]. In the main wild vector, *M. spinolai,* this period is between 9 and 10 months under constant conditions [12, 33], while in environments with RH and T variability, only nymphs are obtained up to N5 status. With greater restriction at low temperature and humidity, they only reach the N2 status in 12 months [24]. The arrest of secondary development in unfavorable conditions (induced diapause) has been observed in both species [24, 33, 40]. Also, some parameters like the net reproductive rate (R_0) are strongly affected. Both species present survival curves with exponential decays and similar mortality rates [24, 28, 33, 41]. The mortality and fertility rates in *T. infestans* present periodic variations during the year even under relatively constant environmental conditions. For example, under laboratory conditions the mean fecundity of *T. infestans* varied from 0.39 eggs/female/week in autumn to 1.63 eggs/female/week in spring, with maximum values of 7.59 eggs/female/week in spring and 5.83 eggs/female/week in summer. Maximum mean mortality and fertility rates were in spring and summer [42].

2.3. Ecophysiology and behavior

Triatoma infestans is a diurnal insect, while all species of the genus *Mepraia* are diurnal. In the laboratory *M. spinolai* moves between 15 and 42°C with a preferred temperature of 24.8°C [43]. *T. infestans* moves between 18 and 42°C with a preferred temperature of 24.2°C [43]. Other authors have found that *T. infestans* preferred temperatures between 26 and 27°C [44] and variations from 28 to 29°C at the beginning of the night, immediately after the ingestion of blood, but 25°C 12 days later [45, 46]. The synchronization of activity patterns to the L/D cycle is similar to other triatomines [47–51]. Other activities synchronous to the L/D cycles are the rhythms of oviposition [52], molt [53], hatching [46], and aggregation [54]. The stimulus for orientation and approach to a potential prey is temperature, displaying the classic pattern of antennal movements-locomotor movement and extension of the proboscis [55, 56]. *T. infestans* decreases the frequency of antennal movements when it is within 30 to 15 cm of its prey, whereas *M. spinolai* always maintains a low frequency, which may be due to a greater distance of perception in this species [57]. Once in contact with its prey, *T. infestans* introduces its proboscis, sucking blood, being able to increase its weight from four to six times in a single ingestion [38, 39, 57]. The volume of blood ingested is estimated between 30 and 70 ml when fed on a species such as *Mesocricetus auratus* [58]. The bite frequency in *T. infestans* has been estimated at 0.0754 bites/day [21]. The bite frequency of *M. spinolai* has been estimated at 0.155 bites/day, with volumes of blood ingestion between 20 and 160 mg. The intake volume has been found to be inversely correlated with the weight prior to intake, which is an indicator of nutritional status. Thus, the volume of the intake is related to the time elapsed since the last feeding and to the degree of distension of the abdomen [59].

T. infestans emits its dejections during the feeding act [60], which takes on average 19.5 min [38, 39, 57], usually between 3 and 4 min from the start of feeding, while in *M. spinolai* this latency is 24.4 min and not necessarily on the prey, which decreases the probability of transmission [38, 39, 57]. The bite rate and the latency between the start of the bite and the dejection are affected by the presence of the *T. cruzi* parasite in the vector; *M. spinolai* showed a higher frequency of bite and a lower latency of dejection in infected individuals [59].

The feeding spectrum of *T. infestans* in Chile was obtained by means of ag-ac reactions and double gel diffusion [60]. The diet of this species is made up of humans 68.4%, cats 6.1%, dogs 3.2%, rabbits 5.9%, rodents 1.6%, Artiodactyla 0.3%, birds 7.2%, and amphibians 0.5%. The proportions for *M. spinolai* are humans 7.4%, cats 3.7%, dogs 12.3%, rabbits 53.1%, rodents 9.9%, Artiodactyla 12.3%, and birds 1.2% [29]. The amplitude of the trophic niche of *M. spinolai* is greater than that of *T. infestans*, and they have a niche overlap of 0.229 [29]. An increase in the amplitude of the niche in times of greater heat has also been demonstrated [29]. Introducing the information of the food profile of 15 species of triatomines with multivariate analysis techniques has shown a clear separation between species of domiciliary habits and peridomiciliary, wild, and stenophagous specialists; *M. spinolai* is among the peridomiciliary species [4]. In a later study, this species was located between wild and peridomiciliary [30].

The average percentages of *T. cruzi* infection in the vectors (trypano-triatomine indices) are *M. gajardoi* 16.92 ± 17.77%, *M. spinolai* 20.88 ± 11.51%, and *T. infestans* 41.83 ± 13.23% [32]. The trypano-triatomine indices of *M. gajardoi* have remained stable over time, although based on a small number of individuals. The same occurs with the *M. spinolai* indices, but *T. infestans* shows an increasing trend.

The high trypano-triatomine indices in *T. infestans* are interesting, since a decrease of these indices was expected once these insects were removed from human habitats. Thus, for example, in Uruguay, the indices were drastically reduced as a result of vector control actions [61]. An explanation for the lack of a decline in these indices in Chile could be that despite the change in diet that involves the elimination of the human environment, *T. infestans* can find rodents and other species with high infection rates that make high trypano-triatomine indices persist. This may be true, since there is a great diversity of infected wild, domestic, and peridomestic mammals, some reaching levels of infection higher than 10% [15, 62], but this is also probably true in Uruguay.

3. *Trypanosoma cruzi* lineages

Lineages of *T. cruzi* have been recognized for a long time. Initially, isoenzymes that differ in gel electrophoresis were classified as zymodemes Z1 and Z2, the first one mainly associated with the wild cycle and the second one with the domestic cycle [63]. Subsequently, biochemical and genetic differentiation was carried out, and two lineages, TcI corresponding to Z1 and TcII corresponding to Z2, were proposed. However, the first TcII was divided into five subgroups a, b, c, d, and e, where TcIIb corresponded to Z2, TcIIa to the new zymodeme Z3 and TcIIc, and d and e to hybrids [64]. Subsequently, subgroups were also recognized in TcI: a, b, c, and d [63, 65]. Currently, it has been simplified into six subgroups, from TcI to TcVI, where TcI corresponds to Z1, TcII to TcIIb (Z2), TcIII to TcIIc, TcIV to TcIIa (Z3), TcV to TcIId, and TcVI to TcIIe.

Only TcII and TcVI have been found in *M. gajardoi* in Chile [66, 67], TcI and TcII in *M. spinolai* [66] and subsequently TcI, TcII, TcV, and TcVI [68], while in *T. infestans*, the most important lineage is TcI circulating in wild (93.3%) and domiciliary (100%) individuals. TcII, TcV, and TcVI have also been detected mainly in nymphs, suggesting differential adaptation of *T. cruzi* lineages between nymph states [69].

It has been proposed that in small wild mammals TcI and TcII would be associated with marsupials and placental mammals, respectively. However, the TcI, TcII, TcV, and TcVI lineages have been detected in the rodent *Octodon degus* in Chile [26, 70]. The same lineages have been detected in wild *Oryctolagus cuniculus* [71], and in 117 individuals of different infected species, TcI, TcII (TcIIb), TcV (TcIId), and TcVI (TcIIe) have been detected with frequencies of 38, 41, 26 and 9%, respectively, in wild mammals. In peridomestic mammals the frequencies of these lineages were 29, 33, 43, and 14%, respectively. More than one lineage was found in 31% of the individuals analyzed, without specific association with marsupials [72, 73]. Thus, it seems that the information on the wild mammal reservoir and the vectors *T. infestans* and *M. spinolai* is quite consistent in pointing to TcI, TcII, TcV, and TcVI as the main circulating lineages, although more studies are still missing in the other wild vectors of the genus *Mepraia*.

4. Reservoir

The animal reservoir is very extensive; it is constituted by mammals of the peridomestic environment such as dogs, cats, goats, rabbits, sheep, horses, donkeys, and cattle, some carnivores, numerous rodents, and some small marsupials. Infection in mammals by *T. cruzi* has been described in around 150 species in America [74] and is widespread in numerous orders; the most important reservoirs are dogs, cats, and goats, due both to high infection rates and to their mobility which establishes a bridge between domestic and wild cycles. Proportions of infection by *T. cruzi* have been reported 14.5% in dogs, 10.7% in cats, 9.4% in goats, 12.1% in rabbits, and 4.8% in sheep [75]. Current studies with PCR in wild mammals have reported percentages of infection between 26 and 59% in the species *Capra hircus* (goat), *Thylamys elegans* (marsupial), *O. degus*, *Phyllotis darwini*, and *Abrothrix olivaceus* (rodents) [72] and large increases in interannual infection rates from 300–400%, which could be explained by a delayed response to the El Niño weather phenomenon after the emergence of small rodents [25].

5. Distribution of the disease

Chagas disease extends in America from the Southern United States at parallel 35°N to southern South America at parallel 34°S on the Chilean side and 45°S on the Argentine side. In this zone, 21 countries report active transmission, with current prevalence very difficult to assess since most of the studies refer to the prevalence in endemic rural areas [15]. The median prevalence in these areas is approximately 8.15%. The lower extreme values probably represent Chagas disease in controlled or urban areas and the maximum Chagas disease prevalence in hyperendemic areas without protection of health systems. Currently, emergence of Chagas disease in Europe has been reported through immigrants and subsequent congenital

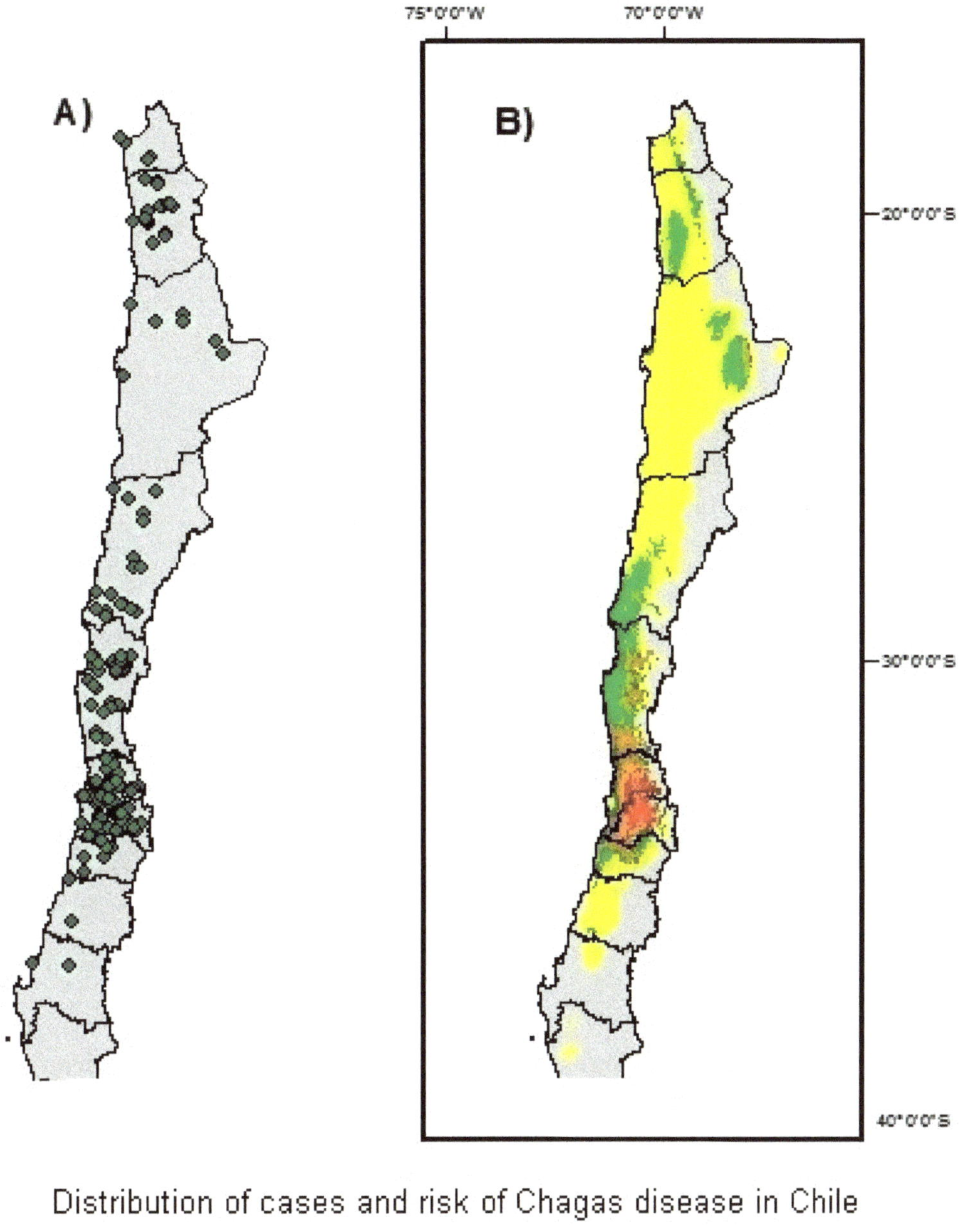

Figure 4. Distribution of cases and the risk of Chagas disease in Chile (modified from [18]).

transmission. For example, Basile et al. [76] reported more than 4000 cases diagnosed in different countries, with the highest number of cases in Spain, but Strasen et al. [77] proposed around 95% underreporting. These latter authors indicated that there could be between 14,000 and 180,000 cases in this continent.

In Chile, Chagas disease is distributed between the Arica and Parinacota Region (18°30′S) and the O'Higgins Region (34°36′S) (**Figure 4**), coinciding in large part with the distribution of the vector domestic *T. infestans* [18]. The highest incidence rates are recorded between Antofagasta and Coquimbo, with Antofagasta, Coquimbo, and Metropolitan Regions concentrating approximately two-thirds of the reported cases (**Table 2**).

Administrative region	Cases	Incidence rate (cases × 10^{-5})
Arica and Parinacota	57	23.8
Tarapacá	64	19.0
Antofagasta	223	35.8
Atacama	67	21.4
Coquimbo	292	37.9
Valparaiso	210	11.5
Metropolitan	313	4.3
O'Higgins	20	2.2
Maule	2	0.2
Bío Bío	11	0.5
Araucanía	1	0.1
Los Ríos	2	0.5
Los Lagos	0	0.0
Aisén	0	0.0
Magallanes	0	0.0
Total country	**1262**	**7.0**

Table 2. Cases and incidence rates of Chagas disease in Chile (2015) (health ministry).

6. Prevalence and incidence

Chagas disease is one of the main neglected diseases that affects the Americas and has now become an emerging disease in some parts of America and Europe [78–81], which has even been compared to the early stage of the HIV/AIDS epidemic [79]. The annual incidence varies between 28,000 and 56,000 people and between 10,000 and 14,000 deaths per year [79], affecting 6–11 million individuals [82] with 65–100 million people at risk in the world [78–80, 83]. The population at risk in Chile is 873,415 people [80, 81]. The latest national health survey (ENS) reports a prevalence of *T. cruzi* infection of 0.7% of the population, with a prevalence of 1.5% in rural areas and 0.6% in urban areas [81], and ministerial reports indicate that home infestation by *T. infestans* is practically nonexistent [80], which contrasts sharply with the data reported in the 1980s and 1990s. For example, between 1937 and 1980, a general prevalence of 16.7% was reported in endemic areas, with a maximum of 43.6% in the Coquimbo Region [11], which did not vary significantly between 1982 and 1985 [84], whereas between 1982 and1989 differences were already reported between rural areas with prevalence of 16.7% and urban areas with prevalence of 1.9% [16]. The same occurs with domiciliary infestation, in which previous reports indicated infestations between 26.8 and 33.2% of dwellings in endemic areas between Arica and the O'Higgins Regions [11, 80].

A study covering 60 years of the disease in Chile of patients referred to the University of Chile and studied through xenodiagnosis revealed an average prevalence of 9.35 ± 0.1% [32]. This prevalence value of 9.35% should be considered as the level for highly endemic zones. It is in the range between 8 and 12% reported by Apt and Reyes in 1986, also based on xenodiagnosis, and is similar to the estimated value for Latin America. This value does not present any variation in the 65 years of study, regardless of the changes in the health systems or interruption of the chain of transmission. Accurate estimation of the prevalence of Chagas disease is a difficult task since it depends not only on the sampling characteristics (random, stratified, etc.), sample size, and bias but also on the screening method used, which in the case of Chagas disease can be by xenodiagnosis, ELISA, immunofluorescence, and/or Western blot.

The values reported by the 2009–2010 ENS based on 4650 volunteers using IgG ELISA show 0.7% average prevalence, with 1.5% in the rural population and 0.6% in the urban population. These values are surprisingly similar to those reported for the urban population in 1982–1989 [85]. In this sense, the prevalence shows an evolution toward the values of an urbanized population.

The incidence in Chile shows a progressive rise from 1985 onward (**Figure 5**), without a slope change attributable to the interruption of the vector transmission chain. On the other hand, there is no appreciable effect attributable to the improvement in detection. For example, supreme decree 158 of 2004 in Chile declares Chagas disease as a notifiable disease, which is not reflected in the trend curve; later in 2008 circular four instructs blood banks to investigate the presence of *T cruzi*; law 1839 of 2009 stipulates the national policy of blood services; and in 2011 in circular B51, number 17 stipulates the surveillance of Chagas disease and establishes ways to record and inform the health authority [80, 81]. The incidence before 2009 had an average value of 2.7 ± 1.29 per 100,000 inhabitants, whereas after 2009 the average is 7.3 ± 2.02

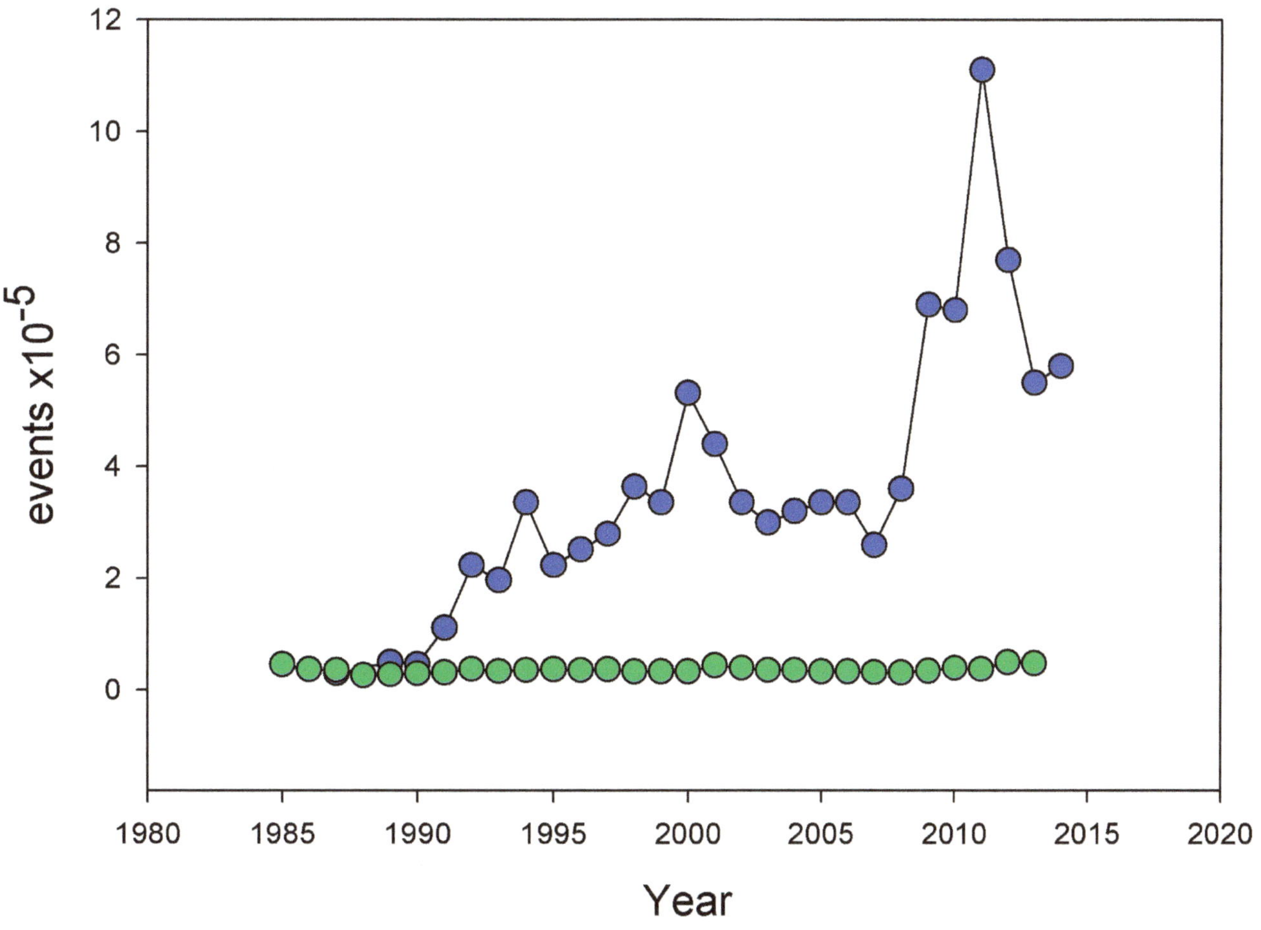

Figure 5. Incidence (blue) and mortality rates (green) of Chagas disease in Chile (Health Ministry).

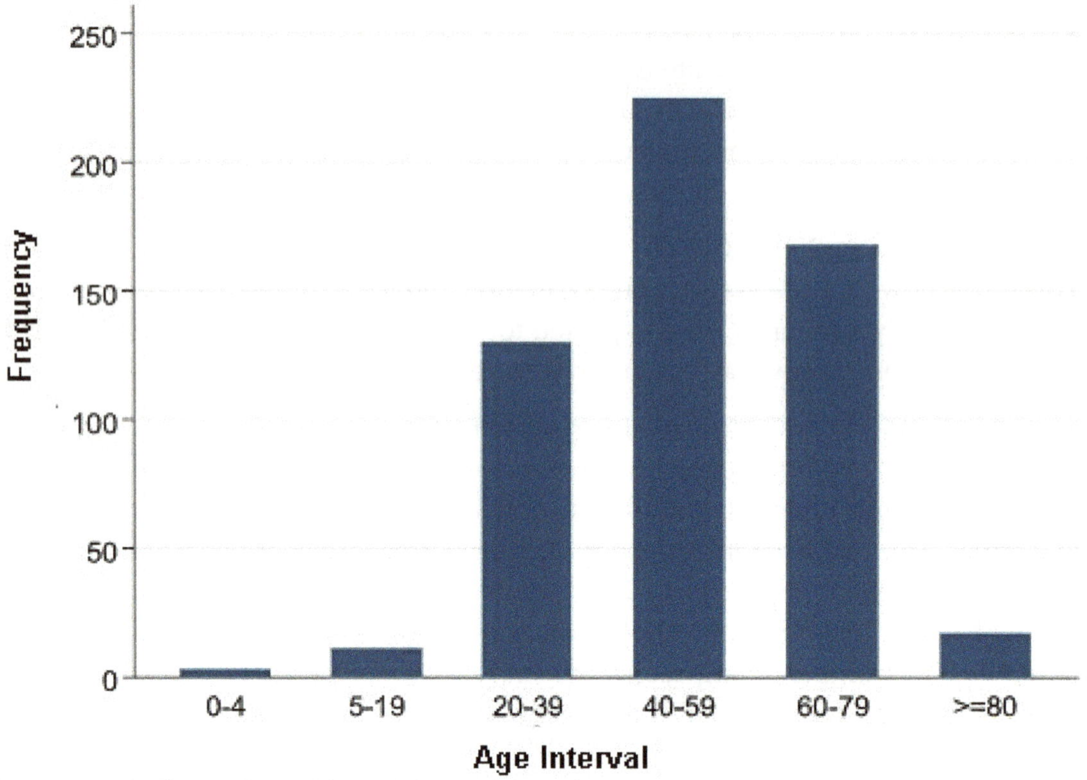

Figure 6. Age distribution of Chagas disease in 2010 (Health inistry).

per 100,000 inhabitants [32], staying relatively stable. One explanation for this temporal dynamics is that the progressive increase was not explained by a particular milestone but by a progressive improvement in the notification attributable to better staff preparation and a better notification system. Another possibility that cannot be ruled out is that this increase is real, and in this case, it should have an impact on mortality rates in the long run, a fact that is not yet evident. If the relative stability detected since 2009 persists, it would indicate that it would be reaching an adequate estimation of the endemic equilibrium, as the models predict [23, 86].

Mortality shows stability over the years (**Figure 5**). The average mortality rate is 0.36 ± 0.55 per 100,000 inhabitants [32]. Chagas disease affects the entire population in Chile, especially people of working age, with the highest rates between 30 and 65 years of age (**Figure 6**) [81].

7. Transfusion and congenital Chagas disease

The seroprevalence of *T. cruzi* in blood donors has been studied in Chile since the 1960s, with a national average of 3.7% reported between 1962 and 1988 [15]. Subsequently, this value has decreased; it was estimated between 0.5 and 1.6% according to information from the ISP between 2000 and 2005, estimated with the ELISA IgG method, and confirmed with IFI [87]. Currently, the seroprevalence of *T. cruzi* in blood donors is estimated at approximately 0.6%. The latest studies in the blood bank of the Clinical Hospital of the University of Chile were 0.4% positive out of a total of 24,568 [87].

A meta-analytic study that considered 13 case studies and 51 observational studies in ten countries estimated the rate of congenital infection was 4.7% with a CI of 3.4–5.7%. This means that in a population of mothers infected with *T. cruzi*, 4.7% of newborns are congenitally infected [88]. In this study it is proposed that in endemic areas the rate is 5% in endemic countries but lower in non-endemic countries (2.7%) and proposes a rate of 2.5% for Chile. In the same year, in a study conducted in Choapa, a highly endemic area, this rate was estimated at 4.7% [89].

8. The reproductive number (R_0)

The transmission of Chagas disease depends mainly on vector and congenital transmission. Accidental and transfusion transmissions are very rare and oral transmission only occurs in particular areas where the contact between man and nature is very close. The reproductive number of an infectious disease (R_0) corresponds to the average number of secondary infections produced by an infected individual. Thus, if R_0 is greater than 1, the disease is established in the population, and if R_0 is less than 1, the disease disappears. In the case of Chagas disease, the main component of the reproductive number is given by vector transmission, and when this is cut off, congenital transmission alone is incapable of perpetuating the disease [86, 90]. There are very few attempts to estimate the R_0 of this disease, an exception being the study by Massad [91], who estimated it at $R_0 = 1.25$ for a region of Brazil. Other estimates based on plausible approximations of many parameters obtained values of $R_0 = 7$ in Colombia [92] and $R_0 = 2.86$ [23] and $R_0 = 1.52$ in Chile [86]. However, recently in a spatial approach, a median value of $R_0 = 1.02$ has been proposed, with an approximate spatial variability between 0 and 5. The reproductive number could vary in different climate change scenarios as consequence of changes in entomological parameters such as biting rate, density, and mortality rate, increasing the Chagas risk area between 13 and 18% [93].

9. Conclusion and the way forward

Chile is in a privileged situation. It has only one domestic vector and probably only one wild vector of epidemiological importance, and the chain of domestic vector transmission by *T. infestans* is cut off. The wild reservoir is made up of small rodents, and the circulating lineages of *T. cruzi* are similar to the rest of America. However, there are some problems that persist: (1) The peri-anthropic reservoir is diverse and has bridging animals between the wild and domestic cycles that facilitate the spread of Chagas disease, such as dogs and goats; (2) housing and education conditions in Northern Chile are limited; (3) there are no control or education campaigns on wild vectors, and human dwellings are built on their territory. In addition there are wild foci of *T. infestans* and vector home intrusion; (4) prevalence, incidence, and trypano-triatomine indices still do not decrease; and (5) climate could change the epidemiological situation.

Given the obvious opportunity to eradicate Chagas disease in two generations, as predicted by the models, the way forward should be focused on (1) strengthening education campaigns of the population; (2) strengthening the monitoring of housing and peridomestic animals; (3) detection, study, and control of wild foci; and (4) reinforcing the study of the effect of climate change on the epidemiology of Chagas disease.

Acknowledgements

The authors acknowledge the financial support of Fondecyt (1150514 to MCL) and the revision of English language to Lafayette Eaton.

Author details

Mauricio Canals Lambarri[1,2*], Andrea Canals Cifuentes[3,4], Salvador Ayala[5], Valentina Tapia-Garay[1] and Dante Cáceres Lillo[1]

*Address all correspondence to: mcanals@uchile.cl

1 Programa de Salud Ambiental, Escuela de Salud Pública, Facultad de Medicina, Universidad de Chile, Chile

2 Departamento de Medicina, Facultad de Medicina, Universidad de Chile, Chile

3 Programa de Bioestadística, Escuela de Salud Pública, Facultad de Medicina, Universidad de Chile, Chile

4 Dirección Académica, Clínica santa María, Chile

5 Departamento de Asuntos Científicos, Instituto de Salud Pública, Chile

References

[1] Rojas A, Sotelo JM, Villarroel F, Contreras MC. La importancia del perro y el gato en la epidemiología de la enfermedad de Chagas. Boletin Chileno De Parasitología. 1973;**28**:42-43

[2] Alcaino H, Ríos A, Apt W, Arrau S. Enfermedad de Chagas en animales sinantrópicos de un área hiperendémica de Chile. Parasitología al Día. 1981;**4**:88

[3] Alcaino H, Arrau S, Apt W, Ríos A. Enfermedad de Chagas en caprinos sinantrópicos de la provincia de Limarí, Chile. Revista Medica De Chile. 1982;**110**:328

[4] Canals M, Ehrenfeld M, Cattan PE. Situación de *Mepraia Spinolai*, vector silvestre de la enfermedad de Chagas en Chile, en relación con otros vectores, desde la perspectiva de sus fuentes de alimentación. Revista Medica De Chile. 2000;**128**:1108-1112

[5] Bacigalupo A, Segura JA, Garcia A, Hidalgo J, Galuppo S, Cattan PE. Primer hallazgo de vectores de la enfermedad de Chagas asociados a matorrales silvestres en la Region Metropolitana, Chile. Revista Médica de Chile. 2006;**134**:1230-1236

[6] Bacigalupo A, Torres-Perez F, Segovia V, Garcia A, Correa JP, Moreno L, et al. Sylvatic foci of the Chagas disease vector *Triatoma infestans* in Chile: Description of a new focus and challenges for control programs. Memórias do Instituto Oswaldo Cruz. 2010;**105**(5):633-641

[7] Bacigalupo A, Correa JP, García A, Cattan PE. Focos silvestres de *Triatoma infestans* en Latinoamérica: análisis y perspectivas para Chile. Parasitología latinoamericana. 2015; **64**(3):33-42

[8] Chagas C. Nova trypanosomíase humana. Estudo sobre a morfología e o ciclo evolutivo do *Schizotrypanum cruzi* n. gen Sp, ajente etiológico de nova entidade mórbida do homen. Memórias do Instituto Oswaldo Cruz. 1909;**1**:159-218

[9] Coura JR. The discovery of Chagas disease (1908-1909): Great successes and certain misunderstandings and challenges. Revista da Sociedade Brasileira de Medicina Tropical. 2013;**46**(4):389-390

[10] Gasic G, Bertín V. Epidemiología de la enfermedad de Chagas en Chile. Revista Chilena de Pediatría. 1940;**11**(8):561-584

[11] Schenone H, Villarroel F, Rojas A, Alfaro E. Factores biológicos y ecológicos en la epidemiología de la enfermedad de Chagas en Chile. Boletín Chileno de Parasitología. 1980;**35**:42-54

[12] Lent H, Jurberg J. Algunas informacoes sobre *T. spinolai*, com um estudo sobre as genitalias externas. Revista Brasileira de Biologia. 1967;**27**:273-288

[13] Frías D, Martinez H, Wallace A. Algunos aspectos taxonómicos de *T. spinolai*. Acta Entomológica Chilena. 1987:155-170

[14] Frías-Lasserre D. A new species and karyotype variation in the bordering distribution of *Mepraia spinolai* (Porter) and *Mepraia gajardoi* Frías *et al* (Hemiptera: Reduviidae: Triatominae) in Chile and its parapatric model of speciation. Neotropical Entomology. 2010;**39**(4):572-583

[15] Apt W, Reyes H. Algunos aspectos de la enfermedad de Chagas en Latinoamérica. Parasitología al Día. 1990;**14**:23-40

[16] Schenone H, Rojas A. Algunos datos y observaciones pragmáticas en relación a la epidemiologia de la enfermedad de Chagas. Boletín Chileno de Parasitología. 1989;**44**: 66-86

[17] Frías-Lasserre D, González C, Reyes C, de Carvalho DB, Oliveira J, Canals M, da Rosa JA. Wing polymorphism and *Trypanosoma cruzi* infection in wild, peridomestic and domestic collections of *Mepraia spinolai* (Hemiptera: Reduviidae) from Chile. Journal of Medical Entomology. 2017;**54**(4):1061-1066

[18] Tapia-Garay V, Figueroa DP, Maldonado A, Frías-Laserre D, Gonzalez CR, Parra A, Canals L, Apt W, Alvarado S, Cáceres D, Canals M. Assessing the risk zones of Chagas′ disease in Chile in a world marked by global climatic change. Memórias do Instituto Oswaldo Cruz. 2018;**113**(1):24-29

[19] Garrido R. Impacto del cambio climático en la distribución geográfica de dos vectores silvestres de la enfermedad de Chagas en Chile, *Mepraia spinolai* y *Mepraia gajardoi* (Hemiptera: Reduviidae) [Tesis Magister en Ciencias Biológicas]. Santiago: Universidad de Chile; 2017. p. 54

[20] Canals M, Cattan PE, Ehrenfeld M. Algunas estimaciones numéricas de la importancia epidemiológica de los vectores de la enfermedad de Chagas en Chile. Parasitología al Día. 1993;**17**:79-86

[21] Canals M, Bustamante RO, Ehrenfeld M, Cattan PE. Assesing the impact of insect vectors on animal populations. Acta Biotheoretica. 1999;**46**:337-345

[22] Cattan PE, Pinochet C, Botto-Mahan C, Acuña MI, Canals M. Abundance of *Mepraia spinolai* in a periurban zone of Chile. Memórias do Instituto Oswaldo Cruz. 2002;**97**(3):285-287

[23] Canals M, Cattan PE. Dinamica de transmisión de la infección de la infección chagásica en Chile: Modelo y simulación. Revista Medica De Chile. 1992;**120**(12):1359-1365

[24] Canals M, Cattan PE, Ehrenfeld M, Torres P. Poblaciones experimentales de *T. infestans*: efectos de condiciones ambientales variables. Parasitología al Día. 1992;**16**(3-4):72-77

[25] Botto-Mahan C, Campos R, Acuna-Retamar M, Coronado X, Cattan PE, et al. Temporal variation of *Trypanosoma cruzi* infection in native mammals in Chile. Vector-Borne and Zoonotic Diseases. 2010;**10**:317-319

[26] Botto-Mahan C, Rojo G, Sandoval-Rodríguez A, Peña F, Ortiz S, Solari A. Temporal variation in *Trypanosoma cruzi* lineages from the native rodent *Octodon degus* in semiarid Chile. Acta Tropica. 2015;**151**:178-181

[27] Schenone H, Contreras MC, Salinas P, Sandoval L, Rojas A, Villarroel F. Epidemiología de la enfermedad de Chagas en chile. Frecuencia de infección humana por *Trypanosoma cruzi* por grupos de edad y regiones. Boletín Chileno de Parasitología. 1995;**50**:84-86

[28] Canals M, Cattan PE, Ehrenfeld M. Sobrevivencia de *Triatoma spinolai* en ambiente habitacional. Parasitología al Día. 1994;**18**(3):82-87

[29] Canals M, Cruzat L, Ehrenfeld M, Molina MC, Ferreira A, Cattan PE. Blood sources of *Mepraia spinolai* (Hemiptera Reduviidae), wild vector of Chagas's disease in Chile. Journal of Medical Entomology. 2001;**38**(2):303-307

[30] Rabinovich JE, Dan Kitron U, Obed Y, Yoshioka M, Gottdenker N, Chaves LF. Ecological patterns of blood-feeding by kissing-bugs. Memórias do Instituto Oswaldo Cruz. 2011;**106**(4):479-494

[31] Molina MC, Cattan PE, Canals M, Cruzat L, Aguillon JC, Ferreira A. A simple immunometric assay to assess the feeding habits of *Mepraia spinolai*, a *Trypanosoma cruzi* vector. Parasitology Research. 2004;**92**:375-379

[32] Canals M, Gonzalez C, Canals L, Canals A, Cáceres D, Alvarado D, et al. Que dicen los números de la evolución temporal de la enfermedad de Chagas? Revista Chilena De Infectologia. 2017;**34**(2):120-127

[33] Ehrenfeld M, Canals M, Cattan PE. Population parameters of *Triatoma spinolai* under different environmental conditions and densities. Journal of Medical Entomology. 1998; **35**(5):740-744

[34] Lehane MJ. Biology of Blood Sucking Insects. Cambridge: Cambridge University Press; 2005

[35] Schofield CJ. Triatominae. Biologia y Control. UK: Eurocomunica Pub; 1994

[36] Wood SF. The laboratory culture of *Triatoma*. Bulletin of the World Health Organization. 1964;**31**:579-581

[37] Rabinovich J, Rossel O. Mathematical models and ecology of Chagas disease. PAHO Pan American Journal of Public Health. 1978;**318**:359-369

[38] Canals M. Thermal ecology of small animals. Biological Research. 1998;**31**:367-374

[39] Canals M, Ehrenfeld M, Solís R, Cruzat L, Pinochet A, Tapia C, Cattan PE. Biología comparada de *Mepraia spinolai* en condiciones de laboratorio y terreno: cinco años de estudio. Parasitología al Día. 1998;**22**:72-78

[40] Jorg ME. Influencia de temperaturas fijas en periodos anuales sobre metamorfosis y fertilidad de *T. infestans*. Boletin Chileno De Parasitologia. 1962;**17**:17-19

[41] Canals M, Cattan PE, Ehrenfeld M. Dinámica comparada de cohortes de *T. infestans* en ambiente habitacional. Revista Medica De Chile 1994;**122**(9):993-997

[42] Canals M, Alvarado S, Cáceres D, Cattan PE. Twenty years of monitoring of mortality and fecundity of *Triatoma infestans* in the laboratory. Parasitología latinoamericana. 2016;**65**(2):54-60

[43] Canals M, Solís R, Valderas J, Ehrenfeld M, Cattan PE. Preliminary studies on temperature selection and activity cycles of *Triatoma infestans* and *T. spinolai*, Chilean vectors of Chagas disease. Journal of Medical Entomology. 1997;**34**:11-17

[44] Di Luciano VS. Orientation of *Triatoma infestans* to environmental temperatures. Journal of Medical Entomology. 1983;**20**:446-454

[45] Lazzari C. Temperature preference in *Triatoma infestans*. Bulletin of Entomological Research. 1991;**81**:273-276

[46] Lazzari C. Circadian rhythm of egg hatching in *T. infestans*. Journal of Medical Entomology. 1991;**28**:740-741

[47] Wiesinger D. Die Bedeutung der Umweltkartoren fur der Saugakt von *T. infestans*. Acta Tropica. 1956;**13**:97-141

[48] Nuñez JA. Food source orientation and activity in *R. prolixus*. Bulletin of Entomological Research. 1982;**72**:252-262

[49] Settembrini BP. Circadian rhythms of locomotion activity in the hematophagous bug *T. infestans*. Journal of Medical Entomology. 1984;**21**:204-212

[50] Lazzari C. Circadian organization of locomotor activity in the hematophagous bug. *T. infestans*. Journal of Insect Physiology. 1992;**38**:895-903

[51] Lazzari CR, Nuñez JA. The response to radiant heat and the estimation of the temperature of different sources in *Triatoma infestans*. Journal of Insect Physiology. 1989;**35**(6):525-529

[52] Ampleford E, Davey K. Egg laying in the insect *R. prolixus* is timed in a circadian fashion. Journal of Insect Physiology. 1989;**35**:183-187

[53] Ampleford E, Steel C. Circadian control of ecdysis in *R. prolixus*. Journal of Comparative Physiology.1982;**147**:281-286

[54] Lorenzo AN, Kenigsten A, Lazzari C. Daily dynamics and factors affecting aggregation in *T. infestans*. Memórias do Instituto Oswaldo Cruz. 1991;**86**:246

[55] Wigglesworth VB, Gillet JD. The function of the antennae in *R. prolixus* and the mechanism of orientation of the host. The Journal of Experimental Biology. 1934;**11**:120-138

[56] Guerenstein PG, Lazzari CR. Host-seeking: How triatomines acquire and make use of information to find blood. Acta Tropica. 2009;**110**(2-3):148-158

[57] Canals M, Solís R, Tapia C, Ehrenfeld M, Cattan PE. Comparison of some behavioural and physiological parameters of the feeding of *Triatoma infestans* KLUG, 1834 and *Mepraia spinolai* PORTER, 1934; vectors of the Chagas's disease in Chile. Memórias do Instituto Oswaldo Cruz. 1999;**94**(5):687-692

[58] Schofield CJ. Population dynamics and control of *T. infestans*. Annales de la Societe Belge de Medicine Tropicale. 1985;**65**:149-164

[59] Friend WG, Smith JB. Factors affecting feeding by blood sucking insects. Annual Review of Entomology. 1977;**22**:309-331

[60] Schenone H, Christensen HA, De Vasquez AM. Fuentes de alimentación de triatomas domésticos y su implicancia epidemiológica en relación a la enfermedad de Chagas en áreas rurales de siete regiones de Chile. Boletín Chileno de Parasitología. 1985;**40**:34-38

[61] Salvatella R. Evolución del índice de infección tripanosómica en *Tríatoma infestans* (KlugJ834) con las acciones de control antivectorial, en dos áreas endémico chagásicas de Uruguay. Revista Médica del Uruguay. 1995;**11**:105-110

[62] Apt W, Reyes H. Aspectos epidemiológicos de la enfermedad de Chagas en Chile. II: Infección en animales, algunas características especiales del problema, el control. Parasitología al Día. 1986;**10**:129-133

[63] Stevens JR, Gibson W. Molecular evolution of trypanosomes. Parasitology Today. 1999; **15**:432-437

[64] -Brisse S, Verhoef J, Tibayrenc M. Characterization of large and small subunit rRNA and mini-exon genes further supports the distinction of six *Trypanosoma cruzi* lineages. International Journal for Parasitology. 2001;**31**:1218-1226

[65] Zingales B, Andrade S, Briones RS, Campbell DA, Chiari E, Fernandes O, et al. A new consensus for *Trypanosoma cruzi* intraspecific nomenclature: Second revision meeting recommends TcI to TcVI. Memórias do Instituto Oswaldo Cruz. 2009;**104**(7):1051-1054

[66] Botto-Mahan C, Sepúlveda M, Vidal M, Acuña-Retamar M, Ortiz S, Solari A. *Trypanosoma cruzi* infection in the sylvatic kissing bug *Mepraia gajardoi* from the Chilean southern pacific ocean coast. Acta Tropica. 2008;**105**:166-169

[67] Toledo A, Vergara F, Campos R, Botto-Mahan C, Ortiz S, Coronado X, Solari A. *Trypanosoma cruzi* genotypes in *Mepraia gajardoi* from wild ecotopes in Northern Chile. The American Journal of Tropical Medicine and Hygiene 2012;**88**(2):285-288

[68] Coronado X, Rozas M, Botto-Mahan C, Ortiz S, Cattan PE, Solari A. Molecular epidemiology of Chagas disease in the wild transmission cycle: The evaluation in the sylvatic vector *Mepraia spinolai* from an endemic area of Chile. The American Journal of Tropical Medicine and Hygiene. 2009;**81**(4):656-659

[69] Bacigalupo A, Segovia V, García A, Botto-Mahan C, Ortiz S, Solari A, Acuña-Retamar M, Torres-Pérez F, Cattan PE. Differential pattern of infection of sylvatic nymphs and domiciliary adults of *Triatoma infestans* with *Trypanosoma cruzi* genotypes in Chile. The American Journal of Tropical Medicine and Hygiene. 2012;**87**(3):473-480

[70] Campos R, Botto-Mahan C, Ortiz S, Coronado X, Solari A. Temporal fluctuation of infection with different *Trypanosoma cruzi* genotypes in the wild rodent *Octodon degus*. The American Journal of Tropical Medicine and Hygiene. 2010;**83**(2):380-381

[71] Botto-Mahan C, Acuña-Retamar M, Campos R, Cattan PE, Solari A. European rabbits (*Oryctolagus cuniculus*) are naturally infected with different *Trypanosoma cruzi* genotypes. The American Journal of Tropical Medicine and Hygiene. 2009;**80**(6):944-946

[72] Rozas M, Botto-Mahan C, Coronado X, Ortiz S, Cattan PE, Solari A. *Trypanosoma cruzi* infection in wild mammals from a chagasic area of Chile. The American Journal of Tropical Medicine and Hygiene. 2005;**73**(3):517-519

[73] Rozas M, Botto-Mahan C, Coronado X, Ortiz S, Cattan PE, Solari A. Coexistence of *Trypanosoma cruzi* genotypes in wild and peridomestic mammals in Chile. The American Journal of Tropical Medicine and Hygiene 2007;**77**(4):647-653

[74] Durán JC, Videla MI, Apt W. Enfermedad de Chagas en una comunidad de pequeños mamíferos simpátricos de la reserva nacional de las chinchillas. Parasitol al Día. 1989;**13**:15-20

[75] Correa V, Zuñiga J, Contreras MC, Valdes JC, Rojas A, Villarroel F, Schenone H. Epidemiología de la enfermedad de Chagas en Chile. Sectores rurales. Infestación domiciliaria por triatominos, tasas de infección de estos por *Trypanosoma cruzi* y nuevos aportes al conocimiento de la infección chagásica en mamíferos domésticos de la IV Región (1982-1983). Boletín Chileno de Parasitología. 1984;**39**:24-27

[76] Basile L, Jamsa JL, Carlier Y, Salamanca DD, Angheben A, Bartoloni A, et al. Chagas disease in European countries: The challenge of a surveillance system. Eurosurveillance. 2011;**16**(37):pii:19968

[77] Strasen J, Williams T, Ertl G, Zoller T, Stich A, Ritter O. Epidemiology of Chagas disease in Europe: Many calculations; little knowledge. Clinical Research in Cardiology. 2013;**103**(1):1-10

[78] Hotez PJ, Bottazzi ME, Franco-Paredes C, Ault S, Periago MR. The neglected tropical diseases of Latin America and the Caribbean: A review of disease burden and distribution and a roadmap for control and elimination. PLoS Neglected Tropical Diseases. 2008;**2**:e300. DOI: 10.1371/journal.pntd.0000300

[79] Hotez PJ, Dumonteil E, Woc-Colburn L, Serpa JA, Bezek S, Edwards MS, et al. Chagas disease: "The new HIV/AIDS of the Americas". PLoS Neglected Tropical Diseases. 2012;**6**(5):e1498. DOI: 10.1371/journal.pntd.0001498

[80] MINSAL. Norma general técnica. Control y prevención nacional de la enfermedad de Chagas. Febrero. Ministerio de Salud de Chile. 2014

[81] MINSAL. Informe Programa Nacional Integral de Enfermedad de Chagas, Julio. Disponible en http://epi.minsal.cl/chagas-materiales-relacionados/ Consultado en 9/2016. 2016

[82] Cucunubá ZM, Okuwoga O, Basáñez MG, Nouvellet P. Increased mortality attributed to Chagas disease: A systematic review and meta-analysis. Parasites &Vectors. 2016;**9**:42. DOI: 10.1186/s13071-016-1315-x

[83] Fuentes R, Maturana M, De la Cruz R. Eficacia de Nifurtimox para el tratamiento de pacientes con enfermedad de Chagas crónico. Revista Chilena de Infectología. 2012;**29**(1): 82-86

[84] Apt W, Reyes H. Aspectos epidemiológicos de la enfermedad de Chagas en Chile. I: Distribución geográfica, índices de infección en vectores y en humanos. Parasitología al Día. 1986; 10: 84-10162.-Apt W. Parasitología humana. Mexico: McGraw-Hill; 2013. 800 pp

[85] Schenone H, Villarroel F, Rojas A. Presencia de *Triatoma spinolai* en viviendas humanas. Boletín Chileno de Parasitología. 1995;**50**(3-4):76-80

[86] Canals M, Caceres D, Alvarado S, Canals A, Cattan PE. Modeling the Chagas disease: From the vectorial to congenital transmission. Biosystems. 2017;**156**:63-71

[87] Apt W, Heitmann I, Jersic MI, Jofré L, Muñoz P, Noemí I, et al. Parte III. Enfermedad de Chagas en donantes de bancos de sangre. Revista chilena de infectología. 2008;**25**(4): 285-288

[88] Howard EJ, Xiong X, Carlier Y, Sosa-Estani S, Buekens P. Frequency of the congenital transmission of *Trypanosoma cruzi*: A systematic review and meta-analysis. BJOG: An International Journal of Obstetrics and Gynaecology. 2014;**121**:22-33

[89] Apt W, Zulantay I, Arnello L, Oddó D, González S, Rodriguez J, et al. Congenital infection by *Trypanosoma cruzi* in an endemic area of Chile: A multidisciplinary study. Transactions of the Royal Society of Tropical Medicine and Hygiene. 2013;**107**:98-104

[90] Raimundo SM, Massad E, Yang HM. Modelling congenital transmission of Chagas, disease. Bio Systems. 2010;**99**:215-222

[91] Massad E. The elimination of Chagas disease from Brazil. Epidemiology and Infection. 2008;**136**:1153-1164

[92] Cordovéz JM, Rendon LM, Gonzalez C, Guhl F. Using the basic reproduction number to assess the effects of climate change in the risk of Chagas disease transmission in Colombia. Acta Tropica. 2014;**129**:74-82

[93] Ayala S. Distribución especial del riesgo de transmisión vectorial de la enfermedad de Chagas basada en la estimación del número reproductivo básico (R0). Tesis Magister en Salud Pública. Facultad de Medicina, Universidad de Chile: 2017; 73 pp

7

Multimodal Treatment for Cancer of the Esophagus

Lucian Mocan, Ofelia Mosteanu, Teodora Pop,
Lucia Agoston-Coldea, Cornel Iancu,
Teodora Mocan and Furcea Luminita

Abstract

There are about 500,000 new cases of cancer of the esophagus and 400,000 esophageal cancer-related deaths recorded annually around the world. The disease is three to four times more frequent in men than in women, being the sixth most common cancer and the fifth most frequent cancer-related death among men. The prognosis of esophageal cancer is quite poor, despite advances in surgical procedures (two-field and three-field lymph node dissection) and perioperative management, which is still controversial. The use of chemotherapy and radiotherapy in combination with surgery might be a new approach for future treatment. Progress in optical technology has led to the development of a new minimally invasive surgical approach for the treatment of esophageal cancer, namely esophagectomy.

Keywords: esophageal cancer, chemotherapy, surgery, radiotherapy, outcome

1. Introduction

There are about 500,000 new cases of cancer of the esophagus and 400,000 esophageal cancer-related deaths recorded annually around the world. The disease is three to four times more frequent in men than in women, being the sixth most common cancer and the fifth most frequent cancer-related death among men [1].

Even though esophageal cancer was not very common in Western populations, the incidence of esophageal adenocarcinoma and its related mortality have increased in the USA and certain European countries [2]. The incidence of adenocarcinomas involving the esophago-gastric junction, the distal esophagus and the gastric cardia has recorded a more significant increase [3]. The transition from squamous cell carcinoma to Barrett's metaplasia-associated adenocarcinoma in Western populations could have been determined by the increase in the incidence of obesity and obesity-induced reflux [4, 5].

There are two main subtypes of the disease, namely esophageal squamous cell carcinoma and esophageal adenocarcinoma. The most common causes of squamous cell carcinoma are tobacco and alcohol, and the most common causes of adenocarcinoma are tobacco, obesity and acid reflux [5]. There has been a major increase in the incidence of adenocarcinoma in North America and Europe, while squamous cell carcinoma is still the most common type of esophageal cancer in Asia [6].

The two subtypes of esophageal cancer have different clinical and biological characteristics. While squamous cell carcinomas occur in the middle or upper third of the esophagus, adenocarcinomas occur in the lower third of the esophagus. Abdominal lymph node metastasis is usually present in adenocarcinomas, and the incidence of cervical or upper mediastinal lymph node metastasis is more frequent in squamous cell carcinomas. Thus, the therapeutic approach is different for each subtype [7].

The prognosis of esophageal cancer is quite poor, despite advances in surgical procedures (two-field and three-field lymph node dissection) and perioperative management, which is still controversial [7]. The use of chemotherapy and radiotherapy in combination with surgery might be a new approach for future treatment. Progress in optical technology has led to the development of a new minimally invasive surgical approach for the treatment of esophageal cancer, namely esophagectomy. Long-term survival in resectable esophageal cancer is also influenced by definitive chemoradiotherapy [8]. Salvage esophagectomy is used in patients with esophageal cancer who were treated with chemoradiation as definitive therapy [9].

Although cancer of the esophagus is among the most common cancers in the world, there are few studies on this malignancy. There have been significant changes in the epidemiology of esophageal cancer in the past 30 years, with a striking increase in incidence in Western populations, where the number of adenocarcinomas has exceeded those of the squamous cell type [6]. On the other hand, squamous cell carcinoma is the most frequent subtype in Asian countries, mainly developing in the middle third of the esophagus, without any dramatic increase in the incidence of adenocarcinoma on this continent. New diagnostic, staging, and therapeutic options have improved survival rates for esophageal cancer.

Early stage adenocarcinoma of the esophagogastric junction (AEG) could be detected based on efficient screening for gastroesophageal reflux disease (GERD) and Barrett's metaplasia, which might be cured using endoscopic ablation or surgery [10].

The infection with *Helicobacter pylori* harboring the cagA gene seems to be associated with a reduced risk of esophageal adenocarcinoma [11, 12].

The potential role of COX-2 inhibitors in the effective chemoprevention of esophageal adenocarcinoma, characterized by COX-2 overexpression, is another aspect to be considered [13]. The types of surgery for cancer of the esophagus are divided based on the complex lymphatic drainage from the esophagus and gastric cardia and their anatomy.

2. Esophageal resection

Hulscher et al. conducted a meta-analysis and obtained a 20% 5-year survival rate [14] following any of the two approaches. However, there were much higher rates of early morbidity and mortality in the case of transthoracic resection. On the other hand, in another study conducted by Hagen et al. [15], better survival rates (41% vs. 14%; $p < 0.001$) were obtained in 30 patients following en bloc esophagectomy compared with 39 patients undergoing transhiatal esophagectomy, suggesting the use of extended en bloc esophagectomy instead of transhiatal resection in the case of carcinoma of the lower third of the esophagus and gastric cardia [15].

Outcomes in esophageal cancer are often poor [16]. The best and most efficient surgical method in patients without evidence of spread to other parts of the body is the combination between esophagectomy and reconstruction surgery [7]. There are three more frequent minimally invasive techniques for esophagectomy: transhiatal esophagectomy, the Ivor Lewis esophagectomy (upper midline laparotomy combined with a right posterolateral thoracotomy), and the McKeown technique (right thoracotomy, upper midline laparotomy, and left neck incision). Several randomized trials compared transhiatal esophagectomy and standard transthoracic esophagectomy, showing no significant differences between them. The differences between transthoracic and transhiatal esophagectomy were examined in three randomized trials [17–21]. The results of these clinical trials showed no significant differences between the two approaches in what concerns patient survival. Hulscher et al. [22] conducted a randomized trial in patients with adenocarcinoma of the esophagus and gastric cardia (106 patients with transhiatal esophagectomy and 114 with transthoracic esophagectomy). There were lower morbidity rates in the case of transhiatal esophagectomy than in transthoracic esophagectomy with extended en bloc lymph node dissection. Despite the absence of statistically significant differences in terms of disease-free, median overall, and quality-adjusted survival, there was an improvement in long-term survival of patients with extended transthoracic resection. Asia, especially Japan, accounts for the majority of the more aggressive surgery records. Five-year survival rates following three-field lymph node dissection were 48.7% in a study conducted by Kato et al. [23] and 55.0% in a study by Akiyama et al. [24].

Esophagectomy can be either transhiatal or transthoracic, performed using the Ivor Lewis technique (combined laparotomy and right thoracotomy) and the modified McKeown procedure, involving laparotomy, right thoracotomy with neck anastomosis, left thoracotomy, or left thoracoabdominal incision [25]. The approach is chosen depending on tumor location and surgeon preferences. Good treatment outcomes result from the complexity of these surgical procedures, the experience of the surgeons, and intensive care resources [26].

A comprehensive randomized study assessing the differences between the transthoracic and the transhiatal approach indicated similar mortality rates for both procedures, whereas morbidity rates were lower for the transhiatal approach. The transthoracic group showed non-significant associations between this procedure and overall and disease-free survival. However, there was an improvement in locoregional disease-free survival following transthoracic esophagectomy in a subgroup of patients who did not present extensive nodal involvement [27].

Long-term survival rates following open esophagectomy do not differ significantly when comparing these surgical procedures, as shown by various meta-analyses and randomized trials [28]. In their study, Tabira et al. [29] recommended the use of three-field lymph node dissection in patients with one to four lymph node metastases. As indicated by Shiozaki et al. [30], neck dissection might be eliminated in patients with carcinoma in the middle or lower third of the esophagus without lymph node metastasis along the recurrent nerve chain. Lerut et al. [31] also proved an improvement in patient survival following three-field lymph node dissection.

When comparing three-field with two-field lymph node dissection for squamous cell carcinoma of the esophagus, Kato et al. obtained 5-year survival rates of 48.7% for the first approach and 33.7% for the second. However, this study was contested due to differences in patient characteristics. Isono et al. [32] conducted a nationwide study and obtained better survival rates when using three-field dissection instead of the two-field approach. Fujita et al. [33] also presented much better survival rates following three-field lymph node dissection ($p < 0.05$) for carcinoma in the upper or middle third of the esophagus spreading to the lymph nodes. Still, there were no differences in mortality, morbidity, and postoperative quality of life between the two approaches [33]. Radical esophagectomy helps remove ≥80 lymph nodes and 5-year survival rates are around 40–60% [34].

3. Minimally invasive surgery

Pulmonary complications after transthoracic esophagectomy are high. The minimally invasive thoracoscopic approach might result in lower morbidity and mortality rates. Being minimally invasive, thoracoscopy should replace the open approach. In a study conducted by Cuschieri et al. [35], the researchers performed right thoracoscopy (esophagectomy and lymph node dissection) in a small group of patients and paved the way for the future use of thoracoscopic esophagectomy. This procedure proved to be feasible and even superior to open surgery. Nevertheless, the first outcomes using this approach were not significantly better than those obtained with the open approach, mainly as a result of the great number of pulmonary complications [36–38]. However, a few medical research centers in Japan found a new stimulus. For example, Akaishi et al. [39] obtained good outcomes in 39 patients with cancer of the esophagus who underwent en bloc esophagectomy with radical lymph node dissection via right thoracoscopy, with the following parameters: 200±41 min operating time, 270±157 ml blood loss, and the number of harvested lymph nodes was 19.7±11. All patients survived and there was a modest decrease in vital capacity in 22 of them, without requiring postoperative ventilation. A significant finding of the study was that pulmonary complications were reduced compared with the open procedure.

In their study, Luketich et al. [40] proved that minimally invasive esophagectomy (MIE) is efficient and safe in the United States. The study was conducted on 1033 consecutive patients and results indicated a significantly lower mortality rate (0.9%), with an 8-day median hospital stay. In a study performed in the United Kingdom, Mamidanna et al. [41] assessed 7502 patients undergoing esophagectomy (E) and MIE ($n = 1.155$) and results showed no differences in terms of 30-day morbidity and mortality. MIE proved to be safe for use by professionals, without supplementary patient safety risks. Despite the low number of annual esophagectomies (2) per medical center, study results were similar and MIE was preferred in terms of perioperative outcomes. On the other hand, there are insufficient and incomplete cancer comparative research data. Certain centers noted higher lymph node retrieval following MIE with lymph node dissection [42–44], whereas others did not find any considerable differences [45]. In a study performed on 168 patients, Palazzo et al. [46] demonstrated that long-term survival was twice better in patients who underwent MIE (hazard ratio—2.0). Despite significant patient and tumor variables, there were concerns related to the ability to reproduce the major differences in results obtained for these groups. Additionally, the small number of patients might assign any variations to defective regulations.

In a study assessing three-field lymph node dissection, Osugi et al. compared 77 patients with squamous cell cancer who underwent minithoracotomy to 72 controls who underwent conventional three-stage treatment. Exceptional outcomes were obtained in terms of lymph node retrieval (33 vs. 32), operating time (227 vs. 186 min), reduced vital capacity (15% vs. 22%, $p = 0.016$), 3-year survival (70% vs. 60%), and 5-year survival (55% vs. 57%) [44]. Resection via thoracoscopy showed almost similar results to open esophagectomy. Moreover, surgical trauma was reduced. The differences in outcome between the first 34 and the next 46 patients who underwent surgery in the same study group demonstrated the impact of the learning curve on obtaining shorter operating times and better results by using this approach. Other advantage is that greater experience helps reduce postoperative pulmonary complications (5% incidence). Reduced blood loss, shorter operating time for thoracoscopy, reduced postoperative respiratory complications and higher lymph node retrieval were all observed in the last group [44]. In a study conducted on 222 patients undergoing thoracoscopic and laparoscopic esophageal resection, Luketich et al. (Ann Surg 2003; 238:486–494) showed an incidence rate of pneumonia of 7.7%. A significant finding was the reduced length of intensive care unit stay (1 day) and hospital stay (7 days) and the 1.4% operative mortality. Quality of life indicator was comparable to baseline scores and population standards. Nguyen et al. [47] assessed 46 consecutive patients and found similar results to Luketich et al. There have also been studies supporting robot-assisted thoracoscopy; however, there is still need for further investigation regarding robotic esophagectomy [48].

The results obtained by Biere et al. [49] in the TIME (Traditional Invasive vs. Minimally Invasive Esophagectomy) trial comparing the outcomes of 115 British patients who underwent either E or MIE showed that besides a decrease in perioperative pulmonary complications, the two procedures were more or less similar. However, the main competence of the trial was to show differences in short-term outcomes, with lower capacity in pointing out other outcomes. Patient outcomes were adapted to a population, improving the ability to perform a multivariate analysis of small differences in survival. There are few data on comparative differences in robot-assisted esophagectomy. In a study conducted on 43 patients who were treated with MIE (of which 11 underwent robot-assisted esophagectomy), Weksler et al. [50] reached the conclusion that robot-assisted and conventional procedures were similar. There were not enough patients included in the study, the results were disorganized, and there were no cancer data. Our study also experiences difficulties due to this aspect when comparing robotic with conventional MIE, but we managed to explain certain confounding variables for our outcomes. The limitations of our study are represented by the inability to determine specific MIE approaches (the McKeown procedure, the Ivor Lewis approach, and the transhiatal procedure). Earlier studies have demonstrated that the three procedures have similar outcomes, even though there are differences in terms of perioperative complications [51]. Another drawback was the difficulty in differentiating between patients who underwent hybrid procedures, such as laparoscopy combined with minithoracotomy, and patients who were treated with total MIE. These limitations pave the way for the occurrence of unknown interactions and confounding variables. Currently, there are two different clinical trials comparing E to MIE patients, namely the French MIRO trial [52] and the British ROMIRO trail [53]. Still, the study that we conducted is the most extensive comparative effectiveness research of MIE assessing long-term survival. As a result, MIE determines poor improvement in perioperative outcomes, with no negative impact on survival rates.

4. Combined modality therapy

4.1. Neoadjuvant chemotherapy

The use of preoperative chemotherapy compared with surgical treatment has been assessed in randomized trials in order to obtain improved surgical outcomes. However, the results are highly disputed. The three meta-analyses built on these randomized trials showed no difference in survival when the endpoint was 1-year survival in six of these trials. On the contrary, in comparison with surgical treatment, 2-year survival rates were improved following preoperative chemotherapy (4.4%) when the endpoint was 2-year survival in seven randomized trials [53]. When the meta-analysis was restricted to four recently randomized trials based on cisplatin and 5-fluorouracil therapy, there was a 6.3% improvement in 2-year survival. Still, this increase did not occur in one meta-analysis where the endpoint was 2-year survival [54]. The impact of preoperative chemotherapy is still uncertain.

4.2. Neoadjuvant chemoradiotherapy

Used in Europe and America since the end of the 1980s, preoperative chemoradiotherapy determined survival rate improvement in patients with cancer of the esophagus. Despite being used on a small scale due to the advanced surgical procedures available in Japan, a randomized trial reported the efficiency of hyperthermochemoradiotherapy in esophageal cancer [55]. Five meta-analyses built on five to seven randomized trials assess the impact of surgery alone, on the one hand, with preoperative chemoradiotherapy used in combination with surgery, on the other hand. There were no improvements in survival rates following preoperative chemoradiotherapy when the endpoint was 1-year or 2-year survival. When the endpoint was 3-year survival, there was an increase in perioperative mortality within 90 days after surgery, contrasted by a decrease in local recurrence and an improvement in 3-year survival rates in analogy to surgery alone (Int J Hyperthermia 1992; 8:289–295). There was a 14% decrease in death risk following preoperative chemoradiotherapy when the endpoint was the hazard ratio of survival curves [56]. Several reports [57–59] of six randomized trials showed higher survival rates following preoperative chemoradiotherapy than after surgery alone. Another report focusing on esophageal adenocarcinoma reported much higher survival rates following preoperative chemoradiotherapy versus surgery alone [60].

A meta-analysis of randomized trials conducted in Europe and America reported no improvement in survival with postoperative chemotherapy following curative resection in patients with cancer of the esophagus. In contrast, a randomized trial conducted in Japan showed that postoperative chemotherapy determined a major improvement in disease-free survival. In conclusion, postoperative chemotherapy recommends itself as an efficient measure to prevent recurrence after surgery.

4.3. Adjuvant radiotherapy

Four randomized trials assessing the differences between surgery alone and postoperative radiotherapy (45–65 Gy) reported no major improvements in survival. However, there was a decrease in local recurrence in the irradiated area following postoperative radiotherapy. No major improvements in survival were observed in a meta-analysis of these randomized trials. In conclusion, postoperative radiotherapy is not a conventional treatment option.

4.4. Postoperative outcome

The incidence of postoperative mortality was assessed in a considerable number of studies [61–65], fewer assessed in-hospital mortality, and 30-day mortality was determined in two studies [66]. Values were higher in patients who were treated with salvage esophagectomy after definitive chemoradiotherapy (23 patients—9.50%) than in patients who treated with planned esophagectomy after neoadjuvant chemoradiotherapy (29 patients—4.07%). Pooling of results validated the much higher incidence of postoperative mortality in the case of salvage esophagectomy (prevalence odds ratios (POR) = 3.02; 95% CI 1.64–5.58; $p < 0.001$).

Author details

Lucian Mocan[1,2*], Ofelia Mosteanu[1,3], Teodora Pop[1,3], Lucia Agoston-Coldea[4], Cornel Iancu[1,2], Teodora Mocan[1,5] and Furcea Luminita[1,2]

*Address all correspondence to: lucian.mocan@umfcluj.ro

1 Regional Institute of Gastroenterology and Hepatology, "Prof. Dr. Octavian Fodor", Cluj-Napoca, Romania

2 Department of Surgery, University of Medicine and Pharmacy, "Iuliu Hatieganu", Cluj-Napoca, Romania

3 Department of Gastroenterology, University of Medicine and Pharmacy, "Iuliu Hatieganu", Cluj-Napoca, Romania

4 Department of Internal Medicine, University of Medicine and Pharmacy, "Iuliu Hatieganu", Cluj-Napoca, Romania

5 Department of Physiology, University of Medicine and Pharmacy, "Iuliu Hatieganu", Cluj-Napoca, Romania

References

[1] Daly JM, Karnell LH, Menck HR. National Cancer Data Base report on esophageal carcinoma. Cancer. 1996;**78**(8):1820-1828

[2] PDQ Screening and Prevention Editorial Board. In: Anonymous, editor. Esophageal Cancer Screening (PDQ(R)): Health Professional Version. In PDQ Cancer Information Summaries. Bethesda (MD): National Cancer Institute; 2002

[3] Hosokawa Y, Kinoshita T, Konishi M, Takahashi S, Gotohda N, Kato Y, Daiko H, Nishimura M, Katsumata K, Sugiyama Y. Clinicopathological features and prognostic factors of adenocarcinoma of the esophagogastric junction according to Siewert classification: Experiences at a single institution in Japan. Annals of Surgical Oncology. 2012;**19**(2):677-683

[4] Spechler SJ. Barrett esophagus and risk of esophageal cancer: A clinical review. JAMA. 2013;**310**(6):627-636

[5] Duits LC, Phoa KN, Curvers WL, Ten Kate FJ, Meijer GA, Seldenrijk CA, Offerhaus GJ, Visser M, Meijer SL, Krishnadath KK, Tijssen JG, Mallant-Hent RC, Bergman JJ. Barrett's oesophagus patients with low-grade dysplasia can be accurately risk-stratified after histological review by an expert pathology panel. Gut. 2015;**64**(5):700-706

[6] Bray F, Ferlay J, Laversanne M, Brewster D, Gombe Mbalawa C, Kohler B, Piñeros M, Steliarova-Foucher E, Swaminathan R, Antoni S. Cancer incidence in five continents: Inclusion criteria, highlights from volume X and the global status of cancer registration. International Journal of Cancer. 2015;**137**(9):2060-2071

[7] Napier KJ, Scheerer M, Misra S. Esophageal cancer: A review of epidemiology, pathogenesis, staging workup and treatment modalities. World Journal of Gastrointestinal Oncology. 2014;**6**(5):112-120

[8] Chen M, Yang Y, Lai C, Chen P, Chen W. Outcome of patients with esophageal cancer: A nationwide analysis. Annals of Surgical Oncology. 2013;**20**(9):3023-3030

[9] Watanabe M, Mine S, Nishida K, Yamada K, Shigaki H, Matsumoto A, Sano T. Salvage esophagectomy after definitive chemoradiotherapy for patients with esophageal squamous cell carcinoma: Who really benefits from this high-risk surgery? Annals of Surgical Oncology. 2015;**22**(13):4438-4444

[10] Wang X, Fan J, Wang A, Leng Y, Li J, Bao Y, Wang Y, Yang Q, Ren Y. Epidemiology of esophageal cancer in Yanting-regional report of a national screening programme in China. Asian Pacific Journal of Cancer Prevention. 2013;**14**(4):2429-2432

[11] Hatakeyama M. Helicobacter pylori CagA and gastric cancer: A paradigm for hit-and-run carcinogenesis. Cell Host & Microbe. 2014;**15**(3):306-316

[12] Kandulski A, Venerito M, Malfertheiner P. Helicobacter pylori and esophageal neoplasia. In: Esophageal Cancer and Barrett's Esophagus. Wiley; 2015. p. 79-86

[13] Yusup G, Akutsu Y, Mutallip M, Qin W, Hu X, Komatsu-Akimoto A, Hoshino I, Hanari N, Mori M, Akanuma N. A COX-2 inhibitor enhances the antitumor effects of che motherapy and radiotherapy for esophageal squamous cell carcinoma. International Journal of Oncology. 2014;**44**(4):1146-1152

[14] Hulscher JB, Tijssen JG, Obertop H, van Lanschot, J, Jan B. Transthoracic versus transhiatal resection for carcinoma of the esophagus: A meta-analysis. The Annals of Thoracic Surgery 2001;**72**(1):306-313

[15] Hagen JA, Peters JH, DeMeester TR. Superiority of extended en bloc esophagogastrectomy for carcinoma of the lower esophagus and cardia. The Journal of Thoracic and Cardiovascular Surgery. 1993;**106**(5):850-858 discussion 858-9

[16] Chen M, Huang J, Zhu Z, Zhang J, Li K. Systematic review and meta-analysis of tumor biomarkers in predicting prognosis in esophageal cancer. BMC Cancer. 2013;**13**(1):1

[17] Chang AC, Ji H, Birkmeyer NJ, Orringer MB, Birkmeyer JD. Outcomes after transhiatal and transthoracic esophagectomy for cancer. The Annals of Thoracic Surgery. 2008;**85**(2): 424-429

[18] Nguyen NT, Follette DM, Wolfe BM, Schneider PD, Roberts P, Goodnight JE. Comparison of minimally invasive esophagectomy with transthoracic and transhiatal esophagectomy. Archives of Surgery. 2000;**135**(8):920-925

[19] Rentz J, Bull D, Harpole D, Bailey S, Neumayer L, Pappas T, Krasnicka B, Henderson W, Daley J, Khuri S. Transthoracic versus transhiatal esophagectomy: A prospective study of 945 patients. The Journal of Thoracic and Cardiovascular Surgery. 2003;**125**(5):1114-1120

[20] Stark SP, Romberg MS, Pierce GE, Hermreck AS, Jewell WR, Moran JF, Cherian G, Delcore R, Thomas JH. Transhiatal versus transthoracic esophagectomy for adenocarcinoma of the distal esophagus and cardia. The American Journal of Surgery. 1996;**172**(5):478-482

[21] Chu K, Law SY, Fok M, Wong J. A prospective randomized comparison of transhiatal and transthoracic resection for lower-third esophageal carcinoma. The American Journal of Surgery. 1997;**174**(3):320-324

[22] Hulscher JB, van Sandick JW, de Boer AG, Wijnhoven BP, Tijssen JG, Fockens P, Stalmeier PF, ten Kate FJ, van Dekken H, Obertop H: Extended transthoracic resection compared with limited transhiatal resection for adenocarcinoma of the esophagus. The New England Journal of Medicine 2002;**347**(21):1662-1669

[23] Kato H, Watanabe H, Tachimori Y, Iizuka T. Evaluation of neck lymph node dissection for thoracic esophageal carcinoma. The Annals of Thoracic Surgery. 1991;**51**(6):931-935

[24] Akiyama H, Tsurumaru M, Udagawa H, Kajiyama Y. Radical lymph node dissection for cancer of the thoracic esophagus. Annals of Surgery. 1994;**220**(3):364-372 discussion 372-3

[25] Boone J, Livestro DP, Elias SG, Borel Rinkes IH, Van Hillegersberg R. International survey on esophageal cancer: Part I surgical techniques. Diseases of the Esophagus. 2009;**22**(3):195-202

[26] Daly JM, Fry WA, Little AG, Winchester DP, McKee RF, Stewart AK, Fremgen AM. Esophageal cancer: Results of an American College of Surgeons patient care evaluation study. Journal of the American College of Surgeons. 2000;**190**(5):562-572

[27] Omloo JM, Lagarde SM, Hulscher JB, Reitsma JB, Fockens P, van Dekken H, ten Kate FJ, Obertop H, Tilanus HW, van Lanschot JJ: Extended transthoracic resection compared with limited transhiatal resection for adenocarcinoma of the mid/distal esophagus: Five-year survival of a randomized clinical trial. Annals of Surgery 2007;**246**(6):992-1000; discussion 1000-1

[28] Pennathur A, Gibson MK, Jobe BA, Luketich JD. Oesophageal carcinoma. The Lancet. 2013;**381**(9864):400-412

[29] Tabira Y, Kitamura N, Yoshioka M, Tanaka M. Significance of three-field lymphadenectomy for carcinoma of the thoracic esophagus based on depth of tumor infiltration, lymph nodal involvement and survival rate. The Journal of Cardiovascular Surgery. 1999;**40**(5):737

[30] Shiozaki H, Yano M, Tsujinaka T, Inoue M, Tamura S, Doki Y, Yasuda T, Fujiwara Y, Monden M. Lymph node metastasis along the recurrent nerve chain is an indication for cervical lymph node dissection in thoracic esophageal cancer. Diseases of the Esophagus. 2001;**14**(3-4):191-196

[31] Lerut T, Nafteux P, Moons J, Coosemans W, Decker G, De Leyn P, Van Raemdonck D, Ectors N. Three-field lymphadenectomy for carcinoma of the esophagus and gastroesophageal junction in 174 R0 resections: Impact on staging, disease-free survival, and outcome: A plea for adaptation of TNM classification in upper-half esophageal carcinoma. Annals of Surgery. 2004;**240**(6):962-974

[32] Isono K, Sato H, Nakayama K. Results of a nationwide study on the three-field lymph node dissection of esophageal cancer. Oncology. 1991;**48**(5):411-420

[33] Fujita H, Kakegawa T, Yamana H, Shima I, Toh Y, Tomita Y, Fujii T, Yamasaki K, Higaki K, Noake T. Mortality and morbidity rates, postoperative course, quality of life, and prognosis after extended radical lymphadenectomy for esophageal cancer. Comparison of three-field lymphadenectomy with two-field lymphadenectomy. Annals of Surgery. 1995;**222**(5):654-662

[34] Nishimaki T, Suzuki T, Suzuki S, Kuwabara S, Hatakeyama K. Outcomes of extended radical esophagectomy for thoracic esophageal cancer. Journal of the American College of Surgeons. 1998;**186**(3):306-312

[35] Cuschieri A, Shimi S, Banting S. Endoscopic oesophagectomy through a right thoracoscopic approach. Journal of the Royal College of Surgeons of Edinburgh. 1992;**37**(1):7-11

[36] Dexter S, Martin I, McMahon M. Radical thoracoscopic esophagectomy for cancer. Surgical Endoscopy. 1996;**10**(2):147-151

[37] Robertson G, Lloyd D, Wicks A, Veitch P. No obvious advantages for thoracoscopic two-stage oesophagectomy. The British Journal of Surgery. 1996;**83**(5):675-678

[38] Law S, Fok M, Chu K, Wong J. Thoracoscopic esophagectomy for esophageal cancer. Surgery. 1997;**122**(1):8-14

[39] Akaishi T, Kaneda I, Higuchi N, Kuriya Y, Kuramoto J, Toyoda T, Wakabayashi A. Thoracoscopic en bloc total esophagectomy with radical mediastinal lymphadenectomy. The Journal of Thoracic and Cardiovascular Surgery. 1996;**112**(6):1533-1541

[40] Markar SR, Karthikesalingam A, Penna M, Low DE. Assessment of short-term clinical outcomes following salvage esophagectomy for the treatment of esophageal malignancy: Systematic review and pooled analysis. Annals of Surgical Oncology. 2014;**21**(3):922-931

[41] Mamidanna R, Bottle A, Aylin P, Faiz O, Hanna GB. Short-term outcomes following open versus minimally invasive esophagectomy for cancer in England: A population-based national study. Annals of Surgery. 2012;**255**(2):197-203

[42] Parameswaran R, Veeramootoo D, Krishnadas R, Cooper M, Berrisford R, Wajed S. Comparative experience of open and minimally invasive esophagogastric resection. World Journal of Surgery. 2009;**33**(9):1868-1875

[43] Singh RK, Pham TH, Diggs BS, Perkins S, Hunter JG. Minimally invasive esophagectomy provides equivalent oncologic outcomes to open esophagectomy for locally advanced (stage II or III) esophageal carcinoma. Archives of Surgery. 2011;**146**(6):711-714

[44] Osugi H, Takemura M, Higashino M, Takada N, Lee S, Ueno M, Tanaka Y, Fukuhara K, Hashimoto Y, Fujiwara Y. Learning curve of video-assisted thoracoscopic esophagectomy and extensive lymphadenectomy for squamous cell cancer of the thoracic esophagus and results. Surgical Endoscopy And Other Interventional Techniques. 2003; **17**(3):515-519

[45] Watanabe M, Baba Y, Nagai Y, Baba H. Minimally invasive esophagectomy for esophageal cancer: An updated review. Surgery Today. 2013;**43**(3):237-244

[46] Palazzo F, Rosato EL, Chaudhary A, Evans NR, Sendecki JA, Keith S, Chojnacki KA, Yeo CJ, Berger AC. Minimally invasive esophagectomy provides significant survival advantage compared with open or hybrid esophagectomy for patients with cancers of the esophagus and gastroesophageal junction. Journal of the American College of Surgeons. 2015;**220**(4):672-679

[47] Nguyen NT, Roberts P, Follette DM, Rivers R, Wolfe BM. Thoracoscopic and laparoscopic esophagectomy for benign and malignant disease: Lessons learned from 46 consecutive procedures. Journal of the American College of Surgeons. 2003;**197**(6):902-913

[48] Bodner JC, Zitt M, Ott H, Wetscher GJ, Wykypiel H, Lucciarini P, Schmid T. Robotic-assisted thoracoscopic surgery (RATS) for benign and malignant esophageal tumors. The Annals of Thoracic Surgery. 2005;**80**(4):1202-1206

[49] Biere SS, van Berge Henegouwen, Mark I, Maas KW, Bonavina L, Rosman C, Garcia JR, Gisbertz SS, Klinkenbijl JH, Hollmann MW, de Lange ES: Minimally invasive versus open oesophagectomy for patients with oesophageal cancer: A multicentre, open-label, randomised controlled trial. The Lancet 2012;**379**(9829):1887-1892

[50] Weksler B, Sharma P, Moudgill N, Chojnacki K, Rosato E. Robot-assisted minimally invasive esophagectomy is equivalent to thoracoscopic minimally invasive esophagectomy. Diseases of the Esophagus. 2012;**25**(5):403-409

[51] Pfister DG, Johnson DH, Azzoli CG, Sause W, Smith TJ, Baker S,Jr, Olak J, Stover D, Strawn JR, Turrisi AT, Somerfield MR, American Society of Clinical Oncology: American Society of Clinical Oncology treatment of unresectable non-small-cell lung cancer guideline: Update 2003. Journal of Clinical Oncology 2004;**22**(2):330-353

[52] Briez N, Piessen G, Bonnetain F, Brigand C, Carrere N, Collet D, Doddoli C, Flamein R, Mabrut JY, Meunier B, Msika S, Perniceni T, Peschaud F, Prudhomme M, Triboulet JP, Mariette C. Open versus laparoscopically-assisted oesophagectomy for cancer: a multicentre randomised controlled phase III trial—The MIRO trial. BMC Cancer. 2011;**11**: 310-2407-11-310

[53] Avery KN, Metcalfe C, Berrisford R, Barham CP, Donovan JL, Elliott J, Falk SJ, Goldin R, Hanna G, Hollowood AA. The feasibility of a randomized controlled trial of esophagectomy for esophageal cancer-the ROMIO (randomized oesophagectomy: Minimally invasive or open) study: Protocol for a randomized controlled trial. Trials. 2014;**15**(1):1

[54] Urschel JD, Vasan H, Blewett CJ. A meta-analysis of randomized controlled trials that compared neoadjuvant chemotherapy and surgery to surgery alone for resectable esophageal cancer. The American Journal of Surgery. 2002;**183**(3):274-279

[55] Sugimachi K, Kitamura K, Baba K, Ikebe M, Morita M, Matsuda H, Kuwano H. Hyperthermia combined with chemotherapy and irradiation for patients with carcinoma of the oesophagus—A prospective randomized trial. International Journal of Hyperthermia. 1992;**8**(3):289-295

[56] Greer SE, Goodney PP, Sutton JE, Birkmeyer JD. Neoadjuvant chemoradiotherapy for esophageal carcinoma: A meta-analysis. Surgery. 2005;**137**(2):172-177

[57] Urba SG, Orringer MB, Turrisi A, Iannettoni M, Forastiere A, Strawderman M. Randomized trial of preoperative chemoradiation versus surgery alone in patients with locoregional esophageal carcinoma. Journal of Clinical Oncology. 2001;**19**(2):305-313

[58] Bosset J, Gignoux M, Triboulet J, Tiret E, Mantion G, Elias D, Lozach P, Ollier J, Pavy J, Mercier M. Chemoradiotherapy followed by surgery compared with surgery alone in squamous-cell cancer of the esophagus. The New England Journal of Medicine. 1997; **337**(3):161-167

[59] Prise EL, Etienne PL, Meunier B, Maddern G, Hassel MB, Gedouin D, Boutin D, Campion JP, Launois B. A randomized study of chemotherapy, radiation therapy, and surgery versus surgery for localized squamous cell carcinoma of the esophagus. Cancer. 1994;**73**(7):1779-1784

[60] Enzinger PC, Mayer RJ. Esophageal cancer. The New England Journal of Medicine. 2003;**349**(23):2241-2252

[61] Chao Y, Chan S, Chang H, Liu Y, Wu Y, Hsieh M, Tseng C, Liu H. Salvage surgery after failed chemoradiotherapy in squamous cell carcinoma of the esophagus. European Journal of Surgical Oncology (EJSO). 2009;**35**(3):289-294

[62] Marks JL, Hofstetter W, Correa AM, Mehran RJ, Rice D, Roth J, Walsh G, Vaporciyan A, Erasmus J, Chang J. Salvage esophagectomy after failed definitive chemoradiation for esophageal adenocarcinoma. The Annals of Thoracic Surgery. 2012;**94**(4):1126-1133

[63] Miyata H, Yamasaki M, Takiguchi S, Nakajima K, Fujiwara Y, Nishida T, Mori M, Doki Y. Salvage esophagectomy after definitive chemoradiotherapy for thoracic esophageal cancer. Journal of Surgical Oncology. 2009;**100**(6):442-446

[64] Morita M, Kumashiro R, Hisamatsu Y, Nakanishi R, Egashira A, Saeki H, Oki E, Ohga T, Kakeji Y, Tsujitani S. Clinical significance of salvage esophagectomy for remnant or recurrent cancer following definitive chemoradiotherapy. Journal of Gastroenterology. 2011;**46**(11):1284-1291

[65] Smithers B, Cullinan M, Thomas J, Martin I, Barbour A, Burmeister B, Harvey J, Thomson D, Walpole E, Gotley D. Outcomes from salvage esophagectomy post definitive chemoradiotherapy compared with resection following preoperative neoadjuvant chemoradiotherapy. Diseases of the Esophagus. 2007;**20**(6):471-477

[66] Takeuchi H, Saikawa Y, Oyama T, Ozawa S, Suda K, Wada N, Takahashi T, Nakamura R, Shigematsu N, Ando N. Factors influencing the long-term survival in patients with esophageal cancer who underwent esophagectomy after chemoradiotherapy. World Journal of Surgery. 2010;**34**(2):277-284

8

Caustic Ingestion in Children

Alfredo Larrosa-Haro, Carmen A Sánchez-Ramírez,
Johnatan M Mesa-Magaña and
Edgar M Vasquez-Garibay

Abstract

Caustic ingestion (CI) is an unfortunate event that occurs in families with a poor prevention culture. Its prevalence is unknown in developing countries; it occurs mainly in children < 5 years and is more common in boys. The chemical caustic agents are alkaline (85%) or acid products stored in food or beverage containers without warning labels and safety caps. The immediate symptoms include salivation, oropharyngeal burns, vomiting and oropharyngeal/retrosternal pain. Upper endoscopy is the first-line tool to identify the type and extension of oesophageal and gastric damage. A barium swallow performed 2–3 weeks after the CI may identify oesophageal stricture. Dysphagia occurs in about one-third of cases. Regarding the nutritional status, children with dysphagia and/or oesophageal strictures may have lower fat reserves or muscle mass than the cases without these complications, meaning impaired nutritional status. All patients should be hospitalized for evaluation and treatment. Hemodynamic stabilization and adequacy of the patient's airway are priorities; vomiting induction and gastric lavage are contraindicated. Methylprednisolone in II-b oesophageal burns for 3 days diminishes the risk of stricture. Selected cases will require oesophageal dilatations, gastrostomy or oesophageal replacement by colon or stomach. There are other promising agents in the management of caustic oesophageal strictures.

Keywords: caustics, oesophageal burns, oesophageal stricture, dysphagia, child malnutrition

1. Introduction

CI in children and adolescents is an unfortunate event that may lead to significant upper gastrointestinal tract damage manifested in the short term as oesophageal burns and in the long term as oesophageal stricture or acquired motility disorders. A high proportion of these patients may evolve to permanent disability associated to feeding difficulties as well as growth and nutritional impairment. The aim of the chapter is to discuss the experience with our CI paediatric patients treated in a paediatric referral hospital in the context of the published data from other authors.

2. Epidemiology

Although is not a public health problem, CI is a significant issue worldwide, particularly in developing countries in which an unsafe environment is a substantial risk factor for child injury [1]. In 1985, Wasserman reported that approximately 5000 children younger than 5 years ingested lye each year in the United States [2]; in 2008, the USA National Poison Data reported over 200,000 exposures to caustic substances [3]. Unfortunately, the true prevalence regarding this health problem is not known in most developing countries and cannot be extrapolated from publications of series of children with CI treated in paediatric hospitals; however, these publications describe demographic, clinical and treatment characteristics of children from low, lower-middle and high-income countries information is scarce specially in lower-middle income countries [1].

Overall, the paediatric population is the most affected; the highest risk age groups are infants and pre-schoolers [4–13]. This may be attributed to the fact that children younger than 6 years are not able to make reasonable decisions about what they should or should not drink in the context of their developmental stage of motor and sensory skills [8]. Regarding gender, the higher frequency trend of CI in males could be attributed to both a gender-related biological and learned gender-role behaviour of boys different from girls in terms of expressing health and disease and their interaction with risk factors [4–7, 13–15]. A recent publication reveals that children with attention deficit/hyperactivity disorder had a higher risk to suffer CI than children without this condition [16].

Reports related to the social, economic, and educational characteristics that may play a role in families of children with CI are scarce [17]. In this context, the authors performed a case-control study in which the aim was to evaluate the association of socio-demographic factors in a group of 94 children and adolescents with CI; the controls were a random sample of children hospitalized or seen as outpatients in the same paediatric referral hospital and period. The sociodemographic variables were studied using a validated questionnaire. CI occurred at home in 63.8% and at a relative's home in 23.4%. Alkaline products were the most frequently ingested (85.1%); containers had no warning labels in 72.3% and no childproof safety caps in 92.6% of the cases. The sociodemographic variables associated with CI included higher family income, mother's lower education, higher proportion of fathers working as independent professionals, extended family, mother's age < 30 years, and mother's working outside home. The fact that both parents work outside the home and that the mother has a low educational level may reflect a lack of awareness and knowledge of the hazards of corrosive substances kept in the house. Family organization classified as extended implies crowded living conditions and enables both parents to work outside home while other family members take care of their children [18]. Other authors have reported that unsafe homes where safety rules regarding caustic substances are lacking have been identified as a substantial risk factor for CI in children [1, 9, 13, 17, 21]. Sarioglu-Buke *et al.* found that children from families where both parents with low educational level and low socioeconomic status had a higher risk for a CI event. Urganci *et al.* found in a series of 1709 cases that 30% of the mothers were illiterate [13]. Contini *et al.* described most CI particularly in developing countries as being due to parent's lack of knowledge of the hazards of corrosive substances kept in the house, especially among illiterate individuals [1]. Risk factors are summarized in **Table 1**.

2.1. Physiopathology

The physical form, concentration, and pH of the corrosive agent play a significant role in the location and type of resultant injuries [2]. Acid substances lead to coagulation necrosis that usually limits acid penetration and results in damage to the epithelium and submucosal layer. Their low viscosity and specific gravity result in rapid transit to the stomach, and gastric injury is more common than oesophageal injury. Their bitter taste and development of pain with ingestion may result in lower volumes of ingestion. The gastric injury may result in gastric outlet obstruction o perforation [19]. The ingestion of alkalis causes liquefaction necrosis with damage of the epithelium and the submucosa layer with deep penetration and may result in perforation [2]. Injury most typically involves the oesophagus, but the gastric injury may also occur.

Haemorrhage, thrombosis and a marked inflammatory response with significant oedema are seen within the first 24 h of injury [19]. The tissue repair phase extends from the end of the first week through the second week after injury and if the insult has been relatively minor, oesophageal function returns gradually. The healing phase begins around the third week when fibroblast proliferation replaces the submucosa and *muscularis mucosae*; at this time, stricture formation begins [2, 19]. Additionally, lower oesophageal sphincter pressure becomes impaired, leading to increased gastroesophageal reflux, which in turn accelerates stricture formation [20].

Age	**Below 6 years old**
Gender	Boys
Alkali or acid caustic substances at home	Improper storage
	Food or drinks storage containers
	Lack of warning labels
	Lack of security caps
Extended families	Both parents working away from home, children cared for other family members and mother with a low education level

Table 1. Risk factors for caustic ingestion in paediatric patients [18, 21].

In most series, the most commonly reported corrosive agents are alkaline products as caustic soda, sodium hypochlorite and household chemicals [13]. It is essential to highlight that most of these products ingested by children were kept in containers that had no warning labels and no childproof safety caps. These key risk factors should be taken care by worldwide governments by means of health education and implementation of legislative and preventive strategies on labeling, formulation, and packaging of corrosive substances [1, 21].

2.2. Clinical manifestations

The ingestion of acid or alkali substances frequently leads to damage to the gastrointestinal tract. The spectrum damage ranges from mild to severe and may affect the mucosa as well as the muscular layer. In a study performed by the authors in a paediatric referral hospital, the aim was to evaluate the association of clinical data with the oesophageal damage of 94 children who suffered CI. The mean age when the CI occurred was 38.4 months (SD 28.7). Thirty-five cases (37.2%) were females. The higher frequency was in infants (40.4%) and pre-schoolers (45.7%). The symptoms recorded were salivation (77.7%), oropharyngeal burns (76.6%), and vomiting (74.5%), oropharyngeal pain (45.7%), and epigastric pain (18.1%). Symptoms of airway involvement included shortness of breath (14.9%) and retrosternal pain (10.6%) [19]; these signs and symptoms are similar to those reported by other authors in paediatric series [3–7, 9, 12, 13, 21].

2.3. Diagnosis

In a number of cases, CI patients may be symptom-free on admission; in spite of this, endoscopy is mandatory as an effective tool to identify both oesophageal and gastric damage [22]. Even more, the presence or absence of symptoms does not predict the injury severity to the gastrointestinal tract, supporting the endoscopic procedure [23, 24]. The degree of the mucosal injury should be determined by a standardized classification; most colleagues use the Zargar's classification: grade 0 = normal; grade I = oedema and erythema; grade II = linear ulcerations and necrotic tissue with whitish plaques; grade II-a = linear ulcerations and necrotic tissue with whitish plaques and deeper and more circumferential; grade III = circumferential injury which may be transmural with mucosal sloughing, multiple deep ulcerations and areas of necrosis (areas of brown-black or greyish discoloration of mucosa were taken as evidence for necrosis); grade III-a = focal necrosis; grade III-b = extensive necrosis; and grade IV = perforation [25]. A study performed in 206 children reported no complications when the endoscope was advanced beyond the first severe burn; this approach could identify additional oesophageal and gastric lesions that could be missed if the endoscopy is discontinued when finding the first circumferential oesophageal burn, as is usually recommended because of perforation risk [23].

In our series, all cases underwent upper endoscopy within 48 h of CI; in 66 of 78 children (84.6%), we identified moderate or severe oesophageal burns, 76.9% had grade II and 7.7% grade III. An endoscopy plus a barium swallow were repeated after 2 or 3 weeks of the CI to assess mucosal healing and to look for strictures; mucosal healing occurred in all cases but 64.5% had oesophageal stricture [21]. Clinical, endoscopic and image data of our cases are summarized in **Table 2**.

	Variable	*n*	%
Symptoms and signs	Salivation	73	77.7
	Oropharyngeal burns	72	74.5
	Vomiting	70	70.3
	Oropharyngeal pain	42	45.7
	Epigastric pain	17	18.1
	Shortness of breath	14	14.9
	Retrosternal pain	10	10.6
	Septic schok[a]	4	4.2
	Dysphagia[b]	23	24.5
Endoscopy	II or III degree esophageal burns[c]	79	84
	Esophageal stricture[d]	46	48.9
Barium swallow	Esophageal stricture	46	48.9

[a]Oesophageal perforation.

[b]Weeks/months after the caustic ingestion.

[c]Admission endoscopy.

[d]Endoscopy performed 2–3 weeks after admission.

Table 2. Clinical data in 94 children with caustic ingestion [21, 38].

In 2012, Uygun *et al.* developed a tool for predicting risk of developing an esophageal stricture without endoscopy called the DROOL score based on the severity and duration of initial signs and symptoms (drooling, reluctance to eat, presence of burns in oropharynx, fever, hematemesis, abdominal tenderness, dyspnea, chest pain and leukocytosis). A DROOL score ≤ 4 was a significant predictor of esophageal stricture with 100% sensitivity and 96% specificity; this score needs further investigation and validation [26]. It has been recently published that a CT scan may offer a more detailed evaluation than early endoscopy in assessing the transmural damage of esophageal and gastric walls and the extent of necrosis; a CT grading system has also been proposed to predict esophageal stricture [27]. These important findings deserve to be validated because this could mean a significant change in the diagnostic approach of these patients.

2.4. Complications

Acute complications such as mediastinitis and oesophageal perforation may occur and they may represent life-threating complications; in selected cases, chest and abdominal radiographs are needed to rule out the presence of free air in the mediastinum or peritoneum. Lateral neck radiographs should be obtained in patients with stridor or hoarseness [28].

Long-term complications frequently include oesophageal stricture and dysphagia [4–9, 11, 13, 18]. In our series, oesophageal stricture occurred in 48.9%; II and III-degree burns were associated with oesophageal stricture ($p = 0.004$) and ingestion of alkaline products ($p = 0.027$). The observation that one-half of patients with stricture did not complain of dysphagia and that some patients with dysphagia had no oesophageal strictures, points to the underlying complexity of the functional and anatomical oesophageal damage induced by the chemical agent as well as to the individual variation in visceral sensitivity [29].

Several studies have reported oesophageal dysmotility after a CI; oesophageal manometry has revealed hypoperistalsis, with normal upper and lower oesophageal sphincter [30, 31]. Rana et al. showed that patients with corrosive injury have prolonged oro-cecal transit time using the lactulose hydrogen breath test, even in the absence of gastric symptoms; this transit time was maximally prolonged in patients with lower third oesophageal scars [32]. Gastric emptying time assessed by radionucleotide scintigraphy after a CI was significantly prolonged in patients with oesophageal stricture, even in the absence of gastric symptoms [33]. Another study reported that oesophageal transit time assessed by scintigraphy was prolonged in one-third of patients with corrosive induced oesophageal strictures, despite having achieved adequate oesophageal dilatation; these authors found that the prolongation of oesophageal transit time correlated with the length of the stricture and that the severity of the dysphagia correlated with the prolongation of total oesophageal transit time [34].

CI with stricture has been associated with increased risk of oesophageal carcinoma with an incidence of 1000 times the expected in normal population; this important finding points the need for endoscopic surveillance 15–20 years after the caustic injury [28, 35].

The severity of the oesophageal damage that occurs frequently in children with CI may limit the normal feeding process leading to malnutrition and growth impairment [18, 22, 36]; it is surprising that there is very little published information regarding the nutritional status. In France, Ganga-Zandzou *et al.* found that the nutritional status in 34 children with oesophageal stricture was not affected [37]; whereas, in Egypt, Hamza *et al.* recorded 15% of malnutrition [15]. In another study performed by the authors, the aim was to evaluate the nutritional status and its association with dysphagia and oesophageal stricture in 62 children with CI. Although the proportion of cases with z-scores of height for age and weight for height below −2SD was low, all anthropometric arm indicators (fat and muscle) of the children with dysphagia and oesophageal strictures were located in the negative area of the z-score curve. In all cases, adiposity z-score values were significantly lower in children with dysphagia or strictures when compared with the cases without these complications. Arm muscle area z-scores showed the same trend. We concluded that children with dysphagia and/or oesophageal strictures associated to CI had lower fat stores and muscle mass than the cases without these oesophageal complications, meaning impaired nutritional status [38]. In this context, both growth and nutritional status surveillance as an effective nutritional intervention protocol should be part of the mid- and long-term monitoring of these patients.

2.5. Treatment

All patients who suffered a CI should be hospitalized and evaluated comprehensively. The clinical history must emphasize the type and amount of caustic and if possible get the product package. Hemodynamic stabilization and adequacy of the patient's airway are priorities. The induction of vomiting or gastric lavage is contraindicated following CI because a re-exposure of the oesophageal mucosa to the caustic agent with further injury may occur [35]. An endoscopic evaluation with an adequate paediatric endoscope performed within the first 24–48 h is essential to evaluate the type and extent of injury to the oesophagus and stomach.

The information about the efficacy of proton-pump inhibitors and H2 blockers to minimize the oesophageal injury in subjects whom ingested caustic is scarce. Cakal *et al.* performed an open clinical trial on 13 adult patients who were admitted due to CI and received omeprazole 80 mg in bolus IV, followed by continuous infusion of 8 mg/hour for 72 h. A control endoscopy was performed 72 h after admission, identifying a significant difference regarding endoscopic healing between the before and after omeprazole infusion ($p = 0.004$); however, this study lacks a control group and is not possible to draw definitive conclusions [39].

The use of corticosteroids is controversial; two meta-analyses did not demonstrate benefits of steroid administration in terms of stricture prevention [40, 41]. In a recent study on 83 children with II-b oesophageal burns, one group received methylprednisolone (1 g/1,73 m/day/3 days), ranitidine, ceftriaxone, and total parenteral nutrition; the control group received the same regimen except methylprednisolone. The outcome variable was oesophageal stricture and it was more frequent in the control group ($p = 0.038$). The duration of total parenteral nutrition was shorter in the steroid intervention group compared with the control group ($p = 0.001$). The authors concluded that high doses of methylprednisolone used for the management of grade II-b oesophageal caustic burns may reduce the risk of stricture [40–42].

The use of antibiotics is controversial and should be considered in each particular case according to the clinical situation, laboratory inflammation values, the extent and type of mucosal damage and the concomitant use of steroids. The indications, dosages, duration and type of antibiotics are usually included in the protocols of each hospital serving this type of patients [19].

During the course of treatment, some patients may require oesophageal dilations and gastrostomy either for retrograde oesophageal dilations or trans-gastrostomy feeding. Topical mitomycin C application has been used recently to improve the results of endoscopic dilatation for short oesophageal strictures and is a promising agent in the management of the long-segment caustic oesophageal strictures, although long-term follow-up is needed to prove its efficacy and to evaluate potential long-term side effects [43]. The use of oesophageal stents and balloon dilators are known options for treating strictures [5, 28, 35].

A small number of cases with strictures refractory to dilation may require oesophageal replacement by a colonic graft or stomach's plasty to set up a gastric tube. Ezemba *et al.* reported a retrospective study of 21 patients who underwent substernal isoperistaltic colonic interposition graft for the management of corrosive oesophageal stricture. The long segment strictures and multiple strictures were the main indications for the procedure; the complications included cervical fistulae (19%), reflux neo-esophagitis (14.3%), graft infarction (9.5%); lethality occurred in 9.5%. In the mid term, dysphagia was completely relieved in 84% of the cases, no regurgitation or nocturnal aspiration was reported [44].

Special attention should be placed on growth, nutritional status and the emotional situation of the affected children and their families. A limited oral intake, decrease in growth velocity and low-fat reserves or muscle mass may require special dietary regimens with adequate energy and micronutrient intake by means of blended or polymeric diets. A CI is a traumatic event that may shake families emotionally, and in some cases, they may require emotional support by family therapists.

Author details

Alfredo Larrosa-Haro[1,2], Carmen A Sánchez-Ramírez[1,2,3], Johnatan M Mesa-Magaña[1] and Edgar M Vasquez-Garibay[2]*

*Address all correspondence to: calicesr26@hotmail.com

1 Servicio de Gastroenterología y Nutrición, UMAE Hospital de Pediatría, Centro Médico Nacional de Occidente, Instituto Mexicano del Seguro Socia, Guadañajara, México

2 Instituto de Nutrición Humana, Departamento de Clínicas de la Reproducción Humana Crecimiento y Desarrollo Infantil, Centro Universitario de Ciencias de la Salud, Universidad de Guadalajara, Guadalajara, México

3 Facultad de Medicina, Universidad de Colima, Colima, México

References

[1] Contini S, Swarray-Deen A, Scarpignato C. Oesophageal corrosive injuries in children: A forgotten social and health challenge in developing countries. Bull World Health Organ. 2009;**87**:950-954. DOI: 10.247/BLT.08.058065

[2] Wasserman R, Ginsburg C. Caustic substances injuries. Journal of Pediatrics. 1985;**107**: 169-174

[3] Elshabrawi M, A-Kader H. Caustic ingestion in children. Expert Review of Gastroenterology & Hepatology. 2011;**5**:637-645. DOI: 10.1586/egh.11.49

[4] Turner A, Robinson P. Respiratory and gastrointestinal complications of caustic ingestion in children. Emergency Medicine Journal. 2005;**22**:359-361. DOI: 10.1136/emj.2004.015610

[5] Riffat F, Cheng A. Pediatric caustic ingestion: 50 consecutive cases and a review of the literature. Diseases of the Esophagus. 2009;**22**:89-94. DOI: 10.1111/j.1442-2050.2008.00867.x

[6] Dogan Y, Erkan T, Cullu F, Kutlu T. Caustic gastro esophageal lesions in childhood; an analysis of 473 cases. Clinical Pediatrics. 2006;**45**:435-438. DOI: 10.1177/0009922806289618

[7] Arévalo-Silva C, Eliashar R, Wohlgelernter J, Elidan J, Gross M. Ingestion of caustic substances: A 15 year experience. Laryngoscope. 2006;**116**:1422-1426. DOI: 10.1097/01.mlg.0000225376.83670.4d

[8] Gundogdu H, Tanyel F, Buyukpamukcu N, Hicsonmez A. Conservative treatment of caustic esophageal strictures in children. Journal of Pediatric Surgery. 1992;**27**:767-770

[9] Bautista A, Estevez E, Varela R, Villanueva A, Tojo R, Cadranel S. A retrospective analysis of ingestion of caustic substances by children. Ten-year statistics in Galicia. European Journal of Pediatrics. 1997;**156**: 410-414

[10] Christesen H. Epidemiology and prevention of caustic ingestion in children. Acta Paediatrica. 1994;**83**: 212-215

[11] Nuutinen M, Uhari M, Karvali T, Kouvalainen K. Consequences of caustic ingestions in children. Acta Paediatrica. 1994;**83**:1200-1205

[12] Demiroren K, Kocamaz H, Dogan Y. Gastrointestinal system lesions in children due to the ingestion of alkali and acid corrosive substances. Turkish Journal of Medical Sciences. 2015;**45**: 184-190

[13] Urganci N, Usta M, Kalyoncu D, Demirel E. Corrosive substance ingestion in children. Indian Journal of Pediatrics. 2014;**81**: 675-679. DOI: 10.1007/s12098-013-1170-0

[14] Jong A, Macdonald R, Elin S, Forte V, Turner A. Corrosive esophagitis in children: A 30-year review. International Journal of Pediatric Otorhinolaryngology. 2001;**57**: 203-211

[15] Hamza A, Abdelhay S, Sherif H, Hasan T, Soliman H, Kabesh A, et al. Caustic esophageal stenosis in children: 30 year experience. Journal of Pediatric Surgery. 2003;**38**: 828-833

[16] Cakman M, Gollu G, Boybeyi O, Kucuk G, Stertcelik M, Gunal Y, et al. Cognitive and behavioral characteristics of children with caustic ingestion. Journal of Pediatric Surgery. 2015;**50**: 540-542. DOI: 10.1016/j.pedsurg.2014.10.052

[17] Sarioglu-Buke A, Corduk N, Atesci F, Karabul M, Koltuksuz U. A different aspect of corrosive ingestion in children: Socio-demographic characteristics and effect family functioning. International Journal of Pediatric Otorhinolaryngology. 2006;**70**:1791-1798. DOI: 10.1016/j.ijporl.2006.06.005

[18] Sánchez-Ramírez CA, Larrosa-Haro A, Vázquez-Garibay E, Macías-Rosales R. Socio-demographic factors associated with caustic ingestion in children and adolescents. International Journal of Pediatric Otorhinolaryngology. 2012;**76**: 253-256. DOI: 10.1016/j.ijporl.2011.11.015

[19] Kay M, Willye R. Caustic ingestion in children. Current Opinion in Pediatrics. 2009;**21**: 651-654. DOI: 10.1097/MOP.0b013e32832e2764

[20] Mutaf O, Genc A, Herek O, Demircan M, Ozcan C, Arikan A. Gastroesophageal reflux: A determinant in the outcome of caustic esophageal burns. Journal of Pediatric Surgery. 1996;**31**:1494-1495

[21] Sánchez-Ramírez CA, Larrosa-Haro A, Vázquez-Garibay E, Larios-Arceo F. Caustic ingestion and oesophageal damage in children: Clinical spectrum and feeding practices. Journal of Paediatrics and Child Health. 2011;**47**:378-380. DOI: 10.1111/j.1440-1754.2010.01984.x

[22] Adedeji T, Tobih J, Olaosun A, Sogebi O. Corrosive oesophageal injuries: A preventable menace. The Pan African Medical Journal. 2013;**15**:11. DOI: 10.11604/pamj.2013.15.11.2495

[23] Temiz A, Oguzkurt P, Ezer S, Ince E, Hicsonmez A. Predictability of outcome of caustic ingestion by esophagogastroduodenoscopy in children. World Journal of Gastroenterology. 2012;**18**:1098-1103. DOI: 10.3748/wjg.v18.i10.1098

[24] Gaudreault P, Parent M, McGuigan M, Chicoine L, Lovejoy F. Predictability of esophageal injury form signs and symptoms: A study of caustic ingestion in 378 children. Pediatrics. 1983;**71**:767-769

[25] Zargar S, Kochhar R, Mehta S, Mehta SK. The role of fiberoptic endoscopy in the management of the corrosive ingestion and modified endoscopic classification of burns. Gastrointestinal Endoscopy. 1991;**37**:165-169

[26] Uygun I, Aydogdu B, Okur M, Arayici Y, Celik Y, Ozturk H, et al. Clinico-epidemiological study of caustic substance ingestion accidents in children in Anatolia: The DROOL score as new prognostic tool. Acta chirurgica Belgica. 2012;**112**:346-354

[27] Ryu H, Jeung K, Lee B, Uhm J, Park Y, Shin M, et al. Caustic injury: Can CT grading system enable prediction of esophageal stricture? Clinical Toxicology. 2010;**48**:137-142. DOI: 10.3109/15563650903585929

[28] Millar A, Cox S. Caustic injury of the esophagus. Pediatric Surgery International. 2015;**31**: 111-121. DOI: 10.1007/s00383-014-3642-3643

[29] Isbister G, Page C. Early endoscopy or CT in caustic injuries: A re-evaluation of clinical practice. Clinical Toxicology. 2011;**49**:641-642. DOI: 10.3109/15563650.2011.604035

[30] Dantas R, Mamede R. Esophageal motility in patients with esophageal caustic injury. The American Journal of Gastroenterology. 1996;**91**:1157-1161

[31] Genc A, Mutaf O. Esophageal motility changes in acute and late periods od caustic esophageal burns and their relation to prognosis in children. Journal of Pediatric Surgery. 2002;**37**:1526-1528

[32] Rana S, Kochhar R, Pal R, Nagi B, Singh K. Orocecal transit time in patients in the chronic phase of corrosive injury. Digestive Diseases and Sciences. 2008;**53**:1797-1800. DOI: 10.1007/s10620-007-0096-7

[33] Mittal B, Kochhar R, Shankar R, Bhattacharya A, Solanki K, Nagi B. Delayed gastric emptying in patients with caustic ingestion. Nuclear Medicine Communications. 2008;**29**: 782-785. DOI: 10.1097/MNM.0b013e328302f4b9

[34] Kochhar R, Mittal B, Kumor S. Segmental and total esophageal transit time in patients with corrosive induced esophageal stricture. Nuclear Medicine Communications. 2007;**28**:920-923. DOI: 10.1097/MNM, 0b013e3282flb966

[35] Shub M. Therapy of caustic ingestion: New treatment and considerations. Current Opinion in Pediatrics. 2015;**27**:609-613. DOI: 10.1097/MOP.0000000000000257

[36] Contini S, Scarpignato C. Caustic injury of the upper gastrointestinal tract: A comprehensive review. World Journal of Gastroenterology. 2013;**19**:3918-3930. DOI: 10.3748/wjg.v19.i25.3918

[37] Ganga-Zandzou P, Devulder C, Michaud L, Ategbo S. Gottrand F, Debeugny P. Long term follow-up of children with esophageal caustic stenosis. Archives de Pédiatrie. 1998;**5**:610-616

[38] Sánchez-Ramírez C, Larrosa-Haro A, Vásquez-Garibay E, Rodríguez-Anguiano A, Cámara-López M. Nutritional status in children with esophageal stenosis and dysphagia associated to caustic ingestion. Nutrición Hospitalaria. 2016;**33**(1):26-30. DOI: 10.20960/nh.v33i1.11

[39] Cakal B, Akbal E, Koklu S, Babali A, Kocal E, Tas A. Acute therapy with intravenous omeprazole on caustic esophageal injury: A prospective case series. Diseases of the Esophagus. 2013;**26**:22-26. DOI: 10.1111/j.1442-2050.2011.01319

[40] Pelclova D, Navrátil T. Do corticoesteroids prevent oesophageal stricture after corrosive ingestion?. Toxicological Reviews. 2005;**24**:125-129

[41] Fulton J, Hoffman R. Steroids in second degree caustic burns of the esophagus: A systematic pooled analysis of fifty years of human data: 1956-2006. Clinical Toxicology. 2007;**45**:402-408. DOI: 10.1080/15563650701285420

[42] Usta M, Erkan T, Cokugras F, Urganci N, Onal Z, Gulcan M, et al. High doses of methylprednisolone in the managment of caustic esophageal burns. Pediatrics. 2014;**133**:1518-1524. DOI: 10.1542/peds.2013-3331

[43] El-Asmar K, Hassan M, Abdelkader H, Hamza A. Topical mitomycin C can effectively alleviate dysphagia in children with long-segment caustic esophageal strictures. Diseases of the Esophagus. 2015;**28**:422-427. DOI: 10.1111/dote.12218

[44] Ezemba N, Eze J, Nwafor I, Etukokwu K, Orakwe O. Colon interpositicon graft for corrosive esophageal stricture: Midterm functional outcome. World Journal of Surgery. 2014;**38**:2352-2357. DOI: 10.1007/s00268-014-2574-3

9

Anatomy of Esophagus

Murat Ferhat Ferhatoglu and Taner Kıvılcım

Abstract

Anatomy knowledge is the basic stone of healing diseases. Arteries, veins, wall structure, nerves, narrowing, curves, relations with other organs are very important to understand esophagial diseases. In this chapter we aimed to explain anatomical fundementals of oesophagus.

Keywords: anatomy, esophagus, parts of esophagus, blood supply of esophagus, innervation of esophagus

1. Introduction

Esophagus is a muscular tube-like organ that originates from endodermal primitive gut, 25–28 cm long, approximately 2 cm in diameter, located between lower border of laryngeal part of pharynx (**Figure 1**) and cardia of stomach. Start and end points of esophagus correspond to 6th cervical vertebra and 11th thoracic vertebra topographically, and the gastroesophageal junction corresponds to xiphoid process of sternum. Five cm of esophagus is in the neck, and it descends over superior mediastinum and posterior mediastinum approximately 17–18 cm, continues for 1–1.5 cm in diaphragm, ending with 2–3 cm of esophagus in abdomen (**Figure 2**) [1, 2]. Sex, age, physical condition, and gender affect the length of esophagus. A newborn's esophagus is 18 cm long, and it begins and ends one or two vertebra higher than in adult. Esophagus lengthens to 22 cm long by age 3 years and to 27 cm by age 10 years [3, 4].

2. Structure of esophagus

Esophagus consists of four histologic layers: mucosa, submucosa, muscularis propia, and adventitia.

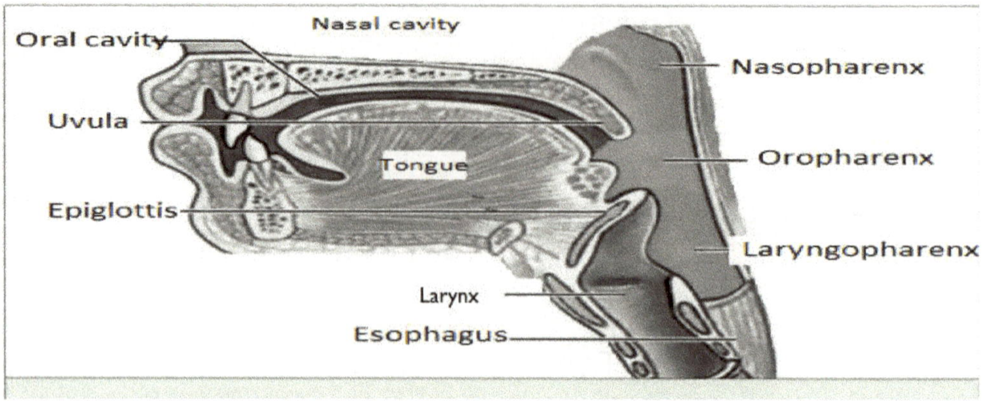

Figure 1. Anatomy of larynx (with permission of Turkish Surgery Association).

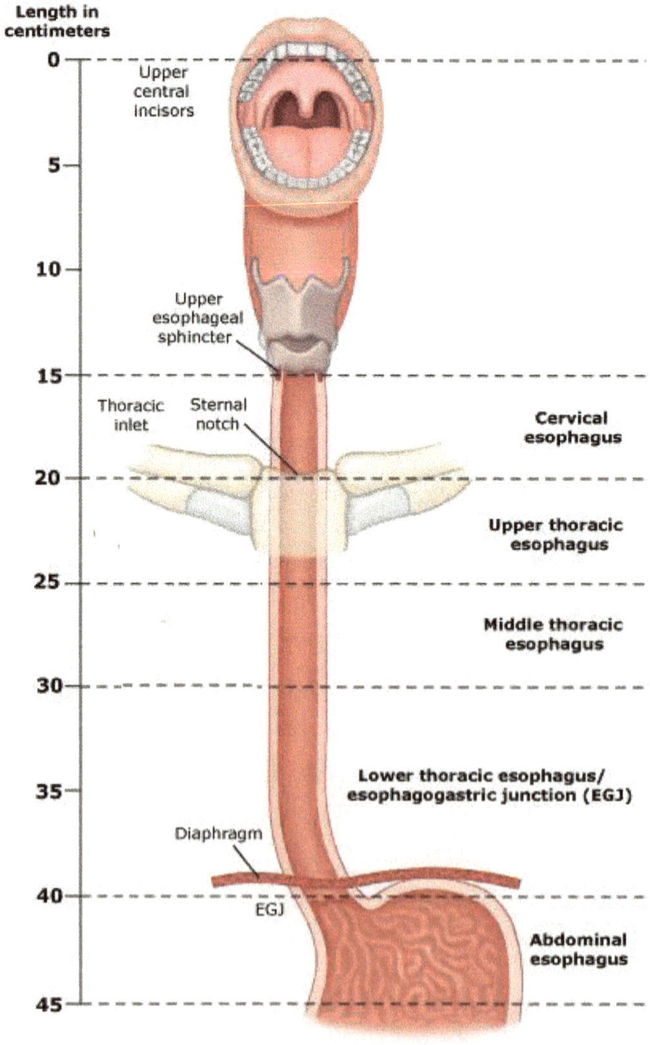

Figure 2. Length of esophageal parts.

2.1. Mucosa

Nonkeratinized stratified squamous epithelium covers all esophageal lumen. Lamina propia and lamina muscularis mucosa are located under this epithelium. Lamina propia consists mostly of loose connective tissue and lamina muscularis mucosa consists of some smooth muscle tissue and elastic fibers. Nonkeratinized stratified squamous epithelium of mucosa transforms simple columnar epithelium in cardia of stomach, occurring at a point called "Z line," an irregular zigzag line. On endoscopy, esophageal mucosa is paler than mucosa of stomach.

2.2. Submucosa

This layer consists of elastic and collagen fibers that form a dense, irregular connective tissue. This layer consists of veins, lymphatics, and meissner plexus.

2.3. Muscularis propia

Both longitudinal and circular muscles form tube-like esophagus: longitudinal muscle fibers are located superficially and the circular muscle fibers are located deeply. Longitudinal fibers begin from posterior face of cricoid cartilage and form a triangle named as "Lamier triangle," which is limited by longitudinal muscle fibers laterally and cricopharyngeus muscle superiorly. Another triangle, called "Killian triangle," is found in this area, and borders of this triangle are formed by inferior constrictor muscle of pharynx and cricopharyngeus muscle. These weaker areas are important for the formation of Zencker's diverticula. Longitudinal muscle fibers are gathered laterally in upper portion of esophagus, but these fibers expand and surround all surfaces at lower sides, becoming strongest in lower third part of esophagus. Circular muscle fibers are located under longitudinal muscle, and the circular muscle is thinner than longitudinal muscle. Circular muscles are not actually circular at all parts of esophagus; these fibers are more elliptic in upper third part and become more circular at lower third part of esophagus. Circular muscle fibers do not make a regular formation, but run in an irregular pattern making a shutter-like system. Spontaneous perforation of esophagus usually occurs in last 2 cm, and this perforation consists of entire esophageal wall, causing mediastinitis because of gastric acid leakage. Upper part of esophagus consists of striated muscle and the lower part consists of smooth muscle fibers. Transition zone differs in all humans, but mostly upper quarter consists only of striated muscle fibers; second quarter consists of both striated and smooth muscle fibers; and lower half consists of only smooth muscle fibers (Aurbach plexus is in this layer).

2.4. Adventitia

This layer surrounds most of the esophagus and consists of loose connective tissue. Because no serosa is found on esophagus, infections, and tumors can spread easily [5, 6].

3. Narrowings and curves of esophagus

Esophagus has seven narrowing points that can be seen using esophagoscopy or barium passage graphy. Four classic narrowings are found in almost all people; three other narrowings are found in certain medical conditions.

First classical narrowing is at the beginning point, and oropharyngeal muscle forms it; this part is the second narrowest point after orifice of appendix vermiformis in alimentary tract. This first narrowing point's luminal diameter is approximately 1.4–1.5 cm, and it is located 15 cm after maxillary central incisor teeth. Topographically, this first point corresponds to corpus of 6th cervical vertebra. This narrowing is named "upper esophageal sphincter." Second narrowing corresponds to plane that is located at superior border of sternum. Anterior and posterior esophageal walls become closer in hyperflexion, and this partial narrowing point occurs. Third narrowing is one of classical narrowings made by aortic arch. This point corresponds to 4th thoracic vertebra topographically and measures 1.5–1.6 cm in width. Point is located 22.5 cm after maxillary central incisor teeth, 7 cm below cricopharyngeus muscle [2]. Fourth narrowing (third classical narrowing) is located at crossing point of esophagus and left main bronchium. This point is located at level of 5th dorsal vertebra, and 27.5 cm after maxillary central incisor teeth and 9 cm below oropharyngeal muscle. Fifth narrowing point is formed if patient has atrial dilatation caused by mitral stenosis. This point is located just below bronchial narrowing. Sixth narrowing, called "Laimer narrowing," is located at second crossing point of esophagus and aorta. This point is located at plane corresponding to upper edge of 10th dorsal vertebral corpus. Laimer narrowing occurs in situation of aortic atherosclerosis. Just above this narrowing, a partial dilatation called "epiphrenic ampulla" or "Vorgamen de Luschka" is found. Last narrowing (and 4th classical narrowing) is made by esophageal hiatus that originates from right crus of diaphragm, and is located at the level of 11th dorsal vertebra and 40 cm after maxillary central incisor teeth; it is 1–1.5 cm in length and1.5–1.8 cm in width. This last narrowing is named "lower esophageal sphincter." Lower sphincter consists of a physiological sphincter mechanism made by muscle fibers of right crus of diaphragm; it provides an antireflux mechanism. When a person is not eating, esophageal lumen is closed above lower esophageal sphincter. Esophagus is primarily median and vertical, but has three slight curves located in neck, behind left bronchus, and at bifurcation of trachea (**Picture 1**).

Esophagus is located at left of midline at level of 1st dorsal vertebra, right of midline at level of 6th dorsal vertebra, and left of midline again at level of 10th dorsal vertebra. Thus, esophagus makes a reverse "S" all the way in front of vertebral column. These narrowings and curves are important landmarks for radiological and endoscopic investigation of abnormalities, cancer diagnosis, and stricture formation after swallowing of chemicals [2, 7].

Esophagus is anatomically divided into three parts: cervical esophagus, thoracic esophagus, and abdominal esophagus.

3.1. Cervical esophagus

Cervical esophagus starts at inferior margin of cricoid cartilage that corresponds to corpus of 6th cervical vertebra. This level is marked by a carotid tubercula named "Chasseing tubercula,"

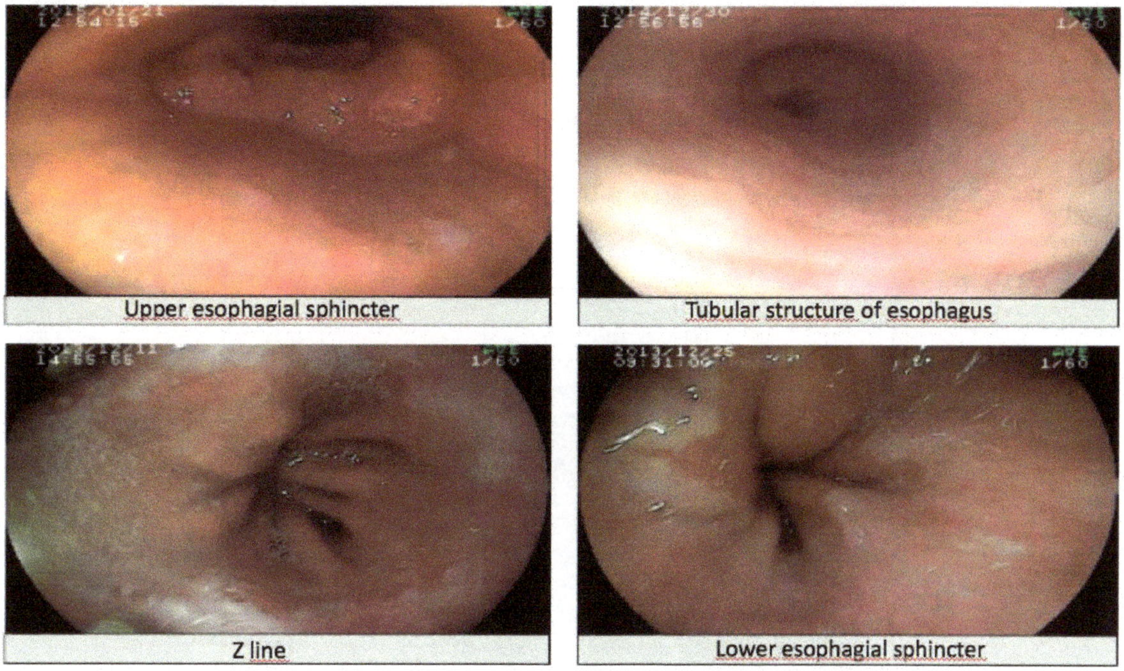

Picture 1. Endoscopic view of esophagus (with the permission of Turkish Surgery Association).

which is an important landmark in cervical esophagectomy. Cervical esophagus ends at inferior edge of first dorsal vertebra that comes up to a horizontal plane of jugular incisura of sternum. The endpoint is the starting point of upper mediastinum, and from this point it is thoracic esophagus. Cervical esophagus is 5–6 cm long, and its luminal diameter is 1.4–1.5 cm at its narrowest point.

3.1.1. Surrounding structures

Esophagus runs in deepest fascial plane of neck, leaning between trachea anteriorly and vertebra posteriorly. Esophagus is attached to prevertebral fascia by sagittal septa, which forms retropharyngeal and retro-esophagial spaces.

Esophagus is covered by larynx and trachea anteriorly (**Figure 3**), but this covering is partial, and an open margin is found on left anterior side, which provides natural surgical access. Esophagus attaches with tracheoesophageal muscle fibers to trachea; it is easy to separate tracheoesophageal plane, except in pathological circumstances. Esophagus's closest structure is carotid artery anterolaterally, which lies 1–2 cm away from it. Inferior thyroid artery, thyroid lobes, and recurrent laryngeal nerves are other important contiguities of esophagus, and ductus thoracicus lies on left side of it. Esophagus connects prevertebral muscles, cervical vertebras, and prevertebral laminas posteriorly. Thoracic duct connects to left "Pirogoff angle," and it makes a slight connection to left side of esophagus.

3.1.2. Importance of surrounding structures

Sagittal septa, which forms retropharyngeal and retro-esophagial spaces, blocks the diffusion of abscess of this area to upper mediastinum, but abscess can diffuse via pretracheal space to the upper mediastinum and can cause a fatal complication. Pretracheal space is important in that it can be perforated, primarily during an esophagectomy.

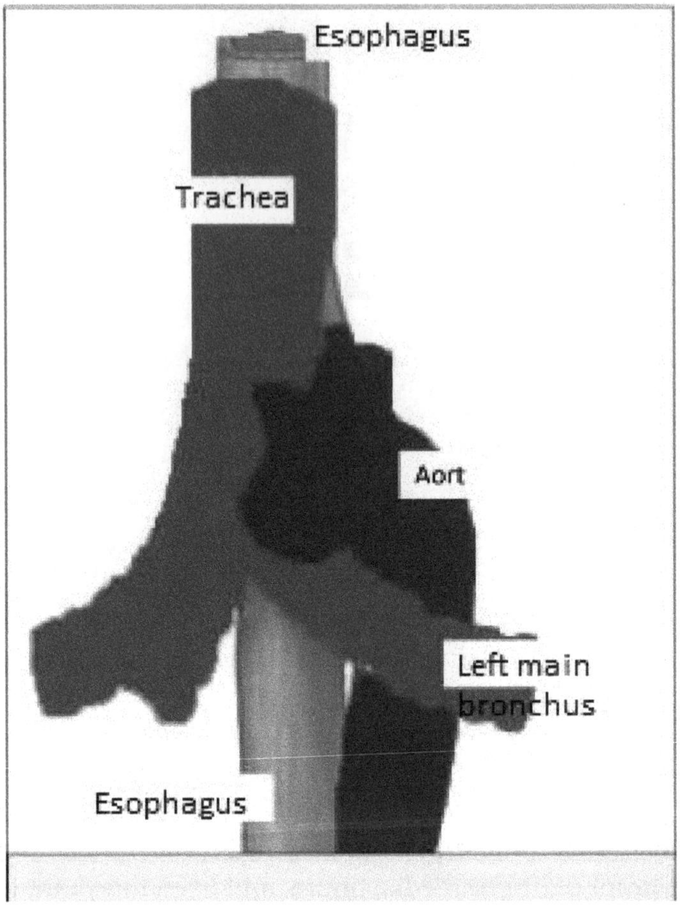

Figure 3. Placement of esophagus relative to other anatomic structures (with permission of Turkish Surgery Association).

Recurrent laryngeal nerve (RLN) lies in tracheoesophageal sulcus, and esophagus is close to this nerve, which is important in case of cervical esophagectomy. Injury of RLN causes unilateral difficulty in swallowing and hoarseness; bilateral injury causes closure of vocal cords in median position, and a tracheostomy becomes necessary. Especially on left side of esophagus, RLN is so close to esophagus that it is easy to injure a nerve with a careless dissection. Thus, dissection should be made close to esophageal muscle fibers to avoid this complication. As previously mentioned, thoracic duct connects to left Pirogoff angle, and it makes a slight connection to left side of esophagus. To avoid harm to thoracic duct, a careful dissection should be made, especially in cervical esophagectomy [8, 9].

3.2. Thoracic esophagus

Measuring 16–18 cm in length, thoracic esophagus is in upper and posterior mediastinum. Running from 1st to 11th dorsal vertebra, it does not fit concavity of vertebral column. However, it changes location to left gradually from start to end. At beginning, it is located between vertebral column and trachea, slightly left of midline and 5 cm left of vertebral column at level of diaphragmatic hiatus (**Figure 4**). Parietal sheet of pleura is tightly connected to both sides of vertebral column, and these connections cause esophageal-pleural recesses that make dissection of esophagus in thorax more difficult. Thus, if a pleural rupture occurs in this area during surgery, fixing rupture can present a challenge for surgeon [2].

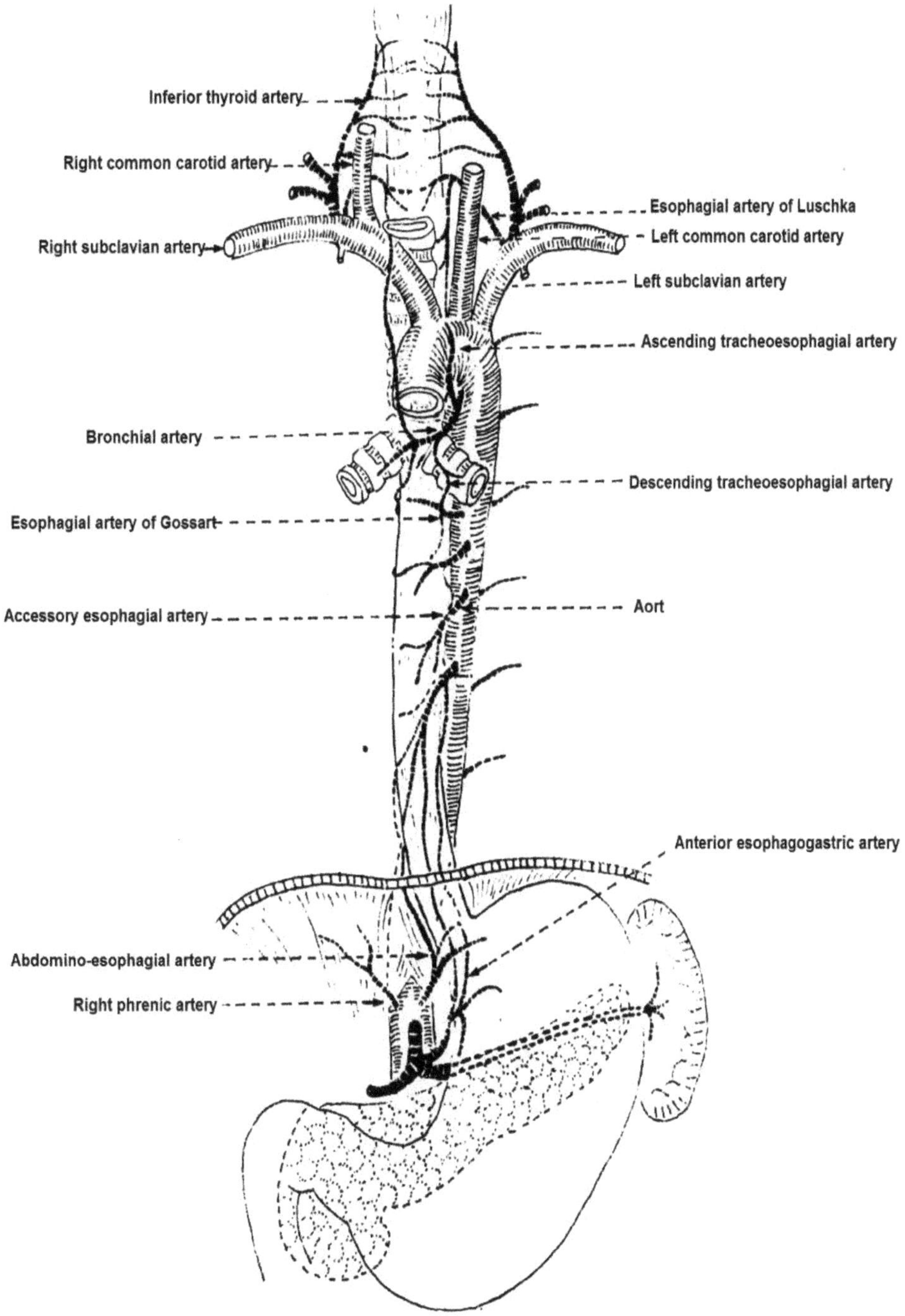

Figure 4. Arteries of Esophagus.

As previously discussed, esophagus within thoracic cavity contains three classical narrowings, two conditional narrowings, and two curves.

3.2.1. Surrounding structures

Most important and challenging structure in this region is thoracic duct, which lies behind esophagus throughout thorax. Thoracic duct is located slightly apart from esophagus in inferior third part of thorax, but it comes closer as esophagus goes upward. Trachea, aortic arch, right pulmonary artery, left main bronchus, plexus of esophagus, pericardium, left atrium, and anterior vagus nerve are found anterior to esophagus. At posterior side, esophagus connects to vertebral column, longus colli muscle, posterior intercostal arteries, azygos vein, hemiazygos vein, anterior wall of aorta, posterior vagal nerve, and pleura. Aortic arch, left subclavian artery, left inferior laryngeal nerve, left vagus nerve, thoracic ductus, and thoracic part of aorta are located on left side of esophagus. Azygos vein, pleura of mediastinum, right main bronchus, and right vagus nerve are located on right side.

3.2.2. Importance of surrounding structures

Close proximity of upper two-thirds of esophagus to thoracic duct increases risk of thoracic duct injury in middle and upper mediastinal dissection of esophagus; thus, careful dissection should be performed in this area.

At a level of diaphragmatic hiatus, a soft areolar tissue connects esophagus to diaphragmatic cruses, and a slight concave area called "portal concavity" allows formation of a hiatal hernia.

The area between aortic arch and esophagus is comprised of aorticoesophagial muscle fibers that include large vessels; dissection of this area is fairly simple, except in the case of tumor invasion. If tumoral invasion occurs among these large vessels, removal is challenging and dangerous.

Upper mediastinum becomes narrower above aortic arch, and esophageal tumors can easily infiltrate left recurrent laryngeal nerve and respiratory system; however, aortic arch and azygos vein block tumors in these areas to infiltrate lower parts of mediastinum.

Lower parts of thoracic esophagus are surrounded by soft areolar tissue. Here esophagus is not touching adjacent organs and descends slightly away from the vertebral column, making dissection and resection easier and tumor infiltration more difficult in this area.

Two weak areas in esophagus that can be vulnerable to pulsing diverticula are upper and lower parts of a cricoid muscle. In addition, another weak area is located on left posterior esophageal wall, very close to diaphragmatic hiatus, spontaneous rupture of esophagus can occur [2, 10].

3.3. Abdominal esophagus

Abdominal esophagus is 1–2.5 cm long and is topographically located at 11thvertebral plane posteriorly. The plane passes through 7th rib cartilage and sternum anteriorly. It passes through esophageal hiatus of diaphragm, which is comprised of muscular fibers of right crus. The anterior side is longer than posterior side of esophagus because diaphragmatic crura are oblique. Anterior and lateral sides are partially covered by visceral peritoneum, and posterior side is nonperitoneal side. Three ligaments connect esophagus to spleen, liver, and diaphragm. They are hepatogastric ligament, gastrosplenic ligament, and gastrophrenic ligament.

3.3.1. Surrounding structures

Following structures are located near abdominal esophagus: posterior side segment of two-thirds of liver, left vagus nerve and esophageal plexus anteriorly, left and right crus of diaphragm, aorta and left inferior phrenic artery posteriorly, caudate lobe of liver at the right side, and fundus of stomach at left side.

Esophageal hiatus is located on right side of midline and is 2 cm in diameter. Topographically, it is located at 10th vertebral plane. Before reaching hiatus, esophagus dilatates at a place called "epithetic ampulla" that is delaying point of morsel when swallowing during radiologic examinations.

Esophagus ends at a place called "cardia of stomach." Right side of esophagus continues as lesser curvate of stomach, and left side angles with greater curvate of stomach, forming "angle of Hiss." A mucosal tongue that descends into stomach is called "Gubaroff valvula." Hiss angle and Gubaroff valvula are important in antireflux mechanism [11].

Phrenoeosophagial ligament is primary part of antireflux mechanism that includes Gubaroff valvula and angle of Hiss (**Figure 5**). This ligament consists of subpleural fascia, pleura,

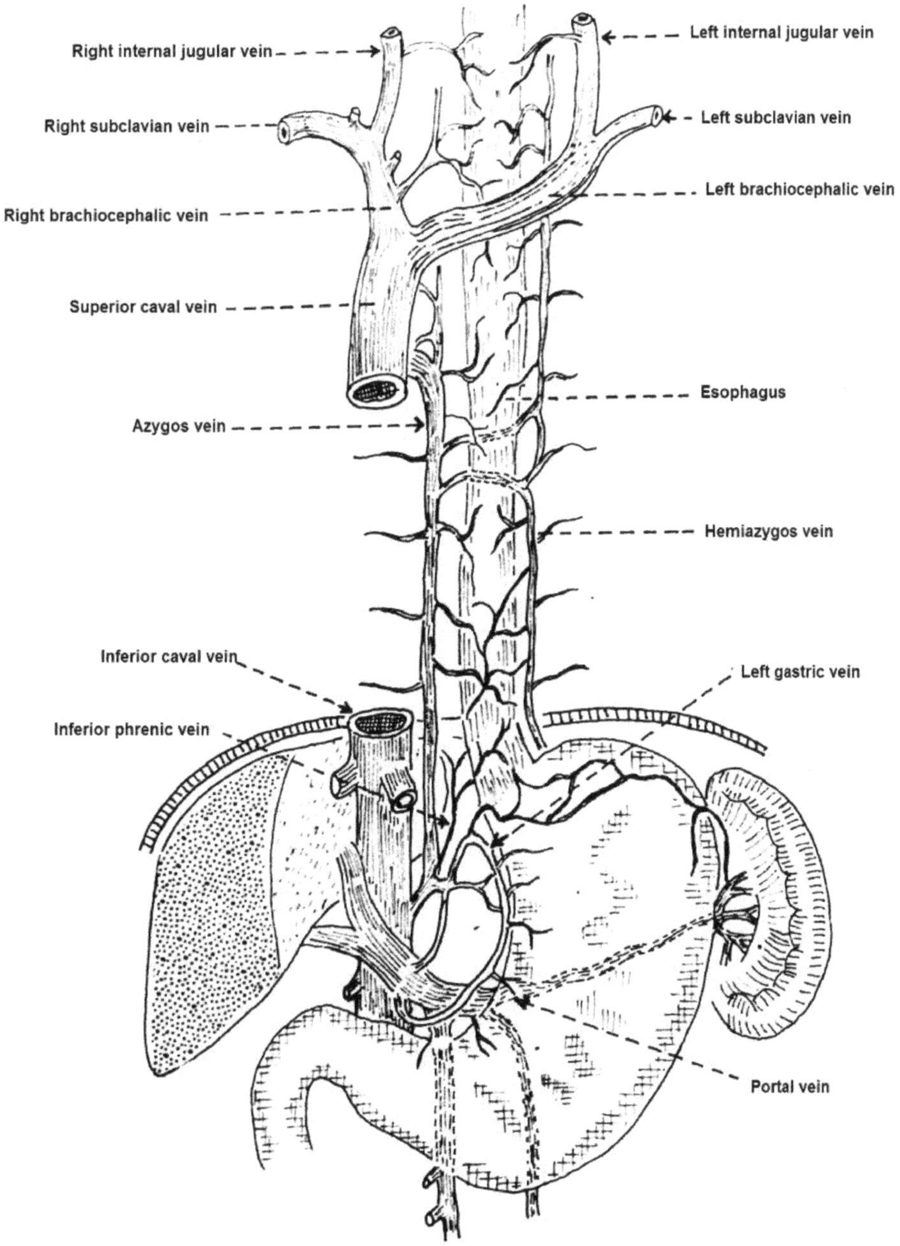

Figure 5. Veins of Esophagus.

phrenoesophageal fascia, and transverse fascia of abdomen and peritoneum. Fibers of this ligament that reach upward are called "Juvara fibers"; downward fibers are called "Rouget fibers." Phrenoesophageal ligament resists vigorous abdominal pressure that pushes stomach to intrathoracic cavity, but it allows esophagus to move upward and downward while swallowing. This ligament makes gastroesophageal junction both flexible and tight [12, 13].

4. Connections that stabilize esophagus

Fibrotic membrane that attaches esophagus to vertebral column is called "Bouteiller membrane." This membrane is tight over diaphragmatic hiatus and limits extreme movements of esophagus. However, under hiatus, membrane is loose and long. Phrenogastric ligament lies between diaphragm and cardia of stomach and both vagus nerves. Vagus nerves hang esophagus to thoracic cavity; thus, cutting vagus nerves elongates esophagus 4–5 cm [2].

4.1. Arteries of esophagus

Inferior thyroid artery provides primary arterial flow to the cervical esophagus, and subclavian artery, main carotid artery, vertebral arteries, ascendant pharyngeal artery, superficial cervical artery, and costocervical trunk are other arterial blood flow providers to cervical esophagus. Thoracic portion of esophagus takes blood flow from aorta, bronchial arteries, and right intercostal arteries. The abdominal esophagus is fed by left gastric artery, short gastric arteries, and descending branch of left phrenic artery. Inferior thyroid artery supplies arterial blood flow to cervical portion of esophagus (**Figure 6**). An excessively low resection of cervical esophagus causes devascularization to this area. In addition, aggressive resection and mobilization or laceration of bronchial artery, or cutting recurrent branches of left gastric artery and inferior phrenic artery causes devascularization at level of tracheal carina. Esophageal arterial blood flow is extremely rich and adequate for anastomosis, but a poor blood supply or careless or over aggressive dissection can cause anastomotic leakage in esophagus [14–16].

4.2. Veins of esophagus

Venous system of esophagus begins at submucosal plexus, which perforates muscular layer and empties into azygos system. Cervical portions of venous drainage empty into inferior thyroid veins. Thoracic portion's venous drainage empties into azygos vein, right brachiocephalic vein and, rarely, vertebral veins on right side, and hemiazygos vein, left brachiocephalic vein and, rarely, vertebral veins on left side. Venous drainage of abdominal portions empties primarily into left gastric veins. Other veins that drain esophageal venous plexus are short gastric veins, splenic vein, left gastroepiploic vein, and branches of an inferior phrenic vein. Lower esophageal veins connect to superior caval venous system by azygos and hemiazygos veins with multiple shunts, and other multiple shunts are located between inferior caval system and lower esophagus (**Figure 7**). Retrograde flow of esophageal venous system causes venous dilatation and varices, and these varices can cause fatal bleeding [2, 14, 17].

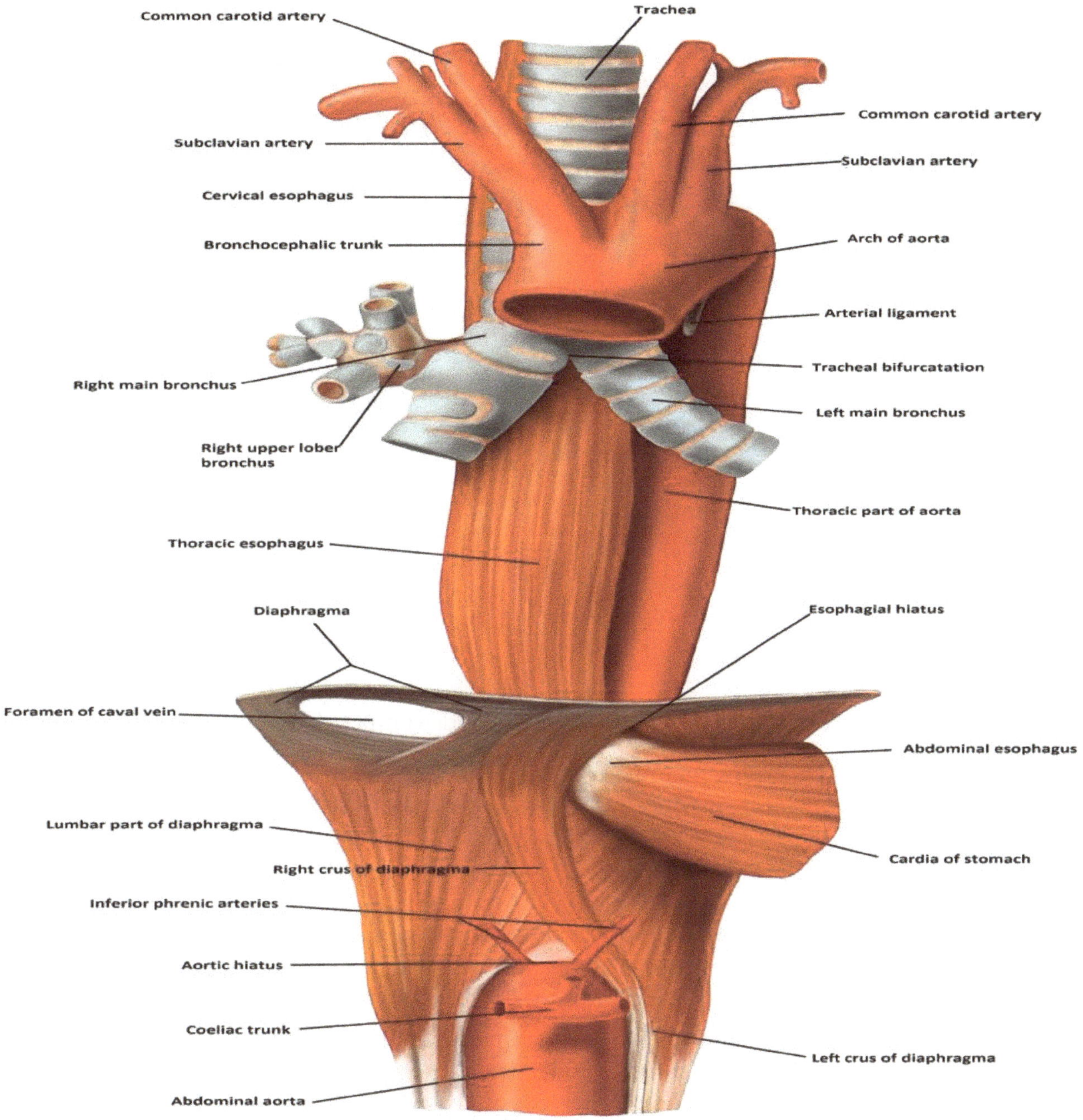

Figure 6. Relation among esophagus, diaphragm, and aorta (with permission from Turkish Surgery Association).

4.3. Lymphatics of esophagus

Lymphatics are located in every layer of esophagus, but primarily at lamina propria, forming a giant network system. Cervical lymphatics empty internal jugular lymph nodes and upper tracheal lymph nodes. An internal jugular lymphatic system that forms deeper cervical lymphatic system connects with lymphatic duct at right side and thoracic duct at left side.

Lymphatics of thoracic esophagus empty posterior parietal, diaphragmatic, tracheal, tracheobronchial, retrocardiac, and infracardiac lymph nodes.

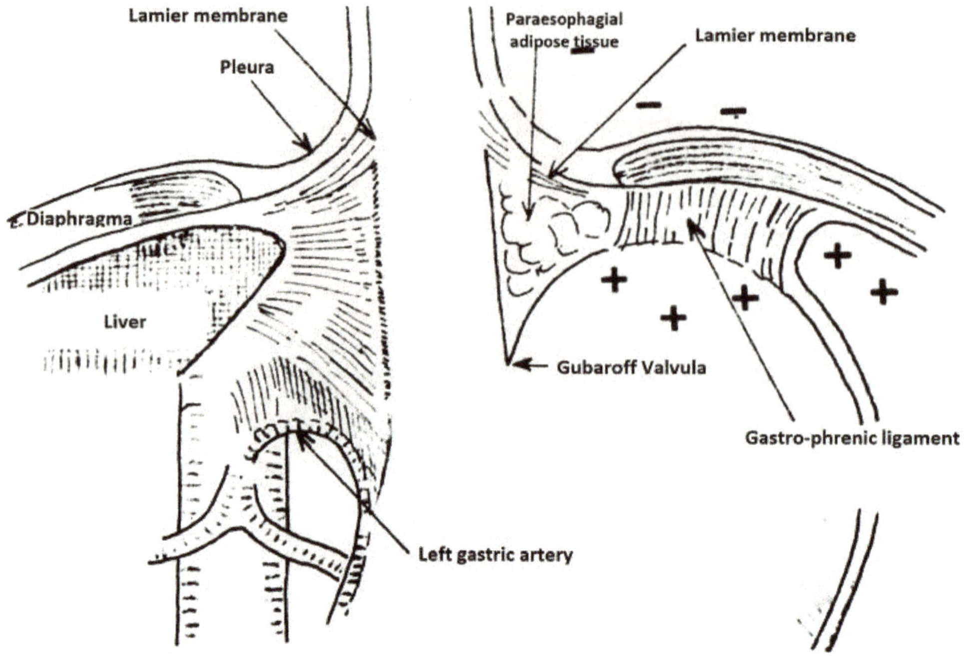

Figure 7. Anti-reflux mechanism of esophagus.

Abdominal parts of lymphatic system empty left gastric, paracardiac lymph nodes, and all these nodes connect to coeliac lymph nodes. Coeliac lymph nodes empty cisterna chyli or thoracic duct.

Posterior parietal lymph nodes include posterior mediastinal and intercostal lymph nodes and connect with thoracic duct or right lymphatic duct. Only posterior part of diaphragmatic lymph nodes are connected to esophageal lymphatic system, and these lymph nodes empty to posterior parietal lymph nodes.

Tracheal or paratracheal lymph nodes are located on two sides of trachea, and tracheobronchial lymph nodes are located around bifurcation of trachea. Tuberculosis, which causes necrosis and fibrosis of tracheobronchial lymph nodes, forms traction diverticula of esophagus. These two lymphatic systems form a broch mediastinal lymphatic chain that empties to thoracic duct or right lymphatic duct (**Figure 8**) [18, 19].

4.4. Innervation of esophagus:

Parasympathetic and sympathetic nerves form esophageal innervation, carrying stimuli to esophageal muscles, glands, veins, and arteries.

4.4.1. Parasymphatic innervation

Parasympathatic fibers that innervate pharynx and upper part of esophagus come from ambiguous nuclei of brain. Esophageal innervation is primarily accomplished by vagus nerves, which end at dorsal vagal nuclei of brain. Cervical esophagus takes thin fibers from both recurrent laryngeal nerves. Both left and right recurrent laryngeal nerves arise from vagus nerves, but on left side, a recurrent laryngeal nerve is closer to aortic arch. On right side,

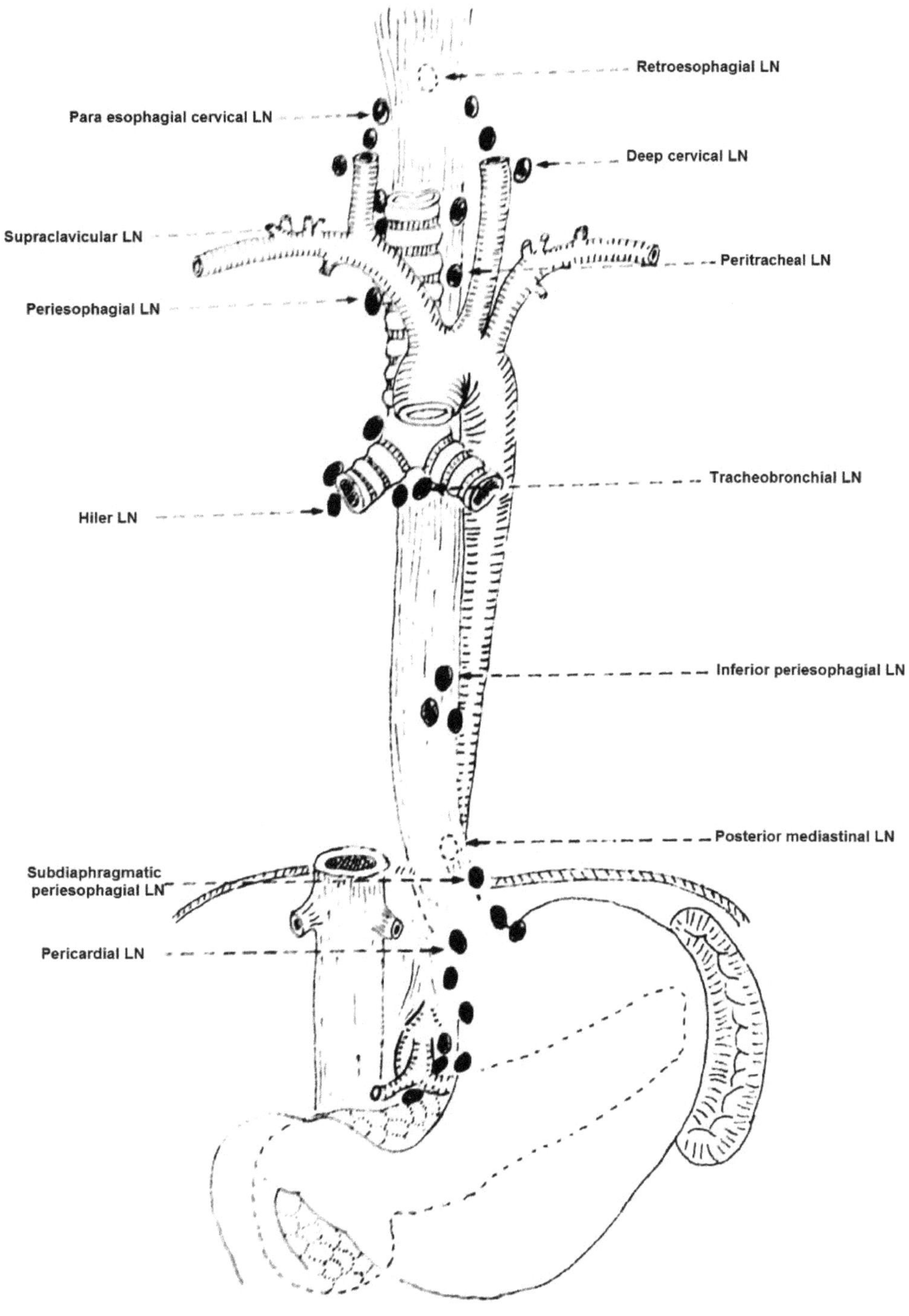

Figure 8. Lymphatics of esophagus.

it is closer to subclavian artery. Finally, left and right recurrent laryngeal nerves run in sulcus between trachea and esophagus. The thoracic esophagus is primarily innervated by vagus nerves, but the upper part of thoracic esophagus takes some fibers from left recurrent laryngeal nerve. Vagus nerve fibers form two to four branches under tracheal bifurcation, and these nerve branches are located on anterior face of esophagus at level of posterior mediastinum. Near esophageal hiatus, these nerve branches unite and form two vagal trunks of esophagus.

Variation of vagal trunks is important during vagotomy. A surgeon should be aware of these variations and be careful because more than one branch can be found in anterior or posterior vagal trunk or both.

4.4.2. Sympathetic innervation

The upper part of esophagus is innervated by pharyngeal plexus, which is fed by upper cervical ganglions, middle cervical ganglions, and sympathetic trunks of vertebral ganglions while running downward. Superior parts of the thoracic esophagus are innervated by stellate ganglion and subclavian ansa. Lower parts of thoracic esophagus are innervated by greater splanchnic nerves that end at coeliac plexus. Left greater splanchnic nerve and right inferior phrenic nerve innervate abdominal esophagus [20, 21].

Author details

Murat Ferhat Ferhatoglu* and Taner Kıvılcım

*Address all correspondence to: erhatferhatoglu@gmail.com

General Surgery Department, Okan University, Istanbul, Turkey

References

[1] Oezcelik A, DeMeester SR. General anatomy of the esophagus. Thoracic Surgery Clinics of North America. 2011;**21**:289-297

[2] Minkari T, Ünal G. Surgical anatomy of esophagus. In: Minkari T, editor. Surgery of Esophagus. 1st ed. Istanbul: Ceylan Publising; 1980. pp. 1-16

[3] Kıyıcı M. Esophagus. In: Kıyıcı M, editor. Atlas of Clinical Gastrointestinal Endoscopy. 1st ed. Istanbul: Nobel Tıp Kitapevleri Ltd, Şti; 2011. pp. 21-22

[4] Floch NR. Topographic relations of rsophagus. In: Floch MH, editor. Netter's Gastroenterology. 2nd ed. Philadelphia: Elsevier Saunders; 2010. pp. 3-4

[5] Lee L. Digestive system. In: Lee L, editor. Lippincott's Pocket Histology. 1st ed. Philadelphia: Lippincott Williams & Wilkins, a Wolters Kluwer; 2014. pp. 137-138

[6] Floch NR. Histology of esophagus. In: Floch MH, editor. Netter's Gastroenterology. 2nd ed. Philadelphia: Elsevier Saunders; 2010. pp. 15-16

[7] Pope CE 2nd. The esophagus: 1967 to 1969. I. Gastroenterology. 1970;**59**(3):460-476

[8] McWay CB, Anson BJ. Anterior regions of neck. In: McWay CB, Anson BJ, editors. Surgical Anatomy. 5th ed. Philadelphia: Saunders Co; 1971. pp. 271-275

[9] Skandalakis JE, Colborn GL, Weidman TA. Surgical anatomy: The Embryologic and Anatomic Basis of Modern Surgery. Vol. 1. Athens (Greece): Paschalidis Medical Publications; 2004

[10] Anadol Z. Anatomy of upper gastrointestinal system endoscopy. In: Karahan Ö, Cingi A editors. Gastrointestinal System Endoscopy. 1st ed. Ankara: Turkish Surgical Association; 2016. pp. 81-83

[11] Barr H, Almond LM. Abdominal esophagus and stomach. In: Standring S, editor. Gray's Anatomy, The Anatomical Basis of Clinical Practice. 41st ed. Philadelphia: Elsevier; 2016. pp. 1111-1112

[12] Pellegrini CA, Way LW. Esophagus and diaphragm. In: Way LW, editor. Current Surgical Diagnosis and Treatment. Norwalk, CT: Stamford Appleton & Lange; 1994. pp. 841-853

[13] Ugalde PA, Pereira ST, et al. Correlative anatomy for esophagus. Thoracic Surgery Clinics of North America. 2011;**21**:307-317

[14] Moore KL, Dalley FA, Agur AMR. Esophagus. In: Moore, editor. Clinically Orianted Anatomy. 7th ed. Philadelphia: Lippincott Williams & Wilkins, a Wolters Kluwer; 2014. pp. 229-230

[15] Floch NR. Arteriel blood supply of esophagus. In: Floch MH, editor. Netter's Gastroenterology. 2nd ed. Philadelphia: Elsevier Saunders; 2010. pp. 7-8

[16] Swigart LL, Siekert RG, et al. The esophageal arteries: An anatomic study of 150 specimens. Surgery, Gynecology & Obstetrics. 1950;**90**:234-243

[17] Patti MG, Gantert W, Way LW. Surgery of the esophagus: Anatomy and physiology. Surgical Clinics of North America.1997;**77**(5):959-970

[18] Sisic L, Blank S, Weichert W, Jager D, Springfeld C, et al. Prognostic impact of lymph node involvement and the extent of lymphadenectomy (LAD) in adenocarcinoma of the esophagogastric junction (AEG). Langenbeck's Archives of Surgery. 2013;**398**:973-998

[19] Tong D, Law S. Extended lymphadenectomy in esophageal cancer is crucial. World Journal of Surgery. 2013;**37**:1751-1756

[20] Floch NR. Innervation of the Esophagus: Parasympathetic and Sympathetic. In: Floch MH editor. Netter's Gastroenterology. 2nd ed. Philadelphia: Elsevier Saunders; 2010. pp. 12-13

[21] Castell DO. Esophageal motility testing. In: Castell DO, Richter JE, Boag D, editors. Anatomy and Physiology of the Esophagus and Its Sphincters. New York: Elsevier Science; 1987. pp. 13-27

10

Lymph Node Dissection along the Recurrent Laryngeal Nerve in Video-Assisted Thoracoscopic Surgery (VATS-E) for Esophageal Squamous Cell Carcinoma

Hiroshi Makino, Hiroshi Yoshida and Eiji Uchida

Abstract

Esophageal carcinoma is the ninth most common cancer in the world, which is frequently seen in Asia and east Africa. Around 80% of all cases occurred in less-developed regions. Two major histological subtypes of esophageal carcinoma, adenocarcinoma and squamous cell carcinoma, are known to differ greatly in terms of risk factor, epidemiology, male to female ratios, and incidence. Lymph node metastasis is a crucial factor in staging and prognosis is associated with surgical treatment and a major lymphatic chain into the neck. Esophageal adenocarcinoma (EAC) is mainly detected at the lower third of the thoracic esophagus or esophago-gastric-junction (EGJ) and metastasizes mainly to lymph nodes of the lesser sac, celiac regions and lower mediastinal. Esophageal squamous cell carcinoma (ESCC) has a predilection for metastasis to the lymph nodes of the cervical region including recurrent laryngeal nerve (RLN) on both sides. Lymph node dissection is vital yet difficult, left-side lymph node dissection especially requires expertise. There are some reports on lymph node dissection in the prone position by video-assisted thoracoscopic surgery of the esophagus (VATS-E) along the left RLN in Japan and China. We also introduce a stripping method for lymph node dissection in this site.

Keywords: recurrent laryngeal nerve, lymph node dissection, video-assisted thoracoscopic surgery (VATS-E)

1. Introduction

Esophageal carcinoma is strongly invasive and is accompanied by numerous malignant tumors. It is mainly seen in Asia and East Africa. In the eastern countries, especially in Japan, extended lymph node dissection, including the abdominal, upper, middle, lower mediastinal, and occasionally cervical lymph nodes, is suggested as a standard surgical method because systematic dissection of metastatic lymph nodes is thought to improve survival and lead to cure.

Consequently, recommending complete lymphadenectomy of the upper mediastinum is an essential component in radical esophagectomy for esophageal squamous cell carcinoma (ESCC). Three-field lymphadenectomy (3FL) is the ultimate surgical procedure in the pursuit of complete lymph node dissection for thoracic esophageal cancer. However, lymph node dissection along the recurrent laryngeal nerve (RLN) is difficult because severance of nerves by electrical devices can easily lead to paralysis [1, 2].

The prone position provides better visualization in the subaortic arch and subcarinal and supraphrenic regions, but the working space in the left upper mediastinum for dissecting the lymph nodes along the left recurrent laryngeal nerve is limited. Some investigators, including us, have shown how to obtain a good operative field in the upper mediastinum for lymph adenectomy. Osugi reported that tracheobronchus must be retracted ventrally to visualize the left side of the trachea and developed the retractor that provides exposure of the entire mediastinum and esophagus in left lateral position [3]. In eastern countries, surgeons also describe lymphadenectomy along the left recurrent laryngeal nerve, but few surgeons in western countries have discussed lymphadenectomy of esophageal adenocarcinoma (EAC). Here, we describe differences in lymph node metastasis between ESCC and EAC and procedures for lymph node dissection along the recurrent laryngeal nerve in ESCC.

2. Etiological differences between esophageal squamous cell carcinoma (ESCC) and esophageal adenocarcinoma (EAC)

Esophageal carcinoma is seen in two major histological subtypes: adenocarcinoma and squamous cell carcinoma (SCC). These subtypes are very different in terms of risk factors and epidemiology. According to GLOBOCAN 2012, there were an estimated 400,000 cases of ESCC and 50,000 cases of EAC of the esophagus in 2012 worldwide [4].

2.1. Global incidence of ESCC

In 2012, the global incidence of ESCC was 5.2 per 100,000 people. Most affected regions were located in Eastern and South-East Asia, followed by sub-Saharan Africa and Central Asia [4]. About 80% of global ESCC cases occur in Central and South-East Asian regions. China alone provided more than 50% of the global cases. Areas of high incidence of ESCC have been identified in Northern Iran, Central Asia, and China (together forming the so-called "esophageal cancer belt") as well as parts of Eastern Africa. ESCC is more common and the rate of ESCC is about 95% in Japan [3].

2.2. Risk factor of ESCC

Generally, chronic inflammation of the esophageal mucosa is postulated to increase the risk of ESCC. Two major risk factors are smoking and alcohol consumption, which have been found to account for more than 75% of all SCC cases in high-income countries [5]. On the other hand, frequent consumption of extremely hot beverages is a common risk factor for ESCC in less-developed regions [4]. Consumption of hot mate drinks in Latin America and hot beverages in Southern China are associated with the risk of ESCC [4, 5].

In Iran, opium use has been found to increase mortality from esophageal cancer by 50%. High-incidence areas in Africa suggest that smoking, occupational exposures and nutritional deficiencies may be responsible for the high burden of ESCC [4].

Alcohol drinking is a well-established risk factor for esophageal cancer. International Agency for Research on Cancer (IARC) referred to acetaldehyde, an oxidative metabolite of ethanol, as a potential causative agent behind alcohol-induced carcinogenesis based on evidence of interaction between alcohol consumption and acetaldehyde dehydrogenase (ALDH2) enzyme gene polymorphisms [6, 7]. Oze et al. showed that acetaldehyde dehydrogenase Glu504Lys polymorphism had strong effect modification with alcohol drinking and concluded that there is convincing evidence that alcohol drinking increases the risk of esophageal cancer in the Japanese population [8]. Half of the Japanese population is heterozygous or homozygous for the *2 allele of ALDH2, showing respectively, peak blood acetaldehyde concentrations in post-alcohol consumption 6- and 19-fold higher than homozygous wide-type individuals [9]. As a result, ALDH2*2/*2 homozygous carriers show facial flushing and nausea after alcohol consumption that deters them from drinking, whereas heterozygotes exhibit less severe reactions [9]. Fang et al. indicated that individuals heterozygous for the *2 variant allele of aldehyde dehydrogenase 2 (ALDH2*1/*2) frequently detected in Asia had an increased risk of esophageal cancer, especially among heavy drinkers, because inactive ALDH2 fails to metabolize acetaldehyde rapidly, leading to excessive accumulation of acetaldehyde in blood and repeated high exposure to acetaldehyde after drinking. Drinking clearly modifies the effect of ALDH2 on esophageal cancer risk in Asians [6].

2.3. Global incidence of EAC

The global incidence of EAC is 0.7 per 100,000 people. Highest incidence rates by region were found in Northern and Western Europe, North America, and Oceania [4]. On the national level, the highest rates were seen in the UK, the Netherlands, Ireland, Iceland, and New Zealand. The burden of AC is the highest in Northern and Western Europe, North America, and Oceania, accounting for 46% of all global AC cases [4, 10, 11].

2.4. Risk factor of EAC

The strongest known risk factor for EAC is gastroesophageal reflux disease and its more severe manifestation, Barrett's esophagus (BE). Obesity promotes the development of gastroesophageal reflux and also acts as an independent risk factor for EAC.

In North America and Northern and Western Europe, prevalence of *Helicobacter pylori* (H pylori) infection is among the lowest and incidence of EAC is higher [4, 10, 11].

Helicobacter pylori (H pylori) lowers gastric acid secretion and decreases gastric esophageal reflux [10, 11]. In more recent years, prevalence of the latter has leveled out in high-prevalence countries such as the Netherlands and the UK [4].

3. Clinical difference between EAC and ESCC

3.1. Location of ESCC and EAC

In 50–60% of cases, ESCC is located in the middle third thoracic esophagus in Thailand, Iran, and Japan [3, 12, 13, 14]. About 60% of SCCs is also located in the middle third of the esophagus in Iran. Several studies have found that ESCC was most commonly located in the lower third of the esophagus, such as studies conducted in Ghana [15].

In 80% of cases, EAC is located at the gastroesophageal junction (GEJ) and 20% in the lower third thoracic esophagus. This entity is capable of producing EAC directly or, more commonly, through an intermediate pre-neoplastic lesion or Barrett's esophagus (BE). BE is a pre-malignant lesion that develops in 6–14% of patients with Gastroesohageal reflux disease (GERD), of which approximately 0.5–1% will develop EAC [10, 11]. Increased incidence of BE in the past 30 years correlates with an increased incidence of EAC during the same period.

4. Clinical difference of lymph node metastasis between ESCC and EAC

4.1. Lymph node metastasis of ESCC

Udagawa et al. showed that it was necessary to dissect the cervical lymph nodes, particularly for tumors located in the upper and middle thoracic esophagus [2]. Bilateral cervical paraesophageal node dissection is predominantly effective and the inclusion of these stations in the regional lymph nodes is justified in the 7th TNM classification. The lower jugular or supraclavicular region lymph nodes are also important. Abdominal lymph node dissection is also effective, but the effectiveness is limited in upper esophageal cancer. The statistical efficacy index (EI) of individual lymph node stations according to the main tumor location, a more precise modification of the range of lymph node dissection is possible. Although mediastinal nodes are important in general, not all are located in the esophageal drainage area. Some specific stations such as pretracheal, left tracheobronchial, and supradiaphragmatic show least efficacy by dissection. The mediastinal node stations can be re-arranged such as recurrent laryngeal, paraesophageal, posterior mediastinal, subcarinal, and subbronchial in order, according to EI. The number of metastatic lymph nodes may be a better prognostic factor than Japanese N grading. The Japanese N-grouping seems to be more efficient for predicting of the radical and safe operation. It is difficult to detect lymph node metastasis clinically. Japanese N-grouping may be also more available in stage assessment because a single obvious distant lymph node metastasis in Japanese N-group can correctly identify a higher staging. Japanese Surgeons are afraid that discussion about lymph node dissection with precision is no longer possible if meticulous node grouping based on detailed data of lymph node stations is once discontinued.

Ma et al. stated that 3FL improves overall survival rate but has more complications. Because of the high heterogeneity among outcomes, definite conclusions are difficult to draw [16].

4.2. Lymph node metastasis of EAC

Sepesi et al. reported 72% of patients presented with clinically involved lymph nodes showed metastasis in the lesser sac (perigastric/perihepatic) [17]. However, 11% of patients had metastatic lymph nodes located at the celiac artery, and 10% had nodal disease in the paratracheal region. Ninety-eight patients demonstrated clinical metastatic involvement in one or two nodal basins (example: perigastric and paratracheal); only about 2% of patients presented nodal disease in three nodal basins. Feith et al. reported the prevalence and number of lymph node metastases according to pT category in patients with primary resected Barrett's carcinoma. A strong correlation between the pT category and the presence and the number of lymph node metastases was detected [18]. Lymph node metastases in more than 95%of the patients was detected in the lower posterior mediastinum, in the bilateral paracardiac region, or in the region of lesser curvature and left gastric artery of the abdomen. Prevalence of lymph node metastases at the various topographic locations in relation to the T category of the underlying Barrett's carcinoma is shown. As T category increases, prevalence of regional lymph node metastases also markedly increases. Lymph node metastases to more distant locations, such as the tracheal bifurcation region, the proximal mediastinum, or celiac axis, lagged behind and were common only in patients with more advanced primary tumors. This suggests that lymphatic spread occurs in an orderly fashion. Patients who had many lymph nodes metastasis had distant lymph node metastasis in the upper mediastinum and tracheal bifurcation area that can be reached by a transthoracic approach [19]. According to an increasing number of lymph nodes metastasis, positive lymph node metastasis in the upper mediastinum and carinal region also increased. Prevalence of lymph node metastases at the celiac axis was also detected with increasing number of lymph nodes metastasis. There was significantly frequent lymph nodes metastasis in the upper mediastinal, carinal or celiac regions among patients with more than three positive regional nodes. Overall, skipping of regional lymph node stations, positive distant nodes in the absence of positive regional nodes, was seen in less than 5% of the patients.

Yamashita et al. reported clinical records of 2807 EGJ carcinoma patients without preoperative therapy in Japan [20]. There are obvious unbalances in terms of lymph node dissection rate according to histology and the main tumor location. Lymph nodes metastasis frequently involved abdominal lymph nodes. Lymph nodes at the right and left cardia, lesser curvature and along the left gastric artery were especially metastasized. Lymph nodes along the greater curvature of the stomach were not frequently metastatic, and advantage of dissection seemed unlikely. Lower mediastinal node dissection may contribute to improved survival for patients with esophagus-predominant EGJ carcinoma. However, due to low dissection rates for nodes of the middle and upper mediastinum, no conclusive results have been obtained regarding the optimal extent of nodal dissection in this region.

5. Lymph node metastasis along the recurrent laryngeal nerve

Extensive lymphadenectomy with esophagectomy for esophageal carcinoma improves the prognosis in Japan. In particular, lymph nodes along the RLN are considered as significantly important lymph nodes those are recommended to be completely dissected. However, lymph node along the RLN dissection complicates high morbidity and mortality. Udagawa et al. showed lymph node metastasis along the rt. RLN and cervical paraesophageal at a rate of 31.9, 22.2%, 19, 13.9%, and 14.7, 12.4% of upper, middle, and lower thoracic esophagus, respectively. Lymph node metastasis along the lt. RLN and cervical paraesophageal was found at a rate of 19.1, 20.1%, 14.1, 8.3%, and 8.1, 5% of upper, middle, and lower thoracic esophagus in Japan, respectively [2]. Ye et al. reported that the recurrent laryngeal nerve lymph node metastasis from esophageal carcinoma is detected at the rate of 34.2% in China [21]. Lymph node metastasis along the recurrent laryngeal nerve was detected, and the rate of lymph node metastasis was 23.4%. The rate of rt. RLN lymph node metastasis was 20.8%, which was slightly higher than the rate of lt. RLN lymph node metastasis which had a rate of 15.8%.

5.1. ESCC

In ESCC, lymph node metastasis is possible to occur in the neck, mediastinum, and abdomen. The location of RLN lymph node is from the upper mediastinum and to the cervical region, where lymph node metastasis is frequently detected in thoracic ESCC. Early, initial and micro metastasis of ESCC often occur and RLN lymph node metastasis has been regarded as an indication for three-field lymphadenectomy in the surgical treatment of ESCC. More importantly, RLN metastasis has been shown to be a strong predictor of poor prognosis in ESCC.

There are many reports about lymph node metastasis along the recurrent laryngeal nerve in Asia. In Japan, Igaki et al. reported that cervical or celiac lymph node metastasis in patients with carcinomas of the lower thoracic esophagus should be distinguished from pathologic M1 status in the UICC-TNM staging system [1].

5.2. EAC

Giacopuzzi et al. reported that in Siewert type I tumors, when standard mediastinal lymphadenectomy is performed, about half of the node-positive patients show positive nodes in mediastinal stations [22]. Specifically, upper and mid mediastinal lymph node metastases (right paratracheal, subcarinal, aortopulmonary window) were reported in up to 25% of patients. When the few studies in which cervical nodes are also removed are considered, a non-negligible incidence of metastases is detectable, but, due to the scarcity of available data and the higher complication rate of three-field dissection, this is not currently thought to be relevant in clinical practice. Mediastinal nodes are involved in about 30% of Siewert type II cases. Although most of the positive nodes occur at lower stations, the rate of metastasis detected in the upper-mid mediastinum after transthoracic esophagectomy ranges between 8 and 22% [22].

6. Lymph node dissection along the recurrent laryngeal nerve

6.1. ESCC

Surgeons in Asia, where the rate of ESCC is higher, perform lymphadenectomy along the recurrent laryngeal nerve. Udagawa et al. reported that cervical lymph node dissection had high efficacy index (EI) in upper and middle thoracic esophageal cancer but a low EI in lower esophageal cancer. Cervical lymphadenectomy for lower esophageal cancer showed some but limited efficacy only in cervical paraesophageal stations [2]. Three-field lymph node dissection may be indicated even for patients with clinical Stage I ESCC requiring surgical intervention because this surgical procedure offers possible cure by removing unsuspected lymph node metastasis. Altorki et al. also mentioned that three-field lymph node dissection with esophagectomy can involve with a low mortality and reasonable morbidity. Unsuspected metastases to the lymph nodes along the RLN and cervical region are present in 36% of patients in spite of histological tumor type or tumor location of the esophagus [23].

Osugi et al. reported that video-assisted thoracoscopic surgery (VATS), a less invasive method that preserves curability, provides comparable results to open radical esophagectomy. Palanivelu et al. demonstrated the lymph node dissection along the recurrent laryngeal nerve in prone position to be effective [24].

6.2. EAC

Lagergren et al. indicated that the extent of lymphadenectomy during surgery for esophageal carcinomas which include 83.5% adenocarcinoma may not influence 5-year all-cause or disease-specific survival [25]. These results challenge current clinical guidelines.

Feith et al. showed that a transthoracic approach followed by an extended lymph node dissection in the upper mediastinum is not recommended in patients with adenocarcinoma of the distal esophagus. Conservative surgical resection due to the virtual absence of lymph node metastasis in the upper mediastinum can cure patients with high-grade dysplasia and pT1a carcinoma. In addition systematic lymph node dissection of the lower posterior mediastinum and upper abdominal compartment can improve the prognosis in patients with more advanced tumors and a limited number of regional lymph node metastases. A transmediastinal approach with a wide splitting of the esophageal hiatus can achieve this radical lymph node dissection in the lower posterior mediastinum and upper abdominal compartment. Multimodal treatment protocols including chemotherapy and irradiation on systemic therapy are considered to be more appropriate for patients with more extensive lymph node metastases [25].

Cuscheri et al. recommended placing the patient prone to clear the posterior mediastinum, thus avoiding lung compression, but did not demonstrate lymph node dissection along the recurrent laryngeal nerve in EAC patients [26].

6.3. Lymph node dissection along the rt. recurrent laryngeal nerve

Thoracoscopic lymph node dissection along the right (rt.) recurrent laryngeal nerve has been more readily demonstrated by various authors. The rt. recurrent laryngeal nerve LN is removed as follows: the location of the right vagal nerve and the right inferior subclavian artery are confirmed. The airway behind the mediastinal pleura is opened to expose the right subclavian artery. The rt. recurrent laryngeal nerve is separated from the right vagal nerve followed by blunt dissection of the right recurrent laryngeal nerve through the vagus nerve trunk at the level of the right subclavian artery. We performed VATS-E in prone position (**Figure 1**). The surrounding LNs and fatty tissues are subsequently removed from the right recurrent laryngeal nerve [27] (**Figure 2**).

To reduce the risk of paralysis, an electric device is used to separate the nodes from the recurrent laryngeal nerve within 2 s [27].

6.4. Lymph node dissection along the lt. recurrent laryngeal nerve

Lymph nodes along RLNs are thought to be significantly involved by carcinoma cells as well as a main lymphatic chain to the neck, and complete dissection of these nodes is recommended. However, a lymphadenectomy, especially along the left RLN by thoracoscopic esophagectomy, is considered to be a burdensome step due to difficult operative exploration at the left upper mediastinum. To achieve a precise dissection of this portion, stable operative views and technical feasibility are necessary. Noshiro et al. mentioned that in their lymphadenectomy procedure along the left RLN, performing a thoracoscopic esophagectomy in the prone position had advantages compared to surgery in the left lateral decubitus position [27]. They introduced such details, during the procedure, the trachea is rolled back carefully and firmly to the right and ventrally by a grasper holding small gauze to explore the left aspect of the trachea and the left bronchus. The tissue, including the left RLN and lymph nodes, is

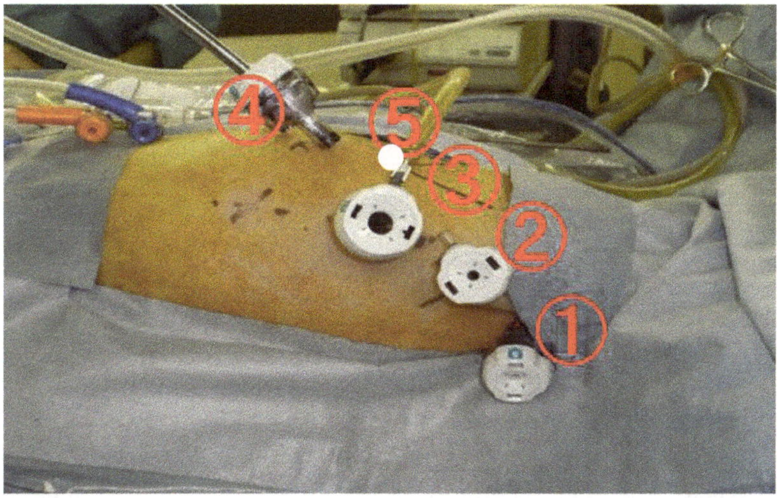

Figure 1. Port site in prone position. 3rd ICS, middle A.L.(1), 5th ICS, posterior A.L.(2), 7th ICS, posterior A.L.(3), 9th ICS, SSCL(4), 7th ICS, SSCL(5). ICS: inter costal space, AL: axillary line, SSCL: subscapular line.

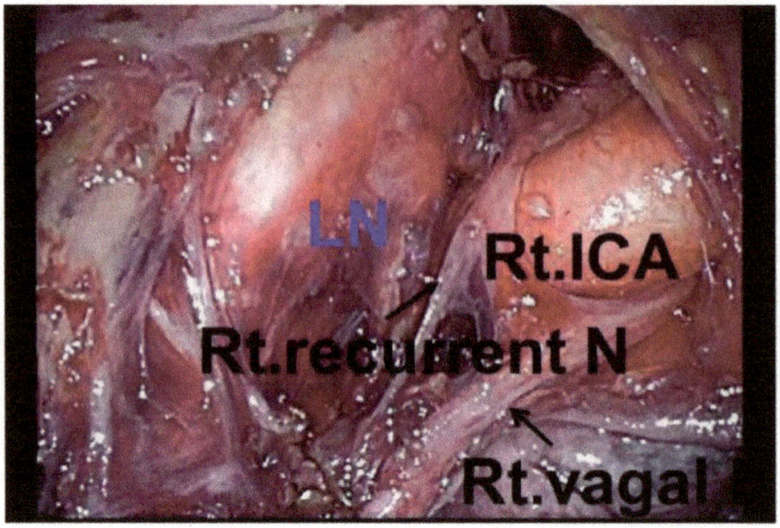

Figure 2. Lymph node dissection along the rt. RLN.

dissected sharply just along the trachea and the left bronchus to make a ventral border of dissection. Finally, the left RLN is sharply isolated from the explored tissue without using an electric device to avoid injury by electricity or heat, and the lymph nodes were consequently dissected in an en-bloc fashion accompanied with the divided thoracic duct.

However, dissecting the lymph nodes along the left RLN during VATS is challenging and requires significant technical skill, and there is limited working space in the left upper mediastinum for dissecting the lymph nodes along the left RLN and expertise in dissection is required. The technique of lymph node dissection along the lt. RLN in VATS-E has been demonstrated by some authors (**Table 1**).

We have previously reported a "Stripping method" to overcome this disadvantage in prone position [28]. Therefore, we considered stripping the esophagus toward the neck to remove the esophagus. Both the esophagus and stomach tube in the upper mediastinum are cut apart from the tumor by a linear stapler after isolating the esophagus (**Figure 3A**). The residual esophagus is stripped in the reverse direction and retracted toward the neck when the stomach

Method		Position
Stripping method	Makino et al. [28, 29]	Prone position
Bascule method	Oshikiri et al. [30]	Prone position
Suspension method	Xi et al. [31]	Prone position
Suspension method	Zheng et al. [32]	Prone position
LN dissection of hybrid position	Kaburagi et al. [33]	Hybrid position
Looping method	Lin et al. [34]	Prone position
Mediastinoscopic LN dissection	Fujiwara et al. [35]	Spine position

Table 1. Methods of lymph node dissection along the RLN.

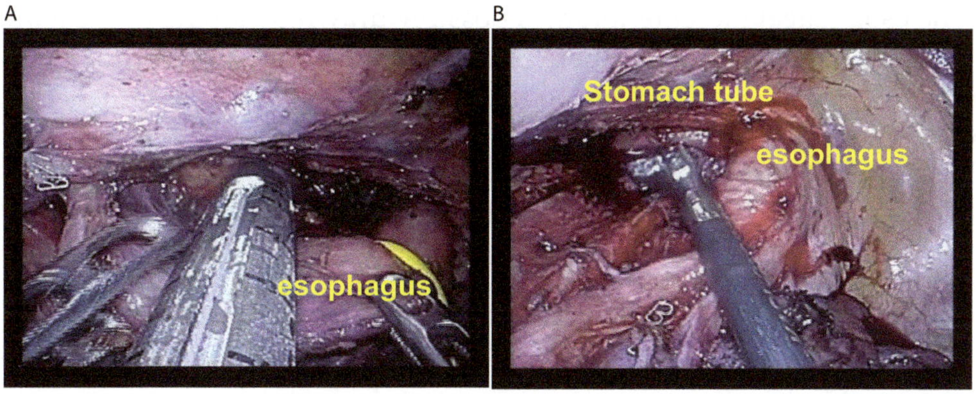

Figure 3. (A) Cutting both the esophagus and stomach tube. (B) Stripping by pulling the stomach tube.

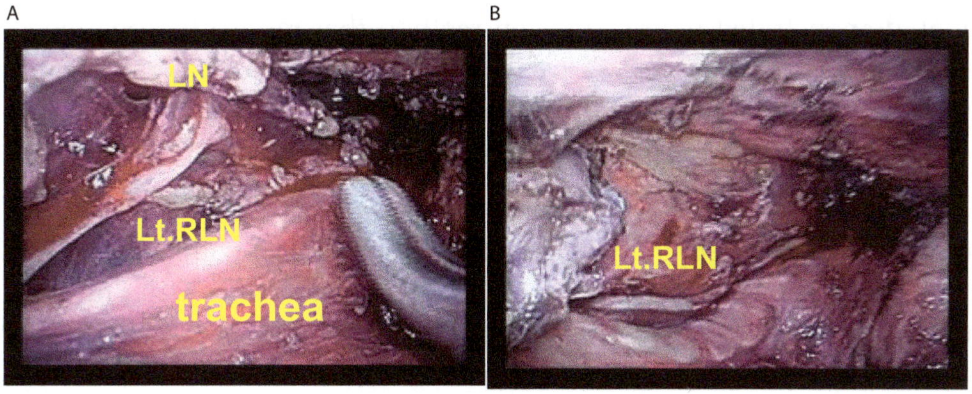

Figure 4. (A) Lymph node dissection along the lt. RLN. (B) After LN dissection along the lt. RLN.

tube is removed through the nose by anesthesiologist (**Figure 3B**). The wide operative field of left upper mediastinum is possible using this stripping technique. Lymph node dissection is performed after stripping the residual esophagus [28, 29] (**Figure 4A**). Moreover, working space is created by compressing the right main bronchus or retracting the trachea using a retractor. Lymph node and fat tissue are ablated from the left edge of the trachea, after which lymph node along the left RLN is dissected (**Figure 4B**). An electrical device is used to separate the node from the nerve, and endoscopic scissors and forceps are used during sharp dissection along the nerve. One hundred patients with esophageal carcinomas underwent VATS-E (27 in left lateral position and 73 in prone position). This original technique of lymphadenectomy along the left RLN has been performed in 54 patients in the prone position VATS-E. The rate of transient recurrent laryngeal nerve palsy is 17.2%, but permanent palsy is only 1.2% [29].

Oshikiri et al. developed the "Bascule method" where the proximal portion of the divided esophagus and tissue that includes the left RLN and lymph nodes are drawn through a gap between the vertebral body and the right scapula [30]. The membranous portion between the esophagus and the trachea like the esophageal mesenteriolum is ablated by traction of the tissue including the left RLN and lymph nodes along the left RLN by the proximal esophagus. The lymph node along the left RLN is distinguished from the left RLN and the tracheoesophageal artery on the posterior side of the left RLN can be detected and easily cut by this traction technique. The esophageal mesenteriolum is possibly drawn by taping of the entire length of the undivided esophagus. However, there is a limit to the amount of retraction. Division of the esophagus increases the amount of retraction possible, allowing for further drawing and development of the operative field.

Xi et al. and Zheng et al. showed an esophageal suspension method in scavenging peripheral lymph nodes of the lt. RLN. In this method, a traction line is used to suspend the incompletely stripped esophagus [31, 32]. Tissues including the left RLN and lymph nodes were extended, which improved operative exposure. Tissue is released in the area close to the trachea and left main bronchus in order to dissect the ventral and cranial borders. The left RLN and LNs are easily recognizable. The lt. RLN to the thyroid gland and the lymph nodes along the left RLN are separated using endoscopic scissors, keeping the remaining lymph nodes attached to the esophagus.

Kaburagi et al. demonstrated hybrid position method that radical lymphadenectomy along the bilateral recurrent laryngeal nerves was performed in the left lateral decubitus position because this approach was superior for lymphadenectomy in the region. Thoracoscopic esophagectomy and other lymphadenectomy were provided in the middle to lower mediastinum in prone position [33].

Lin et al. reported that after looping the esophagus and fixation with a clip, the exposed thorax part of the thread is pulled up by the assistant to lift esophagus [34]. The left RLN is then exposed and separated in the space between lifted esophagus and the trachea. Scissor and isolating forceps are preferred during separation due to safety concerns. During subsequent mobilization of the esophagus and dissection of left RLN lymph nodes, the assistant uses the grasping forceps to compress the trachea so as to better expose the space between esophagus and trachea.

Fujiwara et al. reported that the lymph nodes along the left RLN could be separated from the left RLN trunk using endoscopic scissors under a mediastinoscope, with the nodes remaining attached to the esophagus [35]. First, the nerve trunk is exposed along the anterior plane, then, the lymph nodes are retracted to the left, through beneath the nerve trunk, and separated by dividing the attachment to the nerve trunk. Finally, the subaortic arch lymph nodes are dissected by dividing the attachment to the nerve trunk.

To avoid injury to the lt. RLN by electricity or heat, an electric device should not be used. Wong et al. demonstrated that a more aggressive and thorough nodal dissection may be possible with less concern of RLN injury by the availability of intermittent nerve mapping and continuous intraoperative nerve monitoring (CIONM) [36].

7. Conclusion

In eastern countries ESCC is common and lymph node metastasis along the RLN is frequently seen. Many surgeons in Japan, China and India perform thoracoscopic lymph node dissection along the RLN. The prone position allows for visualization of a dry and wide surgical space without the need for special assistants, but there is difficulty in lymph node dissection along the left RLN. To obtain a good and wide operating field for lymph node dissection along the left RLN, only retraction or rotation of the trachea toward the right is insufficient. With our technique, the residual esophagus can easily be pulled up to the neck after sufficient ablation. In this technique, it is not necessary to retract the esophagus with more holes or to fix the esophagus. Esophageal stripping in lymph node dissection is easier and more effective than other methods.

Lymph node dissection along the left RLN after esophageal stripping is possible in the prone position during VATS-E.

Acknowledgements

The authors like to thank Dr. Hiroshi Maruyama, Dr. Yuta Kikuchi, Dr. Koji Ueda, and Dr. Masafumi Yoshioka for their clinical support.

Author details

Hiroshi Makino[1*], Hiroshi Yoshida[1] and Eiji Uchida[2]

*Address all correspondence to: himiyumo@nms.ac.jp

1 Department of Surgery, Nippon Medical School, Tama-Nagayama Hospital, Tama, Japan

2 Department of Gastrointestinal and Hepato-Biliary-Pancreatic Surgery, Nippon Medical School, Tama, Japan

References

[1] Igaki H, Tachimori Y, Kato H. Improved survival for patients with upper and/or middle mediastinal lymph node metastasis of squamous cell carcinoma of the lower thoracic esophagus treated with 3-field dissection. Annals of Surgery. 2004;**239**(4):483-490

[2] Udagawa H, Ueno M, Shinohara H, Haruta S, Kaida S, Nakagawa M, Tsurumaru M. The importance of grouping of lymph node stations and rationale of three-field lymphoadenectomy for thoracic esophageal cancer. Journal of Surgical Oncology. 2012;**6**:742-747

[3] Osugi H, Takemura M, Higashino N, Takada S, Lee M, Ueno Y, Tanaka Y, Fukuhara K, Hashimoto Y, Fujiwara Y, Kinoshita H. Video-assisted thoracoscopic esophagectomy and radical lymph node dissection for esophageal cancer. Surgical Endoscopy. 2002;**16**:1588-1593

[4] Arnold M, Soerjomataram I, Ferlay J, Forman D. Global incidence of oesophageal cancer by histological subtype in 2012. Gut. 2015;**64**:381-387

[5] José M, Arnal D, Arenas ÁF, Arbeloa ÁL. Esophageal cancer: Risk factors, screening and endoscopic treatment in Western and Eastern countries. World Journal of Gastroenterology. 2015;**21**(26):7933-7943

[6] Fang P, Jiao S, Zhang X, Liu Z, Wang H, Gao Y, Luo H, Chen T, Shi L. Meta-analysis of ALDH2 variants and esophageal cancer in Asians. Asian Pacific Journal of Cancer Prevention. 2011;**12**:2623-2627

[7] Kagemoto K, Urabe Y, Miwata T, Oka S, Ochi H, Kitadai Y, Tanaka S, Chayama K. ADH1B and ALDH2 are associated with metachronous SCC after endoscopic submucosal dissection of esophageal squamous cell carcinoma. Cancer Medicine. 2016;**5**(7):1397-1404

[8] Oze I, Matsuo K, Wakai K, Nagata C, Mizoue T, Tanaka K, Tsuji I, Sasazuki S, Inoue M, Tsugane S. Alcohol drinking and esophageal cancer risk: An evaluation based on a systematic review of epidemiologic evidence among the Japanese population. Japanese Journal of Clinical Oncology. 2011;**41**(5):677-692

[9] Mizoi Y, Yamamoto K, Ueno Y, Fukunaga T, Harada S. Involvement of genetic polymorphism of alcohol and aldehyde dehydrogenases in individual variation of alcohol metabolism. Alcohol and Alcoholism. 1994;**29**(6):707-710

[10] Thrift AP, Whiteman DC. The incidence of esophageal adenocarcinoma continues to rise: Analysis of period and birth cohort effects on recent trends. Annals of Oncology. 2012;**23**:3155-3162

[11] CastroC, Bosetti C, Malvezzi M, BertuccioP, Levi F, Negri E, LaVecchia C, Lunet N. Patterns and trends in esophageal cancer mortality and incidence in Europe (1980-2011) and predictions to 2015. Annals of Oncology. 2014;**25**:283-290

[12] Nun-anan P, Vilaichone R. Late stage and grave prognosis of esophageal cancer in Thailand. Asian Pacific Journal of Cancer Prevention. 2015;**16**:1747-1749

[13] Mansour-Ghanaei F, Heidarzadeh A, Naghipour MR, Joukar F, Valeshabad AK, Fallah MS, Rezvani SM, Sedigh-Rahimabadi M, Rokhshad H, Dadashi A. A 10-year study of esophageal cancer in Guilan province, Iran: The Guilan cancer registry study (GCRS). Asian Pacific Journal of Cancer Prevention. 2012;**13**:6277-6283

[14] Gasmelseed N, Abudris D, Elhaj A, Eltayeb EA, Elmadani A, Elhassan MM, Mohammed K, Elgaili EM, Elbalal M, Schuz J, Leon ME. Patterns of esophageal cancer in the national cancer institute at the University of Gezira, in Gezira State, Sudan, in 1999-2012. Asian Pacific Journal of Cancer Prevention. 2015;**16**:6481-6490

[15] Tettey M, Edwin F, Aniteye E, Sereboe L, Tamatey M, Ofosu-Appiah E, Adzamli I. The changing epidemiology of esophageal cancer in sub-Saharan Africa—The case of Ghana. Pan African Medical Journal. 2012;**13**(6):1-7

[16] Ma GW, Situ DR, Ma QL, Long H, Zhang LJ, Lin P, Rong TH. Three-field vs two-field lymph node dissection for esophageal cancer: A meta-analysis. World Journal of Gastroenterology. 2014;**20**(47):18022-18030

[17] Sepesi B, Schmidt HE, Lada M, Correa AM, Walsh GL, Mehran RJ, Rice DC, Roth JA, Swisher SG, Low DE, Hofstetter WL. Survival in patients with esophageal adenocarcinoma undergoing trimodality therapy is independent regional lymph node location. The Annals of Thoracic Surgery. 2016;**101**:1075-1081

[18] Feith M, Stein HJ, Siewert JR. Pattern of lymphatic spread of Barrett's cancer. World Journal of Surgery. 2003;**27**:1052-1057

[19] Siewert JR, Feith M, Werner M, Stein HJ. Adenocarcinoma of the esophagogastric junction results of surgical therapy based on anatomical/topographic classification in 1,002 consecutive patient. Annals of Surgery. 2000;**232**(3):353-361

[20] Yamashita H, Seto Y, Sano T, Makuuchi H, Ando N, Sasako M, Japanese Gastric Cancer Association and the Japan Esophageal Society. Results of a nation-wide retrospective study of lymphadenectomy for esophagogastric junction carcinoma. Gastric Cancer. 2017;**20**:69-83

[21] Ye K, Xu JH, Sun YF, Lin JA, Zheng ZG. Characteristics and clinical significance of lymph node metastases near the recurrent laryngeal nerve from thoracic esophageal carcinoma. Genetics and Molecular Research. 2014;**13**(3):6411-6419

[22] Giacopuzzi S, Bencivenga M, Weindelmaye J, Verlato G, de Manzoni G. Western strategy for EGJ carcinoma. Gastric Cancer. 2017;(Suppl 1):60-68

[23] Altorki N, Kent M, Ferrara C, Port J.Three-field lymph node dissection for squamous cell and adenocarcinoma of the esophagus. Annals of Surgery. 2002;**236**(2):177-83

[24] Palanivelu C, Prakash A, Senthilkumar R, Senthilnathan P, Parthasarathi R, Rajan PS, Venkatachlam S. Minimally invasive esophagectomy: Thoracoscopic mobilization of the esophagus and mediastinal lymphadenectomy in prone position—Experience of 130 patients. Journal of the American College of Surgeons. 2006;**203**(1):7-16

[25] Lagergren J, Mattsson F,Zylstra J, Chang F, Gossage J, Mason R, Lagergren P, Davies A. Extent of lymphadenectomy and prognosis after esophageal cancer surgery. JAMA Surgery. 2016;**151**(1):32-39

[26] Cuschieri A. Endoscopic subtotal oesophagectomy for cancer using the right thoracoscopic approach. Surgical Oncology. 1993;**2**(Suppl 1):3-11

[27] Noshiro H, Iwasaki H, Kobayashi K, Uchiyama A, Miyasaka Y, Masatsugu T, Koike K, Miyazaki K. Lymphadenectomy along the left recurrent laryngeal nerve by a minimally invasive esophagectomy in the prone position for thoracic esophageal cancer. Surgical Endoscopy. 2010;**24**:2965-2973

[28] Makino H, Nomura T, Miyashita M, Okawa K, Hagiwara N, Uchida E. Esophageal stripping creates a clear operative field for lymph node dissection along the left recurrent laryngeal nerve in prone video-assisted thoracoscopic surgery. Journal of Nippon Medical School. 2011;**78**(3):199-204

[29] Makino H, Yoshida H, Maruyama H, Yokoyama T, Hirakata A, Ueda J, Takada H, Matsutani T, Nomura T, Hagiwara N, Uchida E. An original technique for lymph node dissection along the left recurrent laryngeal nerve after stripping the residual esophagus during video-assisted thoracoscopic surgery of esophagus. Journal of Visualized Surgery. 2016;**2**(166):1-6

[30] Oshikiri T, Yasuda T, Harada H, Goto H, Oyama M, Hasegawa H, Ohara T, Sendo H, Nakamura T, Fujino Y, Tominaga M, Kakeji Y. A new method (the "Bascule method") for lymphadenectomy along the left recurrent laryngeal nerve during prone esophagectomy for esophageal cancer. Surgical Endoscopy. 2015;**29**(8):2442-2450

[31] Xi Y, Ma Z, Shen Y, Wang H, Feng M, Tan L, Wang Q. A novel method for lymphadenectomy along the left laryngeal recurrent nerve during thoracoscopic esophagectomy for esophageal carcinoma. Journal of Thoracic Disease. 2016;**8**(1):24-30

[32] Zheng W, Zhu Y, Guo CH, Zheng B, Han ZY, Chen C. Esophageal suspension method in scavenging peripheral lymph nodes of the left recurrent laryngeal nerve in thoracic esophageal carcinoma through semi-prone-position thoracoscopy. Journal of Cancer Research and Therapeutics. 2014;**10**(4):985-990

[33] Kaburagi T, Takeuchi H, Kawakubo H, Omori T, Ozawa S, Kitagawa Y. Clinical utility of a novel hybrid position combining the left lateral decubitus and prone positions during thoracoscopic esophagectomy. World Journal of Surgery. 2014;**38**:410-418

[34] Lin M, Shen Y, Feng M, Tan L. Minimally invasive esophagectomy: Chinese experiences. Journal of Visualized Surgery. 2016;**2**(134):1-4

[35] Fujiwara H, Shiozaki A, Konishi H, Otsuji E. Mediastinoscope and laparoscope-assisted esophagectomy. Journal of Visualized Surgery. 2016;**2**(128):1-7

[36] Wong I, Tong DKH, Tsang RKY, Wong CLY, Chan DKK, Chan FSY, Law S. Continuous intraoperative vagus nerve stimulation for monitoring of recurrent laryngeal nerve during minimally invasive esophagectomy. Journal of Visualized Surgery. 2017;**3**(9):1-7

11

Prevention and Management of Complications from Esophagectomy

Jacqueline Oxenberg

Abstract

While surgery plays a major role in the treatment and potential cure of esophageal cancer, esophagectomy continues to have a significant amount of morbidity compared to other surgical oncology procedures. Efforts to improve morbidity and mortality from esophagectomy include the Consensus Guidelines for Complications from Esophagectomies, Enhanced Recovery after Surgery protocols as well as others. Although we strive to improve morbidity and mortality after these surgeries, adverse events still occur. They affect not only patient quality of life and increase cost of care for esophageal cancer but also have a negative impact on overall cancer survival. This chapter reviews the prevention of adverse outcomes from esophagectomies as well as discusses the management of many complications that may occur more common to the operation.

Keywords: esophagectomy complications, prevention of esophagectomy complications, management of esophagectomy complications

1. Introduction

Adverse events from esophagectomies directly impact patient quality of life, cancer recurrence/survival, hospital costs and resources, as well as require a great deal of energy from those managing them [1, 2]. Prevention of surgical complications is of utmost importance; however, adverse events from this major surgical procedure still occur, even in high-volume centers or experienced hands. Mortality can range from 7 to 9% while morbidity ranges from 17 to 74% [3]. Prevention, early recognition, and adequate management of complications can decrease mortality [4]. While many studies evaluate postoperative morbidity using even randomized methods, randomized studies on the management of postsurgical complications are by nature extremely limited.

2. Selection of the appropriate patient and surgeon

2.1. The optimal patient

Patient optimization and use of appropriate selection criteria are key to minimizing postoperative morbidity. Unfortunately, those risk factors for the development of esophageal cancer may also put patients at an increased risk for postoperative complications. Risk factors include age, elevated BMI, ECOG score/functional status, dyspnea, diabetes, chronic obstructive pulmonary disease, smoking, alkaline phosphatase level elevations, low serum albumin, and increased complexity score [5–11]. However, age and performance status continue to be the most commonly reported. Neoadjuvant treatments have not been consistently proven to be a risk factor. While fibrosis often occurs after chemoradiation, potentially making surgical resection more difficult, data showing optimal timing to surgery after neoadjuvant chemoradiation and its affect on postoperative morbidity are mixed [12].

2.2. How to optimize the patient

Malnutrition has been reported in 57–80% of patients with esophageal cancer [13, 14]. Many factors can be attributed to malnutrition prior to surgery and include patient factors, chemotherapy, radiation therapy, and tumor-related causes [15]. It is important to recognize that even obese patients can suffer from malnutrition. While laboratory values and anthropometric measurements can be useful, their values can vary and therefore may not be clinically relevant. Therefore, a weight loss of greater than 10% for 6 months or 5% for 1 month is considered malnourished [16].

For the malnourished patient, preoperative optimization of nutrition through the advice of a dietician is key, but other measures should be considered as well if a patient is unable to tolerate at least 50–75% of their caloric needs [15]. The preferred intervention should be handled in a multidisciplinary setting and be initiated as early as possible. This decreases the amount of weight loss, increases chances of completion of neoadjuvant therapies, and decreases hospital admissions [17].

Recommendations to maximize oral nutrition intake include dividing daily oral intake into five to six small meals where the patient is given enough time to eat, eating only foods with a high nutritional content, paying attention to presentation and preparation of meals to make food as desirable as possible, enriching meals and drinks and taking advantage of those days where the patient feels like eating, modifying the consistency of foods to ease swallowing, preventing fatigue, decreasing the risk of aspiration, eating non-irritating soft and smooth foods at room temperature and maintaining oral hygiene for those with mucositis [15]. Patients should also be advised to supplement meals with dietary supplements. The preoperative intake of combined "immunonutrition" products consisting of arginine, glutamine, polyunsaturated omega-3 fatty acids, nucleotides, and antioxidant micronutrients has been shown to decrease postoperative infectious complications and length of hospital stay [15, 18, 19].

For those unable to tolerate adequate nutrition, even with optimization and supplementation, other interventions are needed. These include either stent placement or percutaneous, endoscopic, or surgical placement of feeding gastrostomy or jejunostomy tubes. Esophageal stent placement has the benefit of being placed during endoscopic ultrasound, a common staging procedure. While it may improve dysphagia in the neoadjuvant setting, chest pain can occur and stent migration can be seen in up to 46% of patients [20]. although stent migration can be problematic, it is often a sign of tumor response to neoadjuvant therapy, and therefore the stent may not always need to be replaced. Other reported complications of stent placement in the neoadjuvant setting include perforation, mediastinitis, bowel perforation from migration, tracheo-esophageal fistula, and bleeding [21].

Jejunostomy and gastrostomy tube placement have been proven safe and effective for perioperative nutrition. These can be placed in the laparoscopic, open, endoscopic, or even percutaneous settings. Endoscopic placement may be difficult if a patient has a severe malignant stricture/obstruction, which is often the case when a patient is suffering from severe malnutrition and unable to pass food or liquids through the site of tumor. Gastrostomy tubes have the advantage of bolus feeding, which may improve quality of life. While gastrostomy tube placement has been proven to be safe without increasing the risk of postoperative morbidity, jejunostomy tube placement is often preferred given the stomach is the preferred organ for a neo-esophagus. Jejunostomy tubes are often placed at the time of esophagectomy as well for supportive care. However, some data support that the placement of jejunostomy tubes during esophagectomy is not always necessary [22–24]. Unfortunately, tube feeds cannot be given in boluses with jejunostomy tubes, which, if occurs, can lead to diarrhea and further dehydration. Patients therefore require an ongoing pump connection for feedings.

Smoking cessation is crucial to improving morbidity from esophagectomy. This may be most beneficial if performed greater than 90 days before surgery [25]. Active smoking has also been shown to increase recurrence rates of cancer after esophagectomy [26]. Therefore, smoking cessation counseling and supportive programs are necessary when patients are being assessed for esophagectomy.

2.3. The optimal surgeon/hospital

When deciding the optimal surgeon, it is important to understand that outcomes depend on two major factors: experience and resources. It is well known that with increasing numbers of esophagectomies performed, postoperative morbidity and mortality are improved. In addition, long-term survival can also improve [27]. While data show improved outcomes at higher volume centers, this is inconsistent and may depend further on individual surgeon volumes and hospital resources [28]. Begg et al. described low-volume hospitals as 1–5 esophagectomies/year, medium volume 6–11 esophagectomies/year, and high-volume centers as those performing >11 esophagectomies/year, with an improved mortality with increasing hospital volumes [29]. Later, Birkmeyer et al. divided hospital volumes to <2 esophagectomies/year as low-volume and high-volume centers as >19 esophagectomies/year [30]. The 2003 Leapfrog Group recommended 13 esophagectomies/year as a minimum volume standard [31]. However, esophagectomies at mid-volume centers can also be safely performed, especially with a two-surgeon approach [32]. Hospital type may also be important where improved reoperation rates and mortality are seen when surgery is performed at University centers or institutions centralizing esophageal cancer care [33–35].

of injuries/palsies that are each further separated into unilateral (A) and bilateral (B): Type 1 includes a transient injury requiring no therapy, where only dietary modifications are needed; Type 2 is an injury requiring elective surgical procedures such as thyroplasty or medialization procedures; Type 3 is an injury requiring acute surgical intervention due to aspiration or other respiratory issues that include thyroplasty or medialization procedures. Injury to the left recurrent laryngeal nerve is most common and is mainly associated with esophagectomies that include cervical anastomoses or dissections, McKeown-type operations. Therefore, prevention may include performing thoracic anastomoses or careful dissection and prevention of injury from the above causes. The early recognition of injury and treatment (which may include medialization of the vocal fold) may prevent aspiration and pneumonia and therefore may be of benefit early in the postoperative course [56, 57].

Other causes of respiratory failure or shortness of breath can include ARDS, cardiac causes, pleural effusions, pneumothorax, phrenic nerve injury, or fistula. Other infections can put patients at risk for ARDS (acute respiratory distress syndrome), and cardiac causes may also result in respiratory failure and need for reintubation. If ARDS occurs, the cause should be evaluated, including examining for other infections (urine, leak, etc.). If cardiac in nature, most commonly secondary to atrial fibrillation, heart rate control is usually necessary to alleviate symptoms. Pleural effusions and pneumothorax are common and can be managed with chest tube placement or percutaneous radiologic drainage, depending on the size of the effusion or pneumothorax. If effusions occur simultaneously with anastomotic leak, adequate drainage should be performed to prevent empyema and life-threatening mediastinitis. While phrenic nerve injury is rare, immediate surgical intervention is not always needed. However, patients may require tracheostomy placement for pulmonary conditioning. It is also important to remember that patients are at an increased risk for deep vein thrombosis and even pulmonary embolism. This may occur prior to or even after esophagectomy. Perioperative prophylactic anticoagulation should be administered in the perioperative setting to prevent deep vein thrombosis/pulmonary embolism. Tracheoesophageal fistula should also be considered, especially later in the recovery period or in a complicated postoperative recovery setting.

Impaired lung function is a significant risk factor for pulmonary complications [8]. With preoperative chemoradiation, pneumonitis can occur, making patients at an increased risk for postoperative respiratory failure and pneumonia [8]. While some degree of inflammation is often seen in preoperative imaging, assuring patient lung function has not decompensated is prudent. This can often cause delays in surgery; however, allowing the recovery of lung function may improve postoperative pulmonary failure.

Consistent with the recommendations of the Enhanced Recovery After Surgery pathways, intravenous fluid administration should be minimized to improve time to return of bowel function and decrease the length of hospital stay. Excessive fluid administration/fluid overload should also be considered in all patients with acute respiratory failure since the administration of diuretics may quickly improve symptoms.

3.3. *Anastomotic leak/conduit necrosis*

Anastomotic leak after esophagectomy can be difficult to manage and has a major impact on patient quality of life as well as may affect long-term survival [58, 59]. Incidence varies from 5.7 to 14.3% with a higher incidence in cervical anastomoses versus thoracic [60]. The International Study Group for Rectal Cancer proposed the verbiage of anastomotic leak as, "A defect of the integrity in a surgical joint between two hollow viscera with communication between the intraluminal and extraluminal compartments," which was later validated and expanded to the entire gastrointestinal tract [61]. Lerut et al. with the Surgery Infection Study Group defined anastomotic leak severity as Type 1, a radiological leak without any clinical findings; Type 2 with minor clinical findings of local inflammation (cervical wound) or X-ray showed suppressed leak (thoracic anastomosis); Type 3, a major clinical leak with severe disruption and sepsis; Type 4, conduit necrosis seen by endoscopic confirmation [62]. The Early Complications Consensus Group (ECCG) defined anastomotic leak as a full-thickness GI defect involving esophagus, anastomosis, staple line, or conduit, irrespective of the presentation of the method of identification [3]. Type 1 includes a local defect requiring no change in therapy or treated medically or with dietary modification. Type 2 is a localized defect requiring interventional but not surgical therapy (interventional radiology drainage, stent or bedside opening and packing of incision). Type 3 is a localized defect requiring surgical therapy.

Many patient factors as well as peri- and intraoperative factors can contribute to anastomotic leak. Patients at an increased risk for anastomotic leak include those with increased comorbidities, advanced pathologic stage, prior esophagogastric surgeries, and active smoking [63]. Patient factors can include preoperative malnutrition, diabetes, prolonged hospitalization, hypotension, hypoxemia, preoperative chemotherapy, preoperative chemoradiation, and age. Technical factors also impacting the rate of anastomotic leak include the location of the anastomosis, surgery type, tension on the anastomosis, the type of anastomosis (hand sewn vs. stapled), arterial and venous insufficiency, excessive bleeding, and surgeon experience. While leak incidence may be higher in a single-layer anastomosis, the incidence of stricture may be higher in a double-layer anastomosis [64–66]. While data are mixed, the incidence of leak and stricture may also be lower with a stapled anastomosis [67, 68]. Postoperative factors may include gastric distention, external compression, infection, re-exploration for bleeding, prolonged mechanical ventilation, and continued hypoxemia and hypotension [69]. Technical considerations to decrease the rate of anastomotic leak may include anastomotic support with omentum, pleura, pericardium, and fat tissue. Prospective randomized studies have shown that omental wrapping of the anastomosis may decrease the rate of leak or even stricture [70, 71].

Diagnosis can be made by clinical suspicion if a patient presents with fevers, leukocytosis, empyema, pleural effusion, pneumomediastinum, increased drainage from the chest tube (bile or other gastric contents), the presence of enteric bacteria or bacterial culture or tachycardia. The early detection of anastomotic leaks may also include CRP/ESR elevation, an increase in procalcitonin level, and leukocytosis extending past the second and fifth postoperative days, respectively [72, 73]. While contrast esophagogram can be performed to determine subclinical leaks, caution is advised given the risks of aspiration [4, 74]. A barium swallow can be performed to detect an anastomotic leak; however, its sensitivity can be relatively low and may often be performed too early to detect [75, 76]. The oral intake of methylene blue may be used given it is otherwise nontoxic. CT scan with oral contrast may also be helpful and show contrast extravasation as well as concerning areas for infection.

The etiology of the leak is vital to ascertain where patients with conduit tip necrosis or complete conduit ischemia may require different interventions. This often requires direct visualization with EGD for conduit evaluation as well as evaluation of the defect size. The ECCG defines conduit necrosis into three types, with recommendations for specific treatments: Type 1 includes a focal conduit necrosis that is identified endoscopically, requiring only additional monitoring or nonsurgical therapy; Type 2 includes focal conduit necrosis that is identified endoscopically and is not associated with free anastomotic or conduit leak. Surgical therapy not involving esophageal diversion is performed; Type 3 includes extensive conduit necrosis that is treated with conduit resection and diversion [3].

If a leak occurs, source control with drain placement with or without operative intervention remains key to preventing mortality. For this reason, intraoperative drain placement for detection and source control is common. Management often is determined by anastomotic location; however, mediastinitis can occur with both intrathoracic and cervical anastomoses, a possibly fatal diagnosis for which requires close monitoring and rapid evaluation and treatment. Turkyilmaz et al. created algorithms to help guide treatment for anastomotic leak. For cervical anastomoses, a limited leak that is clinically occult may be managed with antibiotics, dressing changes, and cleansing with oral isotonic fluid. If there is a clinically prominent cervical leak, antibiotics, opening of the cervical wound, drain placement, nasogastric decompression, nutritional support, and cleaning are typically needed. For cervical anastomotic leaks that have intrathoracic complications and clinical sepsis failing to improve, drain placement, stent placement, decortication, resection/diversion or resection/colonic interposition may be needed. For thoracic anastomoses, if a contained leak with less than 30% disruption, injection with fibrin glue, endoclips, or stents can be used for management. However, if the defect is larger, drainage and esophageal stent placement can be performed followed by surgery if stent placement and drainage are unsuccessful (can include primary or supporting tissue repair). However, if the anastomosis has a greater than 70% disruption, surgery including drainage and primary repair should be performed first with esophageal diversion with possible colonic interposition if unable to be performed [69].

With the use of self-expanding metal stents, endoscopic management alone has become possible for anastomotic leaks/disruptions. Covered stents can be placed to control the leak, preventing further seeding into the mediastinum for both cervical and thoracic anastomoses. If well controlled, oral intake may also be safe. However, stent migration can occur, requiring retrieval and replacement [77]. Stent use may be limited in large defects (which may occur from conduit necrosis or staple line disruption). It is also important to understand that lumen caliber differences between the esophagus and gastric conduit can result in the reflux of gastric contents around the distal aspect of a stent. This unfortunately may not be seen with an esophagogram, but rather be noticed with other imaging such as CT after the reflux of contrast and gastric contents occur and may be delayed. Therefore, other options for control have emerged including endoscopic vacuum-assisted closure devices and may even be more effective than stent placement [78–81].

3.4. Fistula

In addition to source control, the awareness and prevention of esophago/gastrotracheal fistula is also necessary. This can occur from infection itself or even the erosion of foreign material (stent, staples, etc.) into the trachea. One should be suspicious in patients with frequent uncontrolled coughing, especially after swallowing, or "Ono's sign" [82]. Workup and diagnosis can include an upper gastrointestinal X-ray with oral contrast or even direct visualization with esophagoscopy or bronchoscopy. Prevention may include a pleural wrap around the anastomosis at the time of original operation or even at the time of reoperation if a leak occurs and anastomotic repair is possible. If reoperation is not performed, stent placement may help control symptoms and healing [83]. However, distal feeding tube placement and resection may be needed. Treatment is necessary to prevent recurring pneumonia.

3.5. Delayed gastric emptying

Delayed or inappropriate gastric emptying can occur secondary to the disruption of vagal nerve complexes to the stomach. This can result in delayed emptying of the stomach, which affects not only patient quality of life and inability to obtain oral nutrition but also can put patients at an increased risk for reflux of gastric contents and even aspiration. The most common options for the management of the pylorus include pyloromyotomy, pyloroplasty, intra-pyloric botulinum toxin injection as well as no intervention. While one multicenter study showed no significant difference between pyloroplasty, botulinum toxin-injection, and no pyloric treatment, one study did show that intra-pyloric botulinum toxin can increase the risk of postoperative reflux and increase the use of promotility agents and endoscopic interventions [84, 85]. While delayed gastric emptying can occur anywhere from 10 to 50%, it also can be successfully managed with prokinetic agents (75%) and endoscopic dilation [86].

3.6. Chyle leak/chylothorax

With the thoracic duct being the largest lymphatic vessel in the body as well as being located in the chest, posterior to the esophagus, injury can occur. Its location, however, often varies. The incidence of chyle leak is rather low (1–4%); however, when it occurs, it can be very problematic [87]. Chyle contains triglycerides in the form of chylomicrons as well as lymphocytes. Chyle leaks can result in malnutrition (with continued protein loss), immune compromise, hypovolemia, electrolyte abnormalities, hypoalbuminemia, lymphopenia, and infection [88]. The ECCG defines a chyle leak into three different types, where output <1 L/day is further classified as "A," and "B" is further classified as >1 L/day [3]. Type 1 leaks can be managed with enteric dietary modifications alone. Type 2 can be managed with total parenteral nutrition. Type 3 requires management with interventional or surgical therapy.

Following esophagectomy, drainage from a chest tube of >500 mL/day is suggestive of a chyle leak; however, the measurement of chylomicrons or triglycerides is most commonly utilized [89]. A measurement of >4% chylomicrons or fluid containing >100–110 mg/dL of triglycerides is typically considered indicative of a chyle leak. Since a chyle leak may present with increased serous or even serosanguinous drainage while fasting, a clinical diagnosis can be made by the oral intake of cream followed by milky drainage from the chest tube/drains.

Prevention unfortunately is difficult. Selective en masse ligation has been shown to reduce the rate of chylothorax [90]. Also, the preoperative oral administration of cream may help identify the thoracic duct to aid in the prevention of its injury or to identify the thoracic duct for prophylactic ligation [91]. The initial management of a chyle leak usually includes drainage as well as TPN and bowel rest. Decreasing oral or enteral fat intake decreases the flow of chyle through the leak, possibly allowing spontaneous closure [92]. Long chain fatty acids should be avoided with diets supported by high percentages of medium-chain triglycerides since they are typically absorbed directly into intestinal cells, bypassing the thoracic duct [87]. If conservative management is not successful, surgical intervention may be necessary, especially if the fistula is of high output. Aggressive surgical intervention should be performed if chyle output is >1.5 L/day for >5–7 days [93]. Surgical intervention includes thoracotomy or thoracoscopic thoracic duct ligation on the side of the chylothorax. This is usually assisted by the preoperative administration of cream or lipophilic dye to help identify the thoracic duct. If the leak can be localized, this may be controlled with clips or suture; however, if the leak is unclear, ligation of the thoracic duct just cephalad to the aortic hiatus is recommended [94–96]. Pleurodesis can also be performed at the time of ligation as well.

Radiologic-guided/percutaneous embolization is becoming more popular, especially for patients who are poor operative candidates. This includes lymphangiography followed by transabdominal percutaneous needle cannulation, although a retrograde subclavian vein approach can be used [97, 98]. Once the cisterna chyli is canalized, a catheter is advanced into the thoracic duct and contrast used to identify the leak. Embolization can then be performed. Since surgical intervention to ligate the thoracic duct using thoracoscopy or a thoracotomy can result in increased morbidity and mortality, thoracic duct embolization has become increasingly more popular when conservative management fails.

Author details

Jacqueline Oxenberg

Address all correspondence to: jcoxenberg@geisinger.edu

Geisinger Wyoming Valley, Wilkes-Barre, PA, USA

References

[1] Kataoka K, Takeuchi H, Mizusawa J, et al. Prognostic impact of postoperative morbidity after esophagectomy for esophageal cancer: Exploratory analysis of JCOG9907. Annals of Surgery. 2017;**265**(6):1152-1157. DOI: 10.1097/SLA.0000000000001828

[2] Lerut T, Moons J, Coosemans W, et al. Postoperative complications after transthoracic esophagectomy for cancer of the esophagus and gastroesophageal junction are correlated with early cancer recurrence: Role of systematic grading of complications using the modified clavien classification. Annals of Surgery. 2009;**250**(5):798-806. DOI: 10.1097/SLA.0b013e3181bdd5a8

[3] Low DE, Alderson D, Cecconello I, et al. International consensus on standardization of data collection for complications associated with esophagectomy: Esophagectomy complications consensus group (ECCG). Annals of Surgery. 2015;**262**(2):286-294. DOI: 10.1097/SLA.0000000000001098

[4] Griffin SM, Lamb PJ, Dresner SM, Richardson DL, Hayes N. Diagnosis and management of a mediastinal leak following radical oesophagectomy. The British Journal of Surgery. 2001;**88**(10):1346-1351. DOI: 10.1046/j.0007-1323.2001.01918.x

[5] Law S, Wong K, Kwok K, Chu K, Wong J. Predictive factors for postoperative pulmonary complications and mortality after esophagectomy for cancer. Annals of Surgery. 2004;**240**(5):791-800. DOI: 10.1097/01.sla.0000143123.24556.1c

[6] Atkins BZ, Shah AS, Hutcheson KA, et al. Reducing hospital morbidity and mortality following esophagectomy. The Annals of Thoracic Surgery. 2004;**78**(4):1170-1176. DOI: 10.1016/j.athoracsur.2004.02.034

[7] Bailey SH, Bull DA, Harpole DH, et al. Outcomes after esophagectomy: A ten-year prospective cohort. The Annals of Thoracic Surgery. 2003;**75**(1):217-222. DOI: 10.1016/S0003-4975(02)04368-0

[8] Avendano CE, Flume PA, Silvestri GA, King LB, Reed CE. Pulmonary complications after esophagectomy. The Annals of Thoracic Surgery. 2002;**73**(3):922-926. DOI: 10.1016/S0003-4975(01)03584-6

[9] Kinugasa S, Tachibana M, Yoshimura H, et al. Postoperative pulmonary complications are associated with worse short- and long-term outcomes after extended esophagectomy. Journal of Surgical Oncology. 2004;**88**(2):71-77. DOI: 10.1002/jso.20137

[10] Raymond DP, Seder CW, Wright CD, et al. Predictors of major morbidity or mortality after resection for esophageal cancer: A society of thoracic surgeons general thoracic surgery database risk adjustment model. The Annals of Thoracic Surgery. 2016;**102**(1):207-214. DOI: 10.1016/j.athoracsur.2016.04.055

[11] Ferguson MK, Martin TR, Reeder LB, Olak J. Mortality after esophagectomy: Risk factor analysis. World Journal of Surgery. 1997;**21**(6):599-604. DOI: 10.1007/s002689900279

[12] Kim JY, Correa AM, Vaporciyan AA, et al. Does the timing of esophagectomy after chemoradiation affect outcome? The Annals of Thoracic Surgery. 2012;**93**(1):207-212; discussion 212-3. DOI: 10.1016/j.athoracsur.2011.05.021

[13] Daly JM, Fry WA, Little AG, et al. Esophageal cancer: Results of American college of surgeons patient care evaluation study. Journal of the American College of Surgeons. 2000;**190**(5):562-573

[14] Dewys WD, Begg C, Lavin PT, et al. Prognostic effect of weight loss prior to chemotherapy in cancer patients. Eastern cooperative oncology group. The American Journal of Medicine. 1980;**69**(4):491-497

[15] Mariette C, De Botton M, Piessen G. Surgery in esophageal and gastric cancer patients: What is the role for nutrition support in your daily practice? Annals of Surgical Oncology. 2012;**19**(7):2128-2134. DOI: 10.1245/s10434-012-2225-6

[16] Nitenberg G, Raynard B. Nutritional support of the cancer patient: Issues and dilemmas. Critical Reviews in Oncology/Hematology. 2000;**34**(3):137-168. DOI: 10.1016/S1040-8428(00)00048-2

[65] Mathisen DJ, Grillo HC, Wilkins EW Jr, Moncure AC, Hilgenberg AD. Transthoracic esophagectomy: A safe approach to carcinoma of the esophagus. The Annals of Thoracic Surgery. 1988;**45**(2):137-143

[66] Postlethwait RW. Complications and deaths after operations for esophageal carcinoma. The Journal of Thoracic and Cardiovascular Surgery. 1983;**85**(6):827-831

[67] Okuyama M, Motoyama S, Suzuki H, Saito R, Maruyama K, Ogawa J. Hand-sewn cervical anastomosis versus stapled intrathoracic anastomosis after esophagectomy for middle or lower thoracic esophageal cancer: A prospective randomized controlled study. Surgery Today. 2007;**37**(11):947-952. DOI: 10.1007/s00595-007-3541-5

[68] Orringer MB, Marshall B, Iannettoni MD. Eliminating the cervical esophagogastric anastomotic leak with a side-to-side stapled anastomosis. The Journal of Thoracic and Cardiovascular Surgery. 2000;**119**(2):277-288. DOI: 10.1016/S0022-5223(00)70183-8

[69] Turkyilmaz A, Eroglu A, Aydin Y, Tekinbas C, Muharrem Erol M, Karaoglanoglu N. The management of esophagogastric anastomotic leak after esophagectomy for esophageal-carcinoma. Diseases of the Esophagus. 2009;**22**(2):119-126. DOI: 10.1111/j.1442-2050.2008.00866.x

[70] Dai JG, Zhang ZY, Min JX, Huang XB, Wang JS. Wrapping of the omental pedicle flap around esophagogastric anastomosis after esophagectomy for esophageal cancer. Surgery (USA). 2011;**149**(3):404-410. DOI: 10.1016/j.surg.2010.08.005

[71] Bhat MA, Dar MA, Lone GN, Dar AM. Use of pedicledomentum in esophagogastric anastomosis for prevention of anastomotic leak. The Annals of Thoracic Surgery. 2006;**82**(5):1857-1862. DOI: 10.1016/j.athoracsur.2006.05.101

[72] Deitmar S, Anthoni C, Palmes D, Haier J, Senninger N, Brüwer M. Are leukocytes and CRP early indicators for anastomotic leakage after esophageal resection? Zentralblatt für Chirurgie. 2009;**134**(1):83-89. DOI: 10.1055/s-0028-1098768

[73] Veeramootoo D, Parameswaran R, Krishnadas R, et al. Classification and early recognition of gastric conduit failure after minimally invasive esophagectomy. Surgical Endoscopy. 2009;**23**(9):2110-2116. DOI: 10.1007/s00464-008-0233-1

[74] Sauvanet A, Baltar J, Le Mee J, Belghiti J. Diagnosis and conservative management of intrathoracic leakage after oesophagectomy. The British Journal of Surgery. 1998;**85**(10):1446-1449. DOI: 10.1046/j.1365-2168.1998.00869.x

[75] Roh S, Iannettoni MD, Keech JC, Bashir M, Gruber PJ, Parekh KR. Role of barium swallow in diagnosing clinically significant anastomotic leak following esophagectomy. Korean Journal of Thoracic and Cardiovascular Surgery. 2016;**49**(2):99-106. DOI: 10.5090/kjtcs.2016.49.2.99

[76] Andreou A, Struecker B, Biebl M, Pratschke J. Routine barium swallow may be unnecessary after resection of esophageal cancer. Journal of the American College of Surgeons. 2015;**221**(4):S145. DOI: 10.1016/j.jamcollsurg.2015.07.347

[90] Lin Y, Li Z, Li G, et al. Selective en masse ligation of the thoracic duct to prevent chyle leak after esophagectomy. The Annals of Thoracic Surgery. 2017;**103**(6):1802-1807

[91] Shackcloth MJ, Poullis M, Lu J, Page RD. Preventing of chylothorax after oesophagectomy by routine pre-operative administration of oral cream. European Journal of Cardio-Thoracic Surgery. 2001;**20**(5):1035-1036. DOI: 10.1016/S1010-7940(01)00928-9

[92] Sriram K, Meguid RA, Meguid MM. Nutritional support in adults with chyle leaks. Nutrition. 2016;**32**(2):281-286. DOI: 10.1016/j.nut.2015.08.002

[93] Browse NL, Allen DR, Wilson NM. Management of chylothorax. The British Journal of Surgery. 1997;**84**(12):1711-1716. DOI: 10.1046/j.1365-2168.1997.02858.x

[94] Martucci N, Tracey M, Rocco G. Postoperative chylothorax. Thoracic Surgery Clinics. Nov. 2015;**25**(4):523-528

[95] Zabeck H, Muley TF, Dienemann HF, Hoffmann H. Management of chylothorax in adults: When is surgery indicated? The Thoracic and Cardiovascular Surgeon. 2011;**59**(4): 243-246

[96] Nair SK, Petko M, Hayward MP. Aetiology and management of chylothorax in adults. European Journal of Cardio-Thoracic Surgery. 2007;**32**(2):362-369. DOI: 10.1016/j.ejcts.2007.04.024

[97] Pamarthi V, Stecker MS, Schenker MP, et al. Thoracic duct embolization and disruption for treatment of chylous effusions: Experience with 105 patients. Journal of Vascular and Interventional Radiology. 2014;**25**(9):1398-1404. DOI: 10.1016/j.jvir.2014.03.027

[98] Guevara CJ, Rialon KL, Ramaswamy RS, Kim SK, Darcy MD. US-guided, direct puncture retrograde thoracic duct access, lymphangiography, and embolization: Feasibility and efficacy. Journal of Vascular and Interventional Radiology. Dec. 2016;**27**(12):1890-1896

12

Congential Diseases of Esophagus

Mehrdad Hosseinpour and Bahareh Ahmadi

Abstract

Esophageal atresia (EA) presents some of the greatest technical hurdles that pediatric has to face. Postnatally, the classical clinical presentation of an infant with EA is an abnormally mucousy infant who is drooling excessive amount of saliva. Diagnosis confirmed when an orogastric tube cannot be passed through the mouth into the stomach. Examination should assess the as cardiac, anal limb. The purpose of the surgery is to divide the trachea esophageal fistula (TEF) and to restore esophageal continuity blind-ending upper esophageal. Achalasia is an uncommon disorder of esophagus dysmotility. Patients typically present with a history of progressively worsening dysphagia that begins with solid foods. The initial diagnosis test in child with dysphasia is usually a contrast esophagogram. Classic findings include a dilated, dysmotile esophagus and a bird's beak deformity at the gastroesophageal junction. The main treatments of achalasia are esophageal myotomy, balloon dilation or botulism toxin. Esophageal diverticula are often first suspected on Chest X ray(CXR) due to presenting symptoms. These lesions can cause wheezing, dyspnea, hemoptysis and recurrent pneumonia due to airway compression and dysphasia due to esophagus compression. These duplications should be further investigated by CT scan or Magnetic resonance imaging (MRI). The preferred method of treatment is thoracoscopy or thoracotomy.

Keywords: esophageal atresia, esophageal diverticula, achalasia

1. Esophageal atresia

1.1. Embryology

Esophageal atresia (EA) and trachea esophageal fistula (TEF) are important human birth defects of unknown etiology and represent a challenge to the pediatric surgeons. The great majority of cases of EA and TEF occur as sporadic events. However, there is emerging evidence of an important role for genetic factors.

Embryologically, the respiratory system is derived from the foregut endoderm with the appearance of the laryngo tracheal groove in the ventral floor of the foregut, just caudal to the level of the pharynx [1].

In broad terms, there have been two contrasting theories to explain how the respiratory foregut separates from the gastrointestinal foregut.

In first theory, the respiratory system develops as a result of rapid outgrowth from the original foregut tube [2], but in an alternative theory, there is active growth of a mesenchymal septum which develops in the coronal plane and, as a result, separates the foregut lumen into ventral (respiratory) and dorsal (gastrointestinal) structures [3]; however, direct evidence of septum formation has been lacking, casting doubt on this theory.

The separate process occurs in human embryo between 28 and 37 days of postfertilization. A number of theories have been put forward for disturbed TE malformation, which themselves reflect the theories of normal development.

In first theory, the normal development of trachea is the result of rapid longitudinal growth of the tracheal primordium away from the foregut, and TE malformation is caused by a failure of tracheal growth, the result of which is a compensatory overgrowth of the undivided foregut with the bronchopulmonary buds originating directly from the foregut [4].

In second theory, failure of separate process of ventral trachea and dorsal esophagus is the main case of TE malformations [5].

Interestingly, EA is not a part of this initial malformation. Atretic proximal esophagus is a result of late rearrangement of the cranial foregut, resulting in a blind-ending structure.

Finally, genetic models show that the expression of some factors is fundamental for separation of anterior foregut and loss of this dorsoventral boundary expression domains disrupts the physical separation of the foregut [3].

1.2. History and classification

The first survivors of EA and TEF were not recorded until 1939 with Leven and Ladd achieving success with staged esophageal repair. Cameron Haight is fully credited with the first successful primary repair and survival of a 12-day-old female neonate [6].

In 1929, Vogt proposed the first anatomical classification of EA and TEF, based on radiological and postmortem findings. **Figure 1** and **Table 1** show a working classification based on the frequency of each anomaly (gross classification).

1.3. Associated anomalies

EA can be divided clinically into isolated EA and syndromic EA, occurring at the same rate. The most frequent associated malformations encountered in syndromic EA are [7]:

Cardiac (20–30%)

Vertebra (10–15%)

Limb (5–19%)

Anorectal (15–25%)

Renal (5–14%)

Nonrandom association has been documented as well. Two of these are the VACTERL (**V**ertebral, **A**norectal, **C**ardiac, **T**racheo-**E**sophageal, **R**enal and **L**imb abnormalities) and CHARGE association (**C**oloboma, **H**eart defects, **A**tresia of choan, developmental **R**etardation, **G**enital hypoplasia and **E**ar deformities).

1.4. Clinical presentation

A newborn with EA is often noted to have difficulty clearing saliva. Episodes of coughing, choking and even transient cyanosis may be observed.

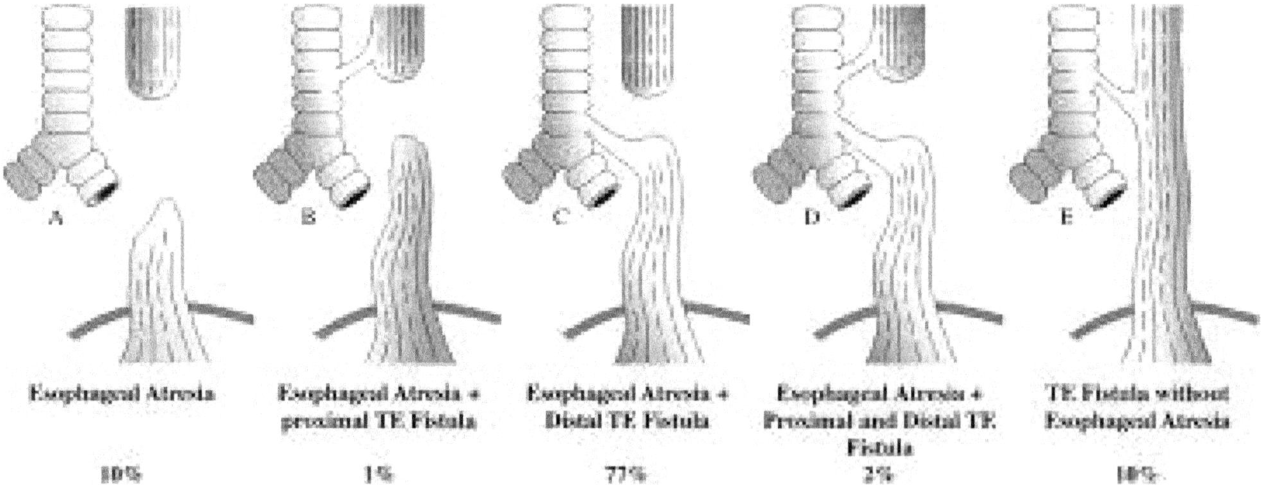

Figure 1. Schematic presentations of EA and TEF.

Type C	**85%**	**EA and distal TEF**
Type A	7%	Isolated EA
Type E	4%	TEF without EA
Type D	3%	EA and proximal and distal fistula
Type B	1%	EA proximal fistula

Table 1. Gross classification of EA and TEF.

1.5. Diagnosis

1.5.1. Antenatal

1. Polyhydramnios
2. Absence of stomach bubble in sonography

1.5.2. Postnatal

The diagnosis of EA and TEF is confirmed by the failure of passage of a firm nasogastric tube. Coiling of the tube can be demonstrated in plain chest and abdominal X-ray (**Figure 2**). Presence of gas-filled intestine loops below the diaphragm is a landmark of associated TEF. In isolated EA, a featureless gasless abdominal X-ray is observed.

1.6. Preoperative preparation

After a complete physical examination, routine blood work including cross match should be performed.

Other evaluations are included as:

1. Preoperative echocardiogram (to assess for major structural abnormalities, the position of aortic arch)
2. VACTERL workup
3. Genetic consultation

1.7. Operative technique

Extrapleural approach through the right fourth intercostal space allows the identification of azygos vein, TEF and upper pouch. Division of TEF and primary anastomosis of the esophagus are essential elements of operative technique. TEF is identified along the vagus nerve. TEF is encircled by tape and divided nearly trachea and closed. One-layer stitch anastomosis is the most standard procedure for end-to-end anastomosis [8].

1.8. Postoperative care

The infant should be nursed in the intensive care unit following repair of EA and TEF. Intravenous fluids and broad spectrum antibiotics are continued. Weaning from ventilation need not to be unduly prolonged in the stable infants with satisfactory anastomosis. In most cases, transanastomotic tube feeding can be commenced after 48 h and slowly increased as tolerated by the infant.

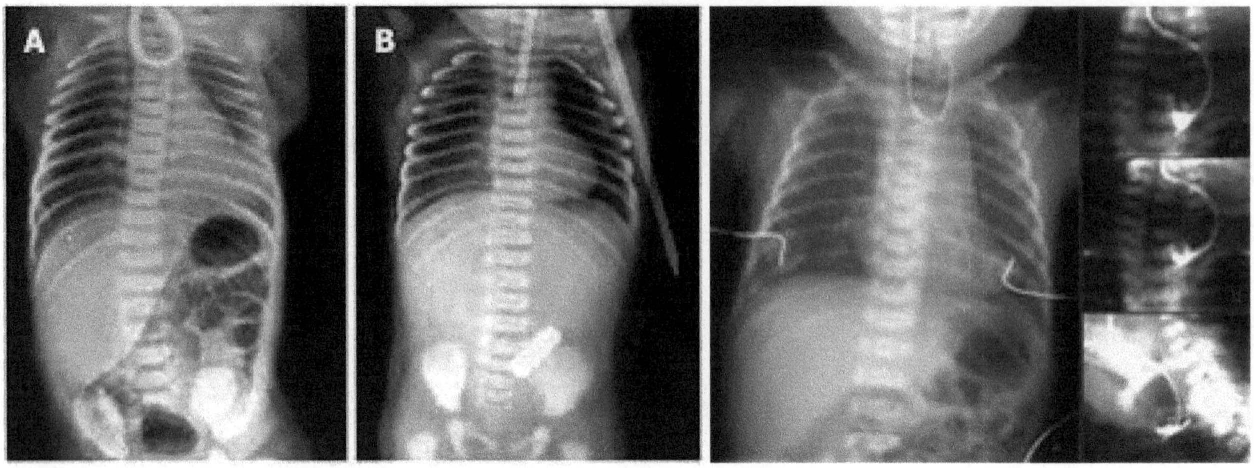

Figure 2. Example of a CXR demonstrating EA.

2. Achalasia

2.1. Embryology

Achalasia is an uncommon disorder of esophageal dysmotility, with an annual incidence of only one in 100,000 individuals.

Achalasia is derived from Greek word, meaning 'no relaxation' of the lower esophageal sphincter (LES). It is suggested that the cause of achalasia is ischemia following excessive rotation of the gut as a volvulus in utero in the embryo which selectively destroys ganglion cells [9]. Other tissues recover but neurons do not regenerate, leaving denervated gut forever.

In normal swallowing, coordinate peristaltic contractions of the esophageal body and transient relaxation of the LES cause the antegrade propulsion of ingested foods.

In patients with achalasia, this normal relaxation fails to occur. Patients with achalasia often have a reduced number of ganglion cells, and the ganglion cells are surrounded by an inflammatory infiltrate. It seems that the primary pathology must be in the wall of the gut and not in the CNS. This ganglion cell loss is best seen in Auerbach's plexus between the esophageal muscle layers.

In second theory, an autoimmune mechanism, which is the progressive partial destruction of the ganglion cells and the inhibitory neurons that normally mediate LES relaxation, is the main cause of Achalasia.

2.2. History

Achalasia/cardiospasm was first described by Sir Thomas Wills in 1672. In 1881, Von Mikulicz described the disease as a functional problem, but Heller (1913) was the first surgeon to perform esophagomyotomy successfully [10].

2.3. Associated anomalies

Achalasia in children has been associated with trisomy 21, triple-A syndrome (achalasia, alacrima and AcTH insensitivity) and familial dysautonomia, but most are sporadic.

2.4. Clinical presentation

In pediatric practice, most achalasia is reported during adolescence, more often in boys. Typical symptoms include dysphagia, vomiting or regurgitation of food, chest pain and weight loss or failure to thrive. Adolescents with achalasia usually suffer from halitosis. In children, respiratory symptoms consistent with aspiration may occur.

Bronchiectasis has also been reported due to recurrent aspiration specially in Down`s syndrome cases.

2.5. Diagnosis

2.5.1. Contrast study

The initial test in the child with dysphagia is usually contrast esophagogram in supine and upright positions. Classic findings include a dilated esophagus and a 'bird beak' deformity at the gastro-intestinal junction (GEJ) (**Figure 3**). In long standing disease, the progressively redundant esophagus can adopted a sigmoid shape.

2.5.2. Manometry

The standard test for achalasia remains manometry. Pressure recording shows absent or diminished peristalsis in the upper esophagus, elevated LES pressures, and minimal or absent LES relaxation.

2.5.3. Endoscopy

Endoscopy may demonstrate pooling of retained fluid within the esophagus and stasis-induced inflammation. Although mild resistance is encountered in endoscopy, but it can be passed in to the stomach, ruling out of mechanical stricture.

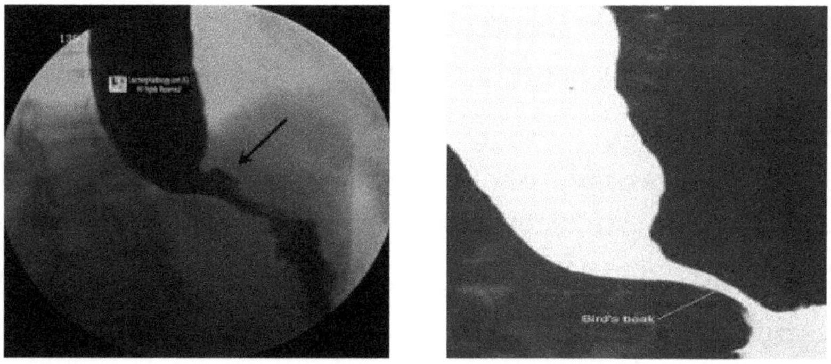

Figure 3. Esophagram demonstrating the 'bird's beak' deformity of achalasia.

2.6. Nonoperative management

2.6.1. Balloon dilation

Balloon dilation of the LES is the most common nonoperative management in achalasia in children; however, symptomatic relief is transient, and thus, repeated dilations are required.

2.6.2. Intrasphincteric toxin injection

Botulinum toxin injection lowers Les pressure by inhibiting acetylcholine release from nerve endings. This effect is also transient, requiring repeated injection [11].

2.7. Operative technique (modified Heller's cardiomyotomy)

Cardiomyotomy for achalasia requires division of the lower esophageal sphincter. This can be accomplished with a thoracic or abdominal approach, open or minimally invasively, with or without a concomitant antireflux procedure [12, 13].

3. Esophageal diverticulum

Esophageal diverticulum is a sac or pouch that protrudes from the esophageal wall, and it is rare in children. It is thought to be caused by an increase in the intraesophageal pressure associated with either distal esophageal motility disorders or periesophageal inflammation [14].

Esophageal diverticulum characterized according to their pathogenesis as either traction or pulsion. Traction diverticulums are true that occur in the mid esophagus secondary to inflammation process in the mediastinum causing an external force on the esophagus.

Pulsion diverticula is a pseudodiverticulum. There are two types of pulsion diverticula: Zenker diverticula and epiphrenic diverticula. Epiphrenic diverticulas occur with increased pressure against the upper and lower esophagus sphincters.

Zenker diverticulum (ZD) is a false diverticulum of the posterior esophagus between the cricopharyng and inferior constrictor. This area of anatomical weakness is known as Killian`s triangle. ZD occurs with high intraluminal pressure created during swallowing [15]. ZD is more likely to occur with increased size of Killian`s triangle [16]. Majority of these cases involve anatomical esophageal deformities or iatrogenic injury in the early postnatal period [17].

Esophageal diverticulum is classified into three categories according to the site of development: pharyngoesophageal diverticulaes, bifurcation diverticulaes and epiphrenic ones [18].

Pediatric esophageal diverticulums were classified according to their physiology by Meadows in 1970 [16]. He described nine types of diverticula in children and infants: cricopharyngeal diverticulum, pulsion diverticulum (Zenker types), duplication of esophagus (epiphrenic and nonepiphrenic), traction diverticulum from the middle third of the esophagus, diverticulum arising in scar tissue, false diverticulum above a congenital stenosis, and traumatic pseudo-diverticulum after trachea esophageal fistula repair. Only nonepiphrenic duplication, traumatic, pulsion and congenital diverticula may involve the pharyngoesophageal junction.

Duplication of the esophagus results from a defect in tabulation of esophagus in division of the embryonic foregut [19]. These duplication cysts consist of double layers of smooth muscle that are covered with epithelium. Two-third of them are located in lower third and one-third in the upper/middle third of esophagus [20]. Mostly, they do not communicate with esophagus wall but the duplication cysts as a separate malformation locate along or in continuity with native esophagus [21].

Esophageal duplication cysts can be associated with other congenital anomalies such as small intestinal duplication, esophageal atresia, trachea esophageal fistula, and spinal abnormalities including scoliosis, hemivertebra and fusion [19, 22].

Traumatic pharyngeal pseudodiverticulum is caused in neonates by traumatic catheterization through the esophagus causing perforation of the pharynx and incorrect insertion of a nasogastric tube [23, 24].

Congenital pharyngoesophageal diverticulum is a true diverticulum that contains all normal esophageal musculomucosal layers. Few cases are reported that allow no valid conclusions as to their etiology [25].

Pulsion diverticulum is rare in children, and the reported cases were 6-month- to 10-year-old children. Some related mechanisms include incoordination between movement of food out of the mouth and relaxation of the cricopharyngeal, motility disorder and developmental muscle weakness [16, 26, 27]. No clinical or radiological differences exist between pharyngo-esophageal diverticulum and pulsion diverticulum; both are posterior diverticulum that only distinguished by histological exams [28].

Chronic impaction of the foreign body has been proposed as the activating factor of pharyngoesophageal diverticula [27]. Foreign body ingestion is frequent in children, especially between 6 months and 3 years of age [29]. Majority of them travel the gastrointestinal tract without any adverse effects [30]. The cricopharyngeal sphincter is a well-known area of upper digestive tract, narrowing where foreign bodies are likely to get blocked. It is hypothesized that chronic impaction of the foreign body at the level of the cricopharyngeal muscle-induced muscle hypertonia responsible for the development of the pouch [28].

3.1. History

(1) Gastrointestinal symptoms: gagging, dysphagia, odynophagia, vomiting, regurgitation, dysphagia, failure to thrive, anorexia, epigastric pain, gastrointestinal hemorrhage, halitosis and poor feeding [31, 32].

(2) Respiratory symptoms: choking, cyanosis [17], dyspnea, wheeze, cough, stridor, respiratory distress [31], recurrent bronchiolitis, pneumonia and aspiration [32].

3.2. Diagnosis

- Barium swallow
- CT scan
- Esophageal endoscopy

3.3. Treatment

The management of esophageal diverticula includes both conservative and surgical treatments. If the child is asymptomatic, conservative treatment and careful follow-up are recommended. However, when the patient has complications related to esophageal diverticula, then surgical treatment is considered [33].

The traditional surgical treatment for esophageal diverticula is either a diverticulectomy or a diverticolopexy. However, in recent years, minimally invasive surgery such as thoracoscopic or laparoscopic treatment has become popular.

Recently, flexible endoscopy using CO_2 laser technique has been developed for the treatment of esophageal diverticula [34].

3.4. Postoperative care

Most of patients show no symptoms and are discharged from the hospital. In some center, esophageal endoscopy is done after months, later to show existence of narrowing or residual diverticulum in esophagus.

Author details

Mehrdad Hosseinpour* and Bahareh Ahmadi

*Address all correspondence to: meh_hosseinpour@yahoo.com

Imam Hossein Children Hospital, Isfahan University of Medical Sciences, Isfahan, Iran

References

[1] Ten Have-Opbroek AAW. Lung development in the mouse embryo. Experimental Lung Research. 1991;**17**:111-130

[2] Sasaki T, Kusafuka T, Okada A. Analysis of the development of normal foregut and tracheoesophageal fistula in an adriamycin rat model using three-dimensional image reconstruction. Surgery Today. 2001;**31**(2):133-139

[3] Ioannides AS, Copp AJ. Embryology of oesophageal atresia. Seminars in Pediatric Surgery. 2009;**18**(1):2-11

[4] Merei J, Hasthorpe S, Farmer P, Huston JM. Relationship between esophageal atresia with tracheoesophageal fistula and vertebral anomalies in mammalian embryo. Journal of Pediatric Surgery. 1998;**33**(1):58-63

[5] Williams AK, Quan QB, Beasly SW. Three dimensional imaging clarifies the process of tracheoesophageal separation in the rat. Journal of Pediatric Surgery. 2003;**38**(2):173-177

[6] Harmon C, Coran A. Congenital anomalies of the oesophagus. In: Coran A, Adzick NS, Krummel T, editors. Paediatric Surgery. Philadelphia: Elsevier; 2012. p. 892

[7] Baird R, Laberge JM. Esophageal atresia and tracheoesophageal fistula. In: Mattei P, editor. Fundamental of Paediatric Surgery. Philadelphia: Springer; 2011. pp. 257-267

[8] Taguchi T. Standard operation for esophageal atresia. In: Taguchi T, Iwanaka T, Okamatsu T, editors. Operative General Surgery in Neonates and Infants. Japan: Springer; 2016. pp. 95-100

[9] Franklin AL, Petrosyan M, Kane TD. Childhood achalasia: A comprehensive review of disease, diagnosis and therapeutic management. World Journal of Gastrointestinal Endoscopy. 2014;**6**(4):105-111

[10] Moreau P. Achalasia. In: Parikh DH, Crabbe DC, Auldist AW, Rothenberg SS, editors. Paediatric Thoracic Surgery. London: Springer; 2009. pp. 335-340

[11] Hurwitz M, Bahar RJ, Ament ME, et al. Evaluation of the use of botulinum toxin in children with achalasia. Journal of Pediatric Gastroenterology and Nutrition. 2000;**30**:509-514

[12] Nau P, Rattner D. Laparoscopic Heller myotomy as the gold standard for treatment of achalasia. Journal of Gastrointestinal Surgery. 2014;**18**(12):2201-2207

[13] Patti MG, Albanese CT, Holcom GW III, et al. Laparoscopic Heller myotomy and Dor fundoplication for esophageal achalasia in children. Journal of Pediatric Surgery. 2001;**36**:1248-1251

[14] Van der Peet DL, Klinkenberg-Knol EC, Berends FJ, Cuesta MA. Epiphrenic diverticula: Minimal invasive approach and repair in five patients. Diseases of the Esophagus. 2001;**14**:60-62

[15] Rush LV, Stingily CR. Congenital diverticulum of the esophagus: Case report. Southern Medical Journal. 1929;**22**:546

[16] Meadows JA. Esophageal diverticula in infants and children. Southern Medical Journal. 1970;**63**:691-694

[17] Lindholm EB, Hansbourg F, Upp JR, Cilloniz R, Lopo J. Congenital esophageal diverticulum—a case report and review of literature. Journal of Pediatric Surgery. 2013;**48**:665-668

[18] Akagi M, Sugano S, Kato I. Two cases of esophageal diverticula. Acta Oto-Laryngologica. 1996;**522**:138-141

[19] Ratan ML, Anand R, Mittal SK, Taneja S. Communicating oesophageal duplication: A report of two cases. Gut. 1988;**29**(2):254-256

[20] Lio R, Aler DG. Duplication cysts: Diagnosis, management, and the role of endoscopic ultrasound. Endoscopic Ultrasound. 2017;**3**(3):152-160

[21] Wootton-Gorges SL, Eckel GM, Poulos ND, Kappler S, Milstein JM. Duplication of the cervical esophagus: A case report and review of the literature. Pediatric Radiology. 2002;**32**:533-535

[22] Sethi GK, Marsden J, Johnson D. Duplication cysts of the esophagus. South Medical Journal. 1974;**67**:616-618

[23] Ducharme JC, Bertrand R, Debie J. Perforation of the pharynx in the newborn: A condition mimicking esophageal atresia. Canadian Medical Association Journal. 1971;**104**(9):785-787

[24] Wang B, Hunter WJ, Bin-Sagheer S, et al. Rare potential pitfall in endoscopic ultrasound-guided fine needle aspiration biopsy in gastric duplication cyst: A case report. Acta Cytologica. 2009;**53**:219-222

[25] Pal K, Alwabari A, Abdulatif M. Traumatic pharyngeal pseudodiverticulum mimicking esophageal atresia. Indian Journal of Pediatrics. 2007;**74**(2):195-196

[26] Theander G. Congenital posterior midline pharyngo-esophageal diverticula. Pediatric Radiology. 1973;**1**(3):153-155

[27] Dokucu AI, Fabre M, Otçu S, Sari UI, Onen A, Oztrk H, et al. Zenker's diverticulum in childhood: A new case. European Journal of Pediatric Surgery. 2000;**10**(3):191-193

[28] Kobayashi T. Esophageal foreign bodies in children. International Journal of Pediatric Otorhinolaryngology. 1984;**7**(2):193-198

[29] Patron V, Gody B, Aubry K, Jegoux F. Endoscopic treatment of pharyngo-esophageal diverticulum in child. International Journal of Pediatric Otorhinolaryngology. 2010;**74**:694-697

[30] Little DC, Shah SR, St Peter SD, Calkin CM, Morrow SE. Esophageal foreign bodies in the pediatric population: Our first 500 cases. Journal of Pediatric Surgery. 2006;**41**:914-918

[31] McGahren ED. Esophageal foreign bodies. Pediatrics in Review. 1999;**20**:129-133

[32] Arana A, Hauser B, Hachimi-Idrissi S, et al. Management of ingested foreign bodies in childhood and review of the literature. European Journal of Pediatrics. 2001;**160**:468-472

[33] Arboya JL, Fazzi JGF, Mayhoral J. Congenital esophageal cysts: Case report and review of the literature. American Journal of Gastroenterology. 1984;**79**:177-182

[34] Nishimoto Y, Taguchi T, Ogita K, Hashizume M. Endoscopic diverticulotomy for symptomatic paediatric esophageal diverticula. Pediatric Surgery International. 2005;**21**:50-53

13

Lymphocytic Esophagitis

Dane Christina Daoud and Mickael Bouin

Abstract

Lymphocytic esophagitis is a new and rare entity, first described in 2006. Histologically, the esophageal mucosa is characterized by a dense peripapillary lymphocytic infiltrate and an intercellular edema without granulocytosis. To this day, it is not yet considered as a disease. Its etiology and clinical significance are still unclear. The predominant symptom is dysphagia and the main endoscopic feature is a normal esophagus. The absence of relationship between lymphocytic esophagitis and specific clinical conditions justifies further studies. Currently, it remains a histologic entity.

Keywords: lymphocyte, esophagitis, dysphagia, Crohn, CD4, CD8, motility

1. Introduction

Lymphocytic esophagitis is a histopathological entity described for the first time in 2006 by Rubio *et al.* [1]. Subsequently, several publications have confirmed the existence of this new condition. Research has allowed us to better characterize the histology of Lymphocytic esophagitis. Unfortunately, clinical presentation and treatment remain poorly understood.

2. Prevalence

Lymphocytic esophagitis is a very rare condition. In 2012, Haque *et al.* estimated its prevalence to 0.1% in the United States [2]. In their cohort that included 129,252 esophageal biopsies, a diagnosis of lymphocytic esophagitis was made in only 119 patients. Since Rubio's first publication, there is a marked increase of its incidence, probably because of pathologists' and gastroenterologists' awareness [3].

Moreover, since it is a novel entity and most of the studies are from North America, world-wide prevalence has not been evaluated.

3. Histology

A small amount of intraepithelial lymphocytes is normally present in the esophagus [4, 5]. A majority of these lymphocytes are CD8 T cells, whereas CD4 are a minority and usually present in the lamina propria. An increase in CD8 T cells is seen in peptic and eosinophilic esophagitis. In addition, this lymphocytosis is generally accompanied by eosinophils and/or neutrophils [5–8].

Compared to other esophageal pathologies, lymphocytic esophagitis is characterized by an isolated lymphocytosis. The main histologic findings are a dense peripapillary intraepithelial lymphocytic infiltrate, an intercellular edema known as spongiosis, as well as the absence or rarity of granulocytes (**Figure 1**) [1]. The intraepithelial lymphocytes express CD3, CD4, and CD8, as shown by immunohistochemistry [1, 9, 11].

Unfortunately, because the histologic criteria are not yet standardized, it can sometimes lead to misdiagnosis. For instance, the presence of rare intraepithelial granulocytes is accepted in lymphocytic esophagitis [1, 2, 10, 11]. However, granulocytes can be found in various esophageal diseases, making diagnosis more difficult [11]. The acceptable number of granulocytes still needs to be better defined.

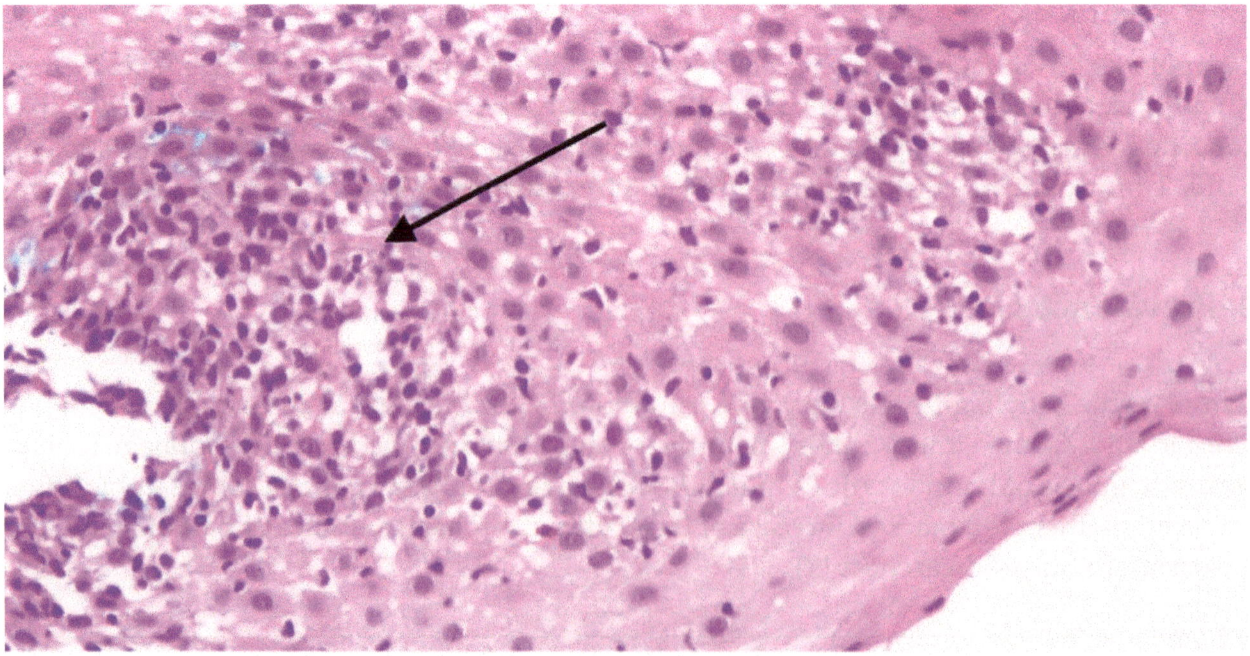

Figure 1. Lymphocytic esophagitic (H&E stain, original magnification ×40). Dense peripapillary lymphocytic infiltrate with spongiosis (arrow). Absence of neutrophils and eosinophils.

Because the lymphocytosis is patchy and uneven, we suggest not to establish a minimum number of intraepithelial lymphocytes [2]. In fact, the various studies about this entity have all used different cutoff, ranging between 10 and 50 lymphocytes per high-power field (HPF) [2, 3, 12, 13].

Furthermore, lymphocytic esophagitis affects the whole esophagus, but predominantly the distal esophagus. Thus, multiple biopsies are necessary to avoid a false negative because the lymphocyte infiltrates are not distributed evenly throughout the entire esophagus [12].

The mucosal involvement is considered mild if the intraepithelial lymphocytosis is only peripapillary and is severe if there is also an interperipapillary lymphocyte infiltration [12].

4. Clinical manifestations

Lymphocytic esophagitis seems to affect mostly women around 60 years old and smokers [2, 3, 10, 11]. The most common symptom is dysphagia [2, 8, 11, 13]. Nausea, vomiting, chest pain, heartburn, and episodes of impactions have also been reported; however, dysphagia remains the principal and most frequent complaint in 53% of cases [2, 3, 12]. Patients with lymphocytic esophagitis do not appear to show weight loss or fever.

The most serious complication is esophageal perforation. In 10 years, two cases of perforation have been reported. One of the two perforations occurred after the removal of a piece of impacted meat, while the second case was a spontaneous microperforation [14, 15].

5. Endoscopic features

Endoscopically, the most frequent findings are a normal esophagus or esophagitis [2, 3, 11]. Up to 33% of cases from the cohort by Haque *et al.* had findings suspicious of eosinophilic esophagitis such as stricture, rings, or felinization without eosinophilic esophagitis on the biopsies [2]. As described later, no other gastrointestinal involvement or association with gastritis or duodenitis has been described, thus stomach and duodenum endoscopic appearance is normal [12].

The endoscopic features are variable and not specific, which makes it impossible to identify and diagnose lymphocytic esophagitis by only relying on symptoms and gastroscopy. It is still a histologic condition, which is why biopsy is essential for the diagnosis.

6. Clinical associations

Some retrospective studies and case reports have tried to identify an association between lymphocytic esophagitis and other clinical conditions. Whether it was inflammatory bowel disease, gastroesophageal reflux disease, celiac disease, asthma, allergies, irritants, or connective tissue diseases (lupus, Behçet's disease), no relationship could be identified [2, 11–13, 16].

Lymphocytic esophagitis is isolated to the esophagus. It does not coexist with other digestive lymphocytosis such as lymphocytic colitis or lymphocytic gastritis. There is no correlation between these distinct entities. In a case series from Purdy *et al.*, some patients had concomitant biopsies from the rest of the digestive tract (stomach, small intestine, or colon). The histologic findings in these biopsies were various and secondary to preexisting conditions. No lymphocytic entity was observed in the rest of the gastrointestinal tract [8].

6.1. Gastroesophageal reflux disease

One of the main research efforts was to identify a relationship between lymphocytic esophagitis and reflux. Unfortunately, no association has been established between these two conditions [2, 12]. Indeed, only 22 out of 119 patients in the cohort from Haque *et al.* had gastroesophageal reflux disease [2].

6.2. Crohn's disease

In the cohort from Rubio *et al.*, 8 of 20 patients had Crohn's disease [1]. However, subsequent studies failed to replicate this association with inflammatory bowel disease [2, 11, 17]. Nevertheless, while it appears that it is not associated with inflammatory bowel disease in adults, lymphocytic esophagitis may be a manifestation of upper gastrointestinal Crohn's disease in the pediatric population [1, 12, 10]. Indeed, seven out of eight Crohn's disease patients from Rubio *et al.* were pediatric cases. Purdy *et al.* confirmed this association with the pediatric Crohn's disease [1].

6.3. Eosinophilic esophagitis

Eosinophilic esophagitis has also been a subject of study and comparison with lymphocytic esophagitis. The clinical and endoscopic manifestations of lymphocytic esophagitis can be confused with those of eosinophilic esophagitis. It is only histology that allows us to differentiate these two entities. Felinization is not pathognomonic of eosinophilic esophagitis, hence the importance of biopsy [2].

In a recent cohort from Rubio *et al.*, out of 311 biopsies with an increased number of intraepithelial lymphocytes, 33 cases were a compound of lymphocytic esophagitis and eosinophilic esophagitis [9]. We can thus ask whether these are two distinct conditions or whether one is the continuum of the other. However, this assumption remains a hypothesis and requires to be studied.

6.4. Motility disorders

Since 2014, an interest for esophageal motility disorders in lymphocytic esophagitis has arisen. Recent studies have demonstrated an association with achalasia and primary esophageal motility disorder (nutcracker esophagus, ineffective esophageal motility, and diffuse spasm) [18].

In 2015, Xue *et al.* noticed that esophageal biopsies in patients with primary esophageal motility abnormalities had CD4 + intraepithelial lymphocytosis. Moreover, Xue evoked the possibility of a new clinical entity that they called "dysmotility-associated LE." We still need further studies to better understand and characterize this association [11].

7. Treatment

Treatment of lymphocytic esophagitis remains controversial. Very few studies addressed this subject. Because it is still a recent and rare entity, a majority of therapeutic trials have been reported in the form of case reports or retrospective studies.

Proton pump inhibitor, topical or oral steroids as well as esophageal dilation or injections of Botox have been tried. All these treatments have been partially effective [3, 13–16, 19–21]. Nevertheless, it is too early to establish which treatment is better and should be recommended.

The use of proton pump inhibitor is based on the belief that lymphocytic esophagitis may be associated with esophageal reflux. However, as mentioned earlier, this association remains unclear and unlikely. Nevertheless, given the low toxicity of proton pump inhibitors, we suggest using them as first line of treatment.

Concerning the efficacy of corticosteroids, it may suggest that lymphocytic and eosinophilic esophagitis belong to the same family.

8. Natural history

Unfortunately, we have very little data on the clinical course of this condition. Cohen *et al.* was the only one who studied this sphere through a survey he sent to 29 patients with lymphocytic esophagitis. In his cohort, patients report an improvement in their symptoms with medical treatment (proton pump inhibitor or anti-TNF for Crohn's cases). Control endoscopies were performed in 22 out of 29 patients and 9 esophageal biopsies showed persistence of lymphocytic esophagitis despite treatment [3].

Current available literature points out that lymphocytic esophagitis is a chronic condition [12]. The risk of esophageal neoplasia is still unknown.

9. Conclusion

Lymphocytic esophagitis is a newly described clinical and histologic condition that will probably be increasingly recognized upon the next years. Recent publications have allowed us to establish clear criteria, thus facilitating the diagnosis. Clinicians need to be aware of this entity because lymphocytic esophagitis may eventually be in the diagnostic algorithm of dysphagia.

Pathologists are increasingly recognizing this condition, which is an asset for research. With larger cohorts, we will be able to further characterize its worldwide epidemiology, clinical associations, as well as treatment and natural history. Single-cell analysis of the intraepithelial lymphocyte subtypes may help in understanding the pathophysiology of the condition and compare subgroups with compound eosinophilic esophagitis and those without. As Haque once said, "it is a condition in search of a disease."

Acknowledgements

We are grateful to Dre Amélie Therrien (Hôpital Saint-Luc, CHUM, Montréal) and Dre Elizabeth Arslanian (Hôpital Saint-Luc, CHUM, Montréal) for the critical review of the manuscript.

Author details

Dane Christina Daoud* and Mickael Bouin

*Address all correspondence to: christina_daoud@hotmail.com

University of Montreal, Saint-Luc Hospital, Montréal, Canada

References

[1] Rubio CA, Sjödahl K, Lagergren J. Lymphocytic esophagitis: A histologic subset of chronic esophagitis. American Journal of Clinical Pathology. 2006;**125**:432–437

[2] Haque S, Genta RM. Lymphocytic oesophagitis: Clinicopathological aspects of an emerging condition. Gut. 2012;**61**:1108–1114

[3] Cohen S, Saxena A, Waljee AK, Piraka C, Purdy J, Appelman H, McKenna B, Elmunzer BJ, Singal AG. Lymphocytic esophagitis: A diagnosis of increasing frequency. Journal of Clinical Gastroenterology. 2012;**46**:828–832

[4] Carmack SW, Lash RH, Gulizia JM, Genta RM. Lymphocytic disorders of the gastrointestinal tract: A review for the practicing pathologist. Advances in Anatomic Pathology. 2009;**16**:290–306

[5] Resnick MB, Finkelstein Y, Weissler A, et al. Assessment and diagnostic utility of the cytotoxic T-lymphocyte phenotype using the specific markers granzyme-B and TIA-1 in esophageal mucosal biopsies. Human Pathology. 1999;**30**:397–402

[6] Podolsky DK, Camilleri M, Fitz JG, Kalloo AN, Shanahan F, Wang TC. Yamada's Textbook of Gastroenterology. United States: John Wiley & Sons Inc. Vol. 2, Set. 6th Edition; 2015. P.49

[7] Lucendo AJ, Navarro M, Comas C, et al. Immunophenotypic characterization and quantification of the epithelial inflammatory infiltrate in eosinophilic esophagitis through stereology: An analysis of the cellular mechanisms of the disease and the immunologic capacity of the esophagus. American Journal of Surgical Pathology. 2007;**31**:598–606

[8] De Jonge PJ, Siersema PD, Van Breda SG, et al. Proton pump inhibitor therapy in gastro-oesophageal reflux disease decreases the oesophageal immune response but does not reduce the formation of DNA adducts. Alimentary Pharmacology & Therapeutics. 2008;**28**:127–136

[9] Rubio CA, Ichiya T, Schmidt PT. Lymphocytic oesophagitis, eosinophilic oesophagitis and compound lymphocytic-eosinophilic oesophagitis. I: Histological and immunohistochemical findings. Journal of Clinical Pathology. 2017;**70**:208–216

[10] Ebach DR, Vanderheyden AD, Ellison JM, et al. Lymphocytic esophagitis: A possible manifestation of pediatric upper gastro-intestinal Crohn's disease. Inflammatory Bowel Diseases. 2011;**17**:45–49

[11] Xue Y, Suriawinata A, Liu X, Li Z, Gabbard S, Rothstein R, Lacy B, Lisovsky M. Lymphocytic esophagitis with CD4 T-cell- predominant intraepithelial lymphocytes and primary esophageal motility abnormalities: A potential novel clinicopathologic entity. American Journal of Surgical Pathology. 2015;**39**:1558–1567

[12] Purdy JK, Appelman HD, Golembeski CP, et al. Lymphocytic esophagitis: A chronic or recurring pattern of esophagitis resembling allergic contact dermatitis. American Journal of Clinical Pathology. 2008;**130**:508–513

[13] Pasricha S, Gupta A, Reed CC, Speck O, Woosley JT, Dellon ES. Lymphocytic esophagitis: An emerging clinicopathologic disease associated with dysphagia. Digestive Disease Science. 2016;**61**:2935–2941

[14] Hendy PJ, Wong DS, Florin TH. Spontaneous oesophageal perforation: An unreported complication of lymphocytic oesophagitis. Gut. 2013;**62**:1668–1669

[15] Mandaliya R, Dimarino AJ, Cohen S. Lymphocytic esophagitis mimicking eosinophilic esophagitis. Annals of Gastroenterology. 2012;**25**:355–357

[16] Figueiredo PC, Pinto-Marques P, Borralho P, Freitas J. Unusual cause for smoldering dysphagia. Lymphocytic esophagitis. Dysphagia. 2014;**29**:283–285

[17] Basseri B, Vasiliauskas EA, Chan O, Wang HL, Basseri RJ, Pimentel M, Soffer E, Conklin JL. Evaluation of peripapillary lymphocytosis and lymphocytic esophagitis in adult inflammatory bowel disease. Gastroenterology & Hepatology (N Y). 2013;**9**:505–511

[18] Putra J, Muller KE, Hussain ZH, Parker S, Gabbard S, Brickley EB, Lacy BE, Rothstein R, Lisovsky M. Lymphocytic esophagitis in nonachalasia primary esophageal motility disorders: Improved criteria, prevalence, strength of association, and natural history. American Journal of Surgical Pathology. 2016;**40**:1679–1685

[19] Zhang Z, Jain D, Brand M. Ringed esophagus secondary to lymphocytic esophagitis. Gastroenterology & Hepatology (N Y). 2016;**12**:237–239

[20] Vangimalla S, Gordon I, Thota PN. Image of the month: Lymphocytic esophagitis in common variable immune deficiency. American Journal of Gastroenterology. 2016;**111**:170

[21] Kasirye Y, John A, Rall C, Resnick J. Lymphocytic esophagitis presenting as chronic dysphagia. Clinical Medicine & Research. 2012;**10**:83–84

14

Nutritional Management of Esophageal Cancer Patients

Dimitrios Schizas, Irene Lidoriki,
Demetrios Moris and Theodore Liakakos

Abstract

Esophageal cancer is associated with malnutrition in the vast majority of patients. This phenomenon is partly attributed to the disease process itself, the location of the tumor and other factors, such as dysphagia which is often accentuated due to chemotherapy/radiotherapy treatment or surgical intervention. The poor nutritional status of these patients is often related to the presence of cancer cachexia, altered metabolism, and tissue wasting. Malnutrition in this patient population affects quality of life, worsens patient's tolerance to chemotherapy and accounts for lower survival. Nutritional management of these patients includes both proper nutritional assessment and support and might prevent, to a certain extent, the manifestation of malnutrition-related consequences. The purpose of this article is to review the current literature in order to focus on the etiology and diagnosis of malnutrition in esophageal cancer patients, emphasizing also on the optimal nutritional support during multimodality treatment.

Keywords: nutritional assessment, nutritional support, perioperative nutritional care, esophageal cancer

1. Introduction

Esophageal cancer is one of the most fatal cancers worldwide as it was ranked ninth for cancer incidence and sixth for cancer death in 2013. In 2013, there were 442,000 new cases of esophageal cancer and 440,000 deaths [1]. There are two main histologic subtypes of esophageal cancer: squamous cell carcinoma and adenocarcinoma, each one of them is related to several risk factors. Among them, modifiable lifestyle factors, such as alcohol consumption, tobacco use, and nutrition should be considered as key points in order to prevent esophageal cancer.

Excess alcohol consumption and consumption of hot food and beverages increase the risk of esophageal squamous cell carcinoma, whereas many components of Western type diet, such as red and processed meat increase the risk of esophageal adenocarcinoma [2–4]. Moreover, obesity, especially central type, and gastroesophageal reflux disease are risk factors toward developing esophageal adenocarcinoma [5, 6]. On the other hand, healthy dietary habits could be a shield against some types of esophageal cancer [7], while nutritional support could be beneficial for the management of these patients after cancer diagnosis.

Esophageal cancer is commonly associated with malnutrition and impaired nutritional intake. Nutritional management of these patients may differ according to the type of therapy and stage of disease, in order to alleviate symptoms, ameliorate nutritional status, and improve quality of life. Furthermore, cancer cachexia affects a great percentage of esophageal cancer patients emerging as a significant factor the multidisciplinary team should deal with [8]. Regarding the perioperative care, the proper type of feeding (i.e. enteral/parenteral nutrition (EN/PN), immunonutrition, oral supplements, etc.) as well as the right time of feeding is a matter of controversy due to lack of consistent evidence for patients undergoing esophagectomy [9]. Special nutritional needs in the long run are also of great significance for patients with both resectable and unresectble disease, bearing in mind that the majority of these patients strive to meet their caloric and protein needs. Considering the treatment approach, nutritional screening and assessment leads to early detection of malnourished patients in need of nutritional support. Taking into account patient's specific needs helps to choose the most suitable routes of delivering nutritional support (nutritional counseling and artificial nutrition). Personalized nutritional support could modify poor nutritional status resulting in reduced postoperative complications and improved survival. Moreover, the implementation of nutritional protocols could reduce toxicity of treatment regimens and in conjunction with nutritional monitoring could have impact on patients' daily living [10]. Therefore, nutritional therapy should be an essential part of a multidisciplinary approach in the clinical setting, in order to improve short- and long-term outcomes.

The aim of the current review is to focus on the etiology of malnutrition, review the various methods of nutritional assessment, and analyze the aspects of nutritional management of esophageal cancer patients as a fundamental part of multimodality therapy.

2. Nutritional status

2.1. Malnutrition rates and weight loss

Esophageal cancer patients often suffer from malnutrition, the manifestation of which is strongly linked to the stage of the disease and therapeutic regimens. Excessive weight loss is partly attributed to the disease process itself and is often deteriorated due to chemotherapy/radiotherapy treatment [11]. Malnutrition occurs in 60–85% of esophageal cancer patients, which is one of the highest reported rates when compared to other malignancies, such as lung, head and neck, stomach, and pancreatic cancers [12]. According to recent publications, 32% of patients who underwent esophagectomy experienced more than 10% weight loss preoperatively [13], while 90% of patients had a 5% weight loss at 3 months postoperatively [14]. It is noteworthy that in many patients weight loss persists for at least 3 years after surgical intervention [15]. Another study revealed that 43.8% of patients with esophageal cancer were underweight based on BMI values, 29.7% of patients were undernourished as indicated from anthropometric measurements and 69% had weight loss within 2 weeks before hospital admission [16]. Chemotherapy and radiotherapy affect nutritional status by promoting weight loss and muscle wasting. More specifically, malnutrition developed in 83.8% of patients after the end of radiotherapy [17] and the number of patients requiring nutritional intervention increased from 56 to 75% during induction chemotherapy [10]. These facts highlight the need of nutritional assessment at several time points in order to identify patients who are candidates for nutritional support.

2.2. Methods of nutritional assessment and impact on clinical outcome

There are various methods of nutritional assessment in the clinical setting providing clinicians with tools for the evaluation of the nutritional status and the estimation of nutritional needs of esophageal cancer patients. One commonly used criterion of malnutrition is the percentage of weight loss in a certain period of time. A weight loss of more than 5% in the previous month or more than 10% in the last 3–6 months is considered significant malnutrition [18]. One retrospective study concluded that weight loss <10% and BMI>18 kg/m^2 were significantly correlated with a better response to chemoradiotherapy, while BMI>18 kg/m^2 was predictive of survival at both univariate and multivariate analysis [19]. Other anthropometric measurements, such as mid-arm circumference and mid upper-arm muscle area can give information about the nutritional status and body composition of these patients.

Biochemical markers, such as plasma proteins are often used as nutritional markers. For instance, albumin is commonly used for the assessment of protein status, but given its long half-life (14–20 days), it has a slow response to dietary interventions and cannot detect subtle changes in nutritional status. Furthermore, albumin reflects an acute phase response and is not always a reliable marker of malnutrition [20]. However, albumin is an independent risk factor for complications after esophagectomy, since patients with hypoalbuminemia have twice the risk of postoperative infection and increased incidence of acute respiratory distress syndrome [21]. A recent review examined the association of serum albumin with postoperative complications in patients undergoing esophagectomy, suggesting that low serum albumin does increase the risk of postoperative complications, but there is still conflicting evidence regarding the prognostic value of this biomarker [22].

Other methods of nutritional assessment include questionnaires that incorporate many factors that impede adequate nutritional intake, as well as laboratory parameters, and unintentional weight loss. For example, Subjective Global Assessment (SGA), a questionnaire based on four parameters of patient's history (percentage of weight loss, changes in habitual diet, presence of significant gastrointestinal symptoms, and changes in patient's functional capacity) and three elements of their physical examination (loss of subcutaneous fat, muscle wasting, and presence of edema or ascites) is one the most commonly used tool for nutritional screening in malnourished hospital patients with cancer. SGA is strongly correlated with performance status in esophageal cancer patients [16] as well as with The Glasgow prognostic score and with complications during cancer treatment [23]. Other tools that have been studied in cancer patients is the Prognostic Nutritional Index (PNI), the Nutritional Risk Screening 2002 (NRS 2002), the Controlling Nutritional Status (CONUT) and the Nutritional Risk Index (NRI). Esophagectomized patients with a high Prognostic Nutritional Index—a tool which includes serum albumin and absolute peripheral lymphocyte count—had a higher prevalence of postoperative complications [24]. These results are in accordance with later studies, indicating that nutritional status preoperatively, expressed as PNI, was significantly related with the occurrence of severe complications and was a predictive factor for long-term survival [25, 26]. Nevertheless, Han-Geurts et al. showed that PNI was not associated with postoperative infectious complications in patients who underwent esophageal resection for malignancy [27]. NRS-2002 is recommended by the European Society for Clinical Nutrition and Metabolism as a standard tool for the assessment of surgical patients [28], but it is not tailored to esophageal cancer patients, thus limiting its prognostic value in this population. The CONUT score, which is calculated by serum albumin concentration, total peripheral lymphocyte count, and total cholesterol concentration, was developed as a screening tool for early detection of patients at risk of malnutrition [29]. Patients classified preoperatively as moderate or severe malnourished had a higher incidence of pulmonary and other severe morbidities, surgical site infections, and reoperation. Consequently, the duration of hospital stay in patients with moderate or severe malnutrition was significantly longer compared to well-nourished or slightly malnourished patients [30]. Similarly, Hirahara et al. [31] and Toyokawa et al. [32] demonstrated that CONUT was significantly associated with cancer death and poorer disease-free survival in patients with resectable esophageal squamous cell carcinoma. NRI is another tool used for the assessment of malnutrition based on serum albumin concentration and weight loss. Increased nutritional risk, derived from NRI, is associated with reduced survival in esophageal cancer patients treated with definitive chemoradiotherapy [10, 33], but is not associated with postoperative infectious complications in patients treated with esophagectomy [27]. The Geriatric Nutritional Risk Index (GNRI) is a new index recently introduced for the assessment of nutritional status of elderly patients. Patients diagnosed with poor nutritional status according to GNRI had significantly higher rate of respiratory complications after esophagectomy and gastric tube reconstruction [34]. In conclusion, there are several nutrition assessment tools for esophageal cancer patients, but since many of the studies mentioned above are of retrospective nature, the gold standard for the evaluation of nutritional status in this cancer subpopulation is yet to be determined (**Table 1**).

Percentage of unintentional weight loss	*Biochemical markers* (albumin, prealbumin, total peripheral lymphocyte count)	*Questionnaires and indices:* SGA, NRS2002, CONUT, NRI, PNI, Glasgow Prognostic Score

Table 1. Nutritional assessment of esophageal cancer patients.

2.3. Sarcopenia and cancer cachexia

Patients with esophageal cancer often witness loss of muscle mass and/or muscle strength, a condition described as sarcopenia. Although there are many different definitions of the term sarcopenia, all of them place emphasis on the impaired physical function following decreased muscle mass [35–37]. Sarcopenia is a component of cancer cachexia, especially in advanced stage cancer patients. Cancer cachexia is a complex syndrome which combines anorexia, early satiety, weakness, anemia, inflammation, weight loss, and loss of muscle mass with or without loss of fat mass [38]. A recent study pointed out that the prevalence of cancer cachexia in advanced esophageal cancer patients was 52.9% [39]. There is lack of consensus on the definition, diagnostic criteria, and classification of cancer cachexia, but the most commonly used definition includes one of the following: Weight loss >5% over past 6 months (in absence of simple starvation); or BMI <20 and any degree of weight loss >2%; or appendicular skeletal muscle index consistent with sarcopenia (males <7.26 kg/m^2; females <5.45 kg/m^2),and any degree of weight loss >2% [40]. Furthermore, assessment of sarcopenia plays an emerging role in cancer patients owing to the fact that CT scanning is a gold standard imaging method of body composition analysis at the tissue-organ level [41]. CT scans can identify reduced muscle mass and predict negative cancer outcomes in people with abdominal malignancies, where traditional methods of assessment are less effective [42]. Handgrip strength is another method used to measure muscle strength, which is directly related to the physiologic status of the individual and reflects patient's nutritional status. It could be easily used in patient's nutritional assessment due to the fact that it is an inexpensive and not time-consuming method.

Sarcopenia and cachexia are prognostic factors for surgical complications, decreased survival, and poor response to chemotherapy. More specifically, patients with weak handgrip strength had higher risk of complications and mortality after elective esophagectomy [43]. Decreased muscle mass, assessed by preoperative computed tomography scans, seems to be an independent predictor of both overall survival (**Figure 1**) [44] and disease-free survival, as significant as tumor stage, in patients following esophagectomy [45, 46]. In addition, sarcopenic patients who underwent esophagectomy had significantly higher rate of respiratory complications compared to nonsarcopenic subjects, but there was no difference in the incidence of overall complications between the two groups [47–49]. Sarcopenia has also impact on chemotherapy outcome since decreased muscle mass is associated with dose-limiting toxicity and pathological chemotherapy response in patients receiving neoadjuvant chemotherapy [50–52]. Therefore, it is imperative to estimate patients' muscle mass not only preoperatively but also before the onset of chemotherapy, bearing in mind that sarcopenia is frequently masqued by obesity making it more difficult to define patients' needs for intervention.

2.4. Mechanisms of malnutrition

Malnutrition, as mentioned above, affects a great percentage of esophageal cancer patients. Most patients are not able to achieve a positive energy balance and in many cases, initial body weight cannot even be maintained. This is ascribed mainly to impaired metabolism and side effects caused by esophagectomy or chemotherapy/radiation treatment. Dysphagia is a very common mechanical cause of malnutrition and is accompanied by dietary changes in order to

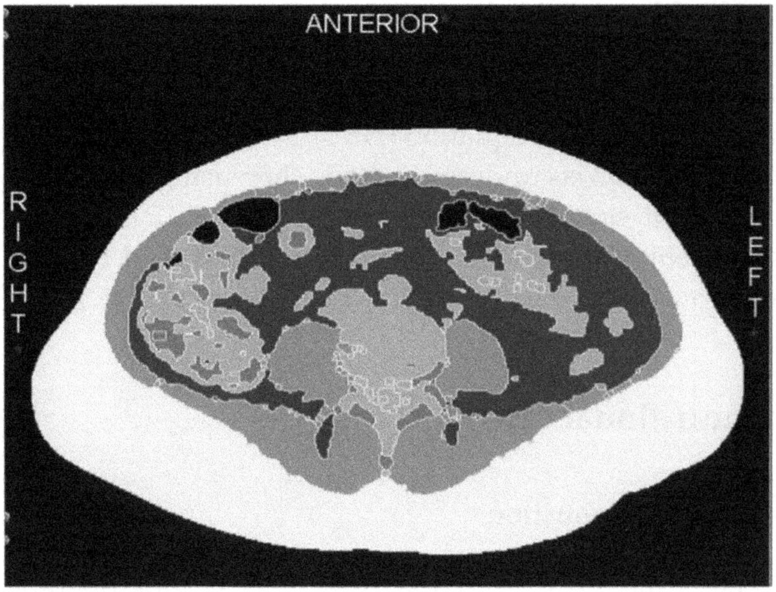

Figure 1. Example of CT scan analysis by the Slice-O-Matic software. Lumbar vertebrae 3 slice with Hounsfield units used to measure area of skeletal muscle, subcutaneous fat and visceral fat. White outer ring, subcutaneous fat; Light grey inner ring, muscle; Dark grey central area, visceral fat. Reproduced from Gibson et al. [42].

avoid foods that worsen symptoms leading to inadequate intake of calories. The surgical procedure often causes deficiencies in macronutrients and micronutrients, with the most prevailing side effects being postprandial dumping syndrome, dysphagia, anorexia, reflux, and early satiety [53–55]. Furthermore, chemotherapy affects rapidly proliferating cells preferentially and, consequently, affects the cells of the gastrointestinal tract. Chemotherapy-related causes of reduced food intake include nausea, vomiting, diarrhea, mucositis, and decreased appetite. Radiotherapy also contributes to malnutrition, and combined with chemotherapy exacerbates patients' nutritional status. Common side effects of radiotherapy include mucositis, esophagitis, odynophagia, mouth and throat soreness, and hypogeusia [56]. Tumor-related causes of malnutrition are also of great significance, but the mechanisms involved are still under investigation. Cancer-induced anorexia may result from circulating factors produced by the tumor or by the host in response to the tumor. For instance, cytokines, such as interleukins (IL) and tumor necrosis factor-alpha (TNF-α) cause anorexia [57], whereas other tumor-secreted factors promote central- and peripheral-mediated cancer cachexia. Tumor growth results in the secretion of pro-inflammatory factors that promote cachexia by signaling anorexia, muscle wasting, and white adipose tissue atrophy. Tumors also secrete both the proteolysis-inducing factor and activin, which promote skeletal muscle degradation and sarcopenia [58, 59].

Even though the mechanisms behind muscle wasting have been widely studied, less is known about the factors implicated in adipose tissue loss in cancer cachectic patients, such as lipid-mobilizing factor, as well as about the derangement in the neuroendocrine regulation of food intake and anorexia [60]. Additionally, changes in carbohydrate, lipid, and protein metabolism account for altered substrate metabolism. Changes in resting energy expenditure (REE) are considered one of the causes of nutritional depletion in cancer. In particular, measured REE by indirect calorimetry (IC) was elevated in patients with newly detected esophageal cancer, compared to healthy individuals [61]. A cross-sectional study involved 30 patients admitted with a diagnosis of squamous cell carcinoma who underwent IC before starting cancer therapy. The basal energy expenditure (BEE) was evaluated using IC and was also estimated using the Harris-Benedict Equation (HBE). The results showed that BEE of patients with squamous cell carcinoma was underestimated when using the HBE [62]. However, current evidence is inconsistent, since some studies suggest that REE is normal and is not affected by stage of disease [63–65]. Consequently, more research should be conducted in order to shed light on this controversial field.

3. Perioperative nutritional care

3.1. Enteral versus parenteral nutrition

Esophagectomy is one of the most invasive and time-consuming operations among gastrointestinal surgical procedures. It induces a strong stress response in the human body [66]. Consequently, patients' nutritional status is deteriorated after surgery, making postoperative nutritional care very important. The use of enteral nutrition (EN) postoperatively is a matter of debate, while scientific research attempts to define the role of enteral and parenteral nutrition (PN) on the clinical outcome of patients undergoing esophagectomy. Enteral feeding is considered the method of choice for the nutritional support of cancer patients with functioning gastrointestinal tract. Enteral nutrition is advantageous over parenteral nutrition for the following reasons: it provides all the necessary micro- and macronutrients in a more intact form, maintains gut mucosal integrity, inhibits the cytokine response, reduces the secretion of stress hormones, inhibits bacterial translocation, has a decreased risk of complications, and is less expensive [67]. Nevertheless, enteral nutrition is often avoided in order to minimize strain to the anastomoses, and reduce the risk of postoperatively impaired gastrointestinal motility. Another concern involves the return of gut motility or peristalsis and the ability of the gut to absorb nutrients. Surgical advances have increased the integrity of all anastomoses, making early oral enteral feeding after surgery a feasible option.

A randomized control trial investigated the outcomes of PN or EN after thoracoscopic esophagectomy. The rate of weight loss at postoperative day (POD) 14 was significantly lower in the EN group than in the PN group. Prealbumin levels at POD 10 showed no differences between the two groups. However, the incidence of postoperative pneumonia was higher in the PN group than in the EN group [68]. The results of another randomized clinical trial showed that there was no significant difference between EN and PN groups in terms of postoperative serum albumin, prealbumin, or transferrin. However, complement component 3 (C3) and 4 (C4) levels were significantly higher in the EN group compared with the PN group, while C-reactive protein level was significantly lower in the enteral feeding group. Bowel movements were restored sooner and costs of treatment were lower in the EN group. Postoperative complications did not differ significantly between the two groups [69]. Results from a recent meta-analysis of 10 randomized controlled trials concerning cancer patients following esophagectomy indicated that early postoperative enteral nutrition could significantly decrease pulmonary complications and anastomotic leakage compared with parenteral nutrition. On the eighth postoperative day, the EN group had higher levels of albumin and prealbumin compared with the PN group, suggesting that postoperative EN support is more effective in maintaining patients' nutritional status than PN support. No difference was observed in digestive complications between these two approaches. However, this meta-analysis is characterized by heterogeneity issues, especially regarding the postoperative nutritional status [70]. Furthermore, others suggest that combination of enteral and parenteral feeding is more beneficial, since total parenteral nutrition (TPN) could lead to hyperglycemia in stressed patients. A combination of EN and TPN might have some benefits when compared to TPN alone, such as improvement of intestinal integrity and stimulation of incretin production contributing to improved glucose control in patients undergoing esophagectomy [71]. Moreover, supplemental parenteral nutrition after esophagectomy contributes to better coverage of patients' calorie requirements, since large amounts of enteral nutrition are not usually tolerated in the first postoperative days [72].

The European Society for Parenteral and Enteral Nutrition (ESPEN) guidelines for nutritional support recommend that interruption of nutritional intake is unnecessary after surgery in most patients and in patients who require postoperative artificial nutrition, enteral feeding, or a combination of enteral and supplementary parenteral feeding is the first choice. Also this combination should be considered in patients in whom more than 60% of energy needs cannot be met via the enteral route. Postoperative parenteral nutrition is beneficial in undernourished patients in whom enteral nutrition is not feasible or not tolerated. In addition, postoperative parenteral nutrition is beneficial in patients with postoperative complications impairing gastrointestinal function that are unable to receive and absorb adequate amounts of oral/enteral feeding for at least 7 days [28]. Moreover, the American Society for Parenteral and Enteral Nutrition (ASPEN) guidelines for critically ill patients recommends that patients who have undergone major upper gastrointestinal tract surgery and EN is not feasible, PN should be initiated (only if the duration of therapy is anticipated to be more than 7 days). Unless the patient is at high nutrition risk, PN should not be started in the immediate postoperative period, but should be delayed for 5–7 days [73]. In conclusion, although enteral nutrition seems to be a safe and feasible option postoperatively in terms of immunological parameters and postoperative complications, no firm conclusion can be drawn regarding postoperative nutritional markers that reflect patients' nutritional status.

3.2. Time of feeding

3.2.1. Early enteral nutrition

The initiation of enteral feeding after esophagectomy remains a controversial topic and many studies examine whether or not early enteral feeding affects negatively or positively the postoperative outcome. One study that investigated early enteral feeding after esophagectomy included 208 patients who received enteral nutrition postoperatively and were divided into three groups (Group 1, 2, and 3) based on whether they received EN within 48 h, 48–72 h or more than 72 h, respectively. The postoperative complications, length of hospital (LOH) stay, days for first fecal passage, cost of hospitalization, and the difference in serum albumin values pre- and postoperatively were all recorded. Group 1 had the lowest thoracic drainage volume, the earliest first fecal passage, and the lowest LOH and hospitalization expenses of all the three groups. The incidence of pneumonia was higher in Group 3. Finally, all postoperative outcomes of nutritional status were worst in Group 3 [74]. Similarly, one systematic review demonstrated that early oral EN was associated with reduced length of stay and did not increase complication rates [75]. More randomized clinical trials are required to confirm the results from retrospective studies that indicated that early EN promotes early recovery of intestinal movement and better recovery from systemic inflammation [66]. In addition, current literature is inconclusive with respect to the right time of EN administration postoperatively, that is, EN initiation within 24 h versus EN initiation during 24–72 h [76, 77].

3.2.2. Enhanced recovery after surgery (ERAS)

Early enteral nutrition is an essential part of fast-track surgery protocols in order to maximize the effects of enhanced recovery. Fast-track programs incorporate new methods regarding anesthesia, nutritional care, pain control, and surgical techniques in the preoperative, intraoperative, and postoperative period, aiming to promote postoperative rehabilitation of patients [78]. ESPEN guidelines recommend that all cancer patients undergoing either curative or palliative surgery should be managed within an enhanced recovery program postoperatively; within this program every patient should be screened for malnutrition and if deemed at risk, given additional nutritional support [79]. Nutritional aspects of ERAS could be summarized as follows: limitation of preoperative fasting, preoperative fluid and carbohydrate loading, and initiation of oral diet on the first postoperative day [80]. A recently published review demonstrated that utilization of enhanced recovery programs in esophageal cancer patients was associated with a reduction in the incidence of anastomotic leak, pulmonary complications, and length of hospital stay, but no significant change was observed in postoperative mortality or readmission rate. Nevertheless, there was significant heterogeneity between the studies in terms of enhanced recovery protocols, surgical approach, and utilization of neoadjuvant therapies that should be taken into account [81]. Results from a randomized controlled clinical study showed that the implementation of a fast-track protocol improved postoperative clinical recovery and cellular and humoral immunity of patients undergoing esophagectomy for esophageal cancer (**Table 2**) [82]. In this context, the implementation of fast-track programs in esophagectomy patients is promising, but the majority of patients included in the studies are relatively healthy patients. More randomized controlled studies and evidence-based research are required in order to justify the routine use of fast-track protocols in esophageal cancer patients [83].

3.3. Perioperative immunonutrition

Immunonutrition is one of the most debated topics in nutritional support of esophageal cancer patients. The term immunonutrition includes formulas that contain immune-modulating substances, such as arginine, glutamine, ribose nucleic acid, and omega-3-fatty acids. A recent review concluded that postoperative enteral immunonutrition could be promising in improving humoral immunity in patients undergoing esophagogastric resection, but this improvement is not related to a reduced hospital stay, nor does it reduce the rate of infections. The authors reported that there is heterogeneity regarding the types of operations undertaken (two studies included patients undergoing esophagectomy, three studied patients undergoing gastrectomy,

Day	FTS pathway
POD1	Jejunostomy tube feeding 500 ml (starting at 20 ml/h) Early postoperative mobilization program (>2 h out of bed) Physical therapy and nebulizers Remove urine catheter Head of bed put at 30° Supply albumin Chest tube to suction Promoted to lung recruitment
POD2	Jejunostomy tube feeding 1000 ml (40 ml/h) Chest tube to suction Expand mobilization (>4 h out of bed) Continue physical therapy and nebulizers Continue supply albumin
POD3	Jejunostomy tube feeding 1500 ml (60–80 ml/h) Remove chest tube Remove epidural catheter Expand mobilization (>6 h out of bed) Continue physical therapy and nebulizers Continue supply albumin
POD4	Gastrograffin opacification of upper gastrointestine If swallow shows no leak, advance patient to oral drink Jejunostomy tube feeding 1500 ml (60–80 ml/h) Continue physical therapy and nebulizers Education on aspiration precaution Education on chewing and swallowing
POD5	Jejunostomy tube feeding 1500 ml (60–80 ml/h) Advance patient to a full liquid diet Continue aspiration precautions Continue physical therapy and nebulizers
POD6	Increase liquid diet Decrease jejunostomy tube feeding (500 or 1000 ml) Continue aspiration precautions Continue physical therapy and nebulizers
POD7	Remove jejunostomy tube Full liquid diet Discharge home on soft diet and liquid diet Continue aspiration precautions

Note: FTS: Fast track surgery. Adapted from Chen et al. [82].

Table 2. Daily guideline of postoperative care of patients with fast-track surgery pathway.

and one had patients undergoing both operations). Additionally, the included randomized clinical trials used different formulations of enteral immunonutrition and standard enteral nutrition, further limiting the accuracy of the results. Moreover, not all studies reported the same outcomes as far as inflammatory and immunological markers are concerned. Therefore, the authors suggest that there is no convincing evidence in terms of routine immunonutrition in patients undergoing esophageal resection for cancer [84].

On the other hand, preoperative nutritional supplementation with immune-enhancing formulas was associated with reduced infectious complications, duration of hospitalization, improved short-term survival and less mortality in patients with esophageal cancer. These results highlight the possible need to provide immunonutrients before surgery to obtain sufficient levels at the time of surgical stress when there is an increased need for stimulation of the immune system [85]. One meta-analysis that included studies with patients that underwent esophagectomy, gastrectomy and pancreatectomy, demonstrated that patients who received immunonutrition postoperatively, had a significantly lower risk of wound infection and shorter length of hospital stay. No significant effect of immunonutrition on other postoperative morbidities and mortality was noticed [86]. The reduction in hospital stay and/or in postoperative complications seems to compensate for the higher cost of immunonutrition compared to standard enteral feeding in a cost-effectiveness analysis [87]. According to ESPEN guidelines on nutrition in cancer patients, upper gastrointestinal tract cancer patients undergoing surgical resection should receive oral/enteral immunonutrition in the context of traditional perioperative care [79]. Furthermore, ASPEN guidelines suggest the routine use of an immunemodulating formula (containing both arginine and fish oils) in the surgical intensive care unit for the postoperative patient who requires enteral nutrition therapy [73].

Synbiotics, which are a combination of prebiotics and probiotics, are speculated to have beneficial effects on human health, but little is known about their clinical value in patients who have undergone esophagectomy. Administration of synbiotics prevented postoperative deterioration of the intestinal microfloral environment and suppressed excessive inflammatory response, possibly by exerting immunomodulatory effects and by inhibiting bacterial translocation [88, 89]. Additionally, synbiotics led to decreased incidence of severe diarrhea and lower interruption or reduction of enteral nutrition. Passage of flatus postoperatively occurred significantly earlier in patients who received synbiotics than in the control group, suggesting that synbiotics maintain intestinal motility [88]. Taking all the aforementioned things into consideration, larger scale studies are needed in order to define whether or not immunonutrition has beneficial effects on the postoperative outcome of esophageal cancer patients. Future research should focus on the optimal dose of specific immunonutrients, on the timing (preoperatively and/or postoperatively) and duration of immunonutrition delivery and clarify which is the target group the intervention should be addressed to.

3.4. Type of feeding

Enteral feeding postoperatively seems to be the method of choice for uncomplicated esophageal cancer patients. Enteral feeding options after surgery include mainly nasoenteric tubes and jejunostomy catheters, in order to bypass recently constructed anastomoses. However there is no general agreement regarding the best method for postoperative feeding, and the optimal access route remains questionable. Tube-related complications include occlusion, catheter displacement and local cellulitis at the site of insertion. More severe complications include leakage into the peritoneal cavity resulting in peritonitis, volvulus at the point of fixation to the anterior abdominal wall, aspiration pneumonia, necrotizing fasciitis or jejunal necrosis at the site of catheter insertion and septicemia [90, 91].

A retrospective analysis of 90 patients who underwent esophagectomy demonstrated that early enteral nutrition can be administered using three different routes (nasojejunal tube, jejunostomy tube, and pharyngostomy tube) with similar results regarding tube-related complications, length of stay, and 30-day morbidity [92]. Another study of esophageal cancer patients with dysphagia examined the effects of jejunostomy feeding on weight loss and treatment outcomes. The palliative group of patients was able to maintain a stable weight despite the presence of cancer cachexia. This was also evident in the esophagectomy group of patients despite the catabolic effect of the operation, indicating the effectiveness of the jejunostomy feeding catheter as a means of nutritional support. The feeding catheter was well tolerated by the majority of patients (86.8%) and the most frequently occurred complications included catheter clogging (10.1% of the study population) and catheter dislodgement (3.1% of the study population) [93]. A randomized clinical study that compared nasoenteric tubes to jejunostomy feeding in upper gastrointestinal tract cancer patients showed that the length of enteral feeding use was less in the nasoenteric group and parenteral feeding was required more frequently than in jejunostomy feeding group. Complications related to the different feeding routes were similar between the two groups [94]. A recent review investigated the best route for enteral nutrition following esophagectomy (oral intake, jejunostomy, or nasojejunal tube feeding) in terms of postoperative complication rates, percentage of patients meeting their nutritional needs, weight loss, tube feeding complications, mortality, patient satisfaction, and length of hospital stay. Complications and catheter efficacy did not differ between postoperative nasojejunal tube feeding and jejunostomy tube feeding. Moreover, jejunostomy feeding patients were able to meet their short-term nutritional requirements, but data concerning long-term outcomes and patients satisfaction were scarce. This review concluded that the best route for the delivery of early enteral nutrition postoperatively is still unclear [75].

ESPEN guidelines on enteral nutrition in surgical patients recommends that tube feeding should be applied in patients who cannot start early oral nutrition, including those undergoing gastrointestinal surgery for cancer and patients with obvious undernutrition at the time of surgery, in whom oral intake will be inadequate (<60%) for more than 10 days. Initiation of tube feeding should start within 24 h after surgery with a low flow rate (i.e. 10–20 ml/h) due to limited intestinal tolerance. Placement of a needle catheter jejunostomy or nasojejunal tube is recommended for all candidates for tube feeding undergoing major abdominal surgery. When anastomoses of the proximal gastrointestinal tract have been performed, enteral nutrition should be delivered via a tube placed distally to the anastomosis [95].

Postoperative nutritional management of esophageal cancer patients can be summarized as in **Figure 2**.

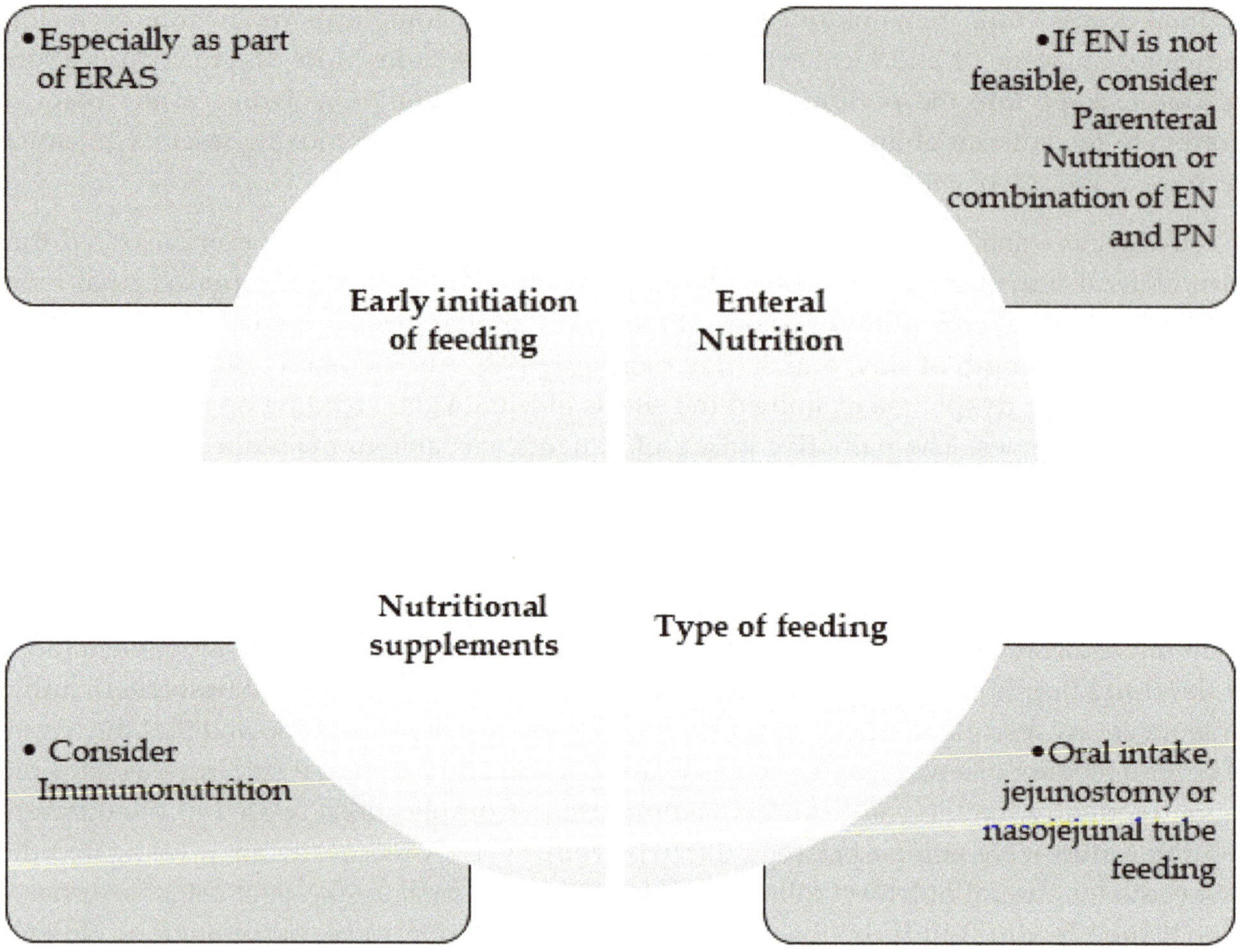

Figure 2. Postoperative nutritional management of esophageal cancer patients.

4. Nutritional care during chemoradiotherapy

4.1. Nutrition issues during chemotherapy and radiotherapy

Currently, perioperative chemotherapy is frequently administered for the treatment of resectable advanced esophageal cancer. The neoadjuvant administration of chemotherapy or chemoradiotherapy preoperatively results in reduced tumor size before surgery. Perioperative chemotherapy improves significantly disease-free survival and overall survival rates compared to surgery alone. However, a great percentage of these patients are not able to complete the planned postoperative chemotherapeutic regimens. This is mainly caused because of postoperative complications and impaired nutritional and physical status [96–98]. Gastrointestinal disorders caused by chemotherapy itself, including nausea, vomiting, diarrhea, and anorexia, negatively affect patients' quality of life and make completion of chemotherapy difficult. Neoadjuvant chemotherapy induces changes in body composition which, in turn have negative impact on clinical outcomes. Results from a small cohort of esophageal cancer patients showed that 26% of patients were sarcopenic before the initiation of neoadjuvant chemotherapy and this percentage increased to 43% after its completion. There was a significant loss of fat mass and skeletal muscle mass which was associated with risk of circumferential resection margin positivity [50]. In another study, sarcopenia was present in 56 and 67% of patients before and after neoadjuvant chemoradiotherapy, respectively. This decrease in muscle mass was predictive of postoperative mortality in the stage III–IV subgroup of patients [99]. Furthermore, most of the radiotherapy-related toxicities are strongly associated with patient's nutritional status. Esophagitis is the main toxicity during radiotherapy in esophageal cancer patients. These patients often suffer from pain and difficulties in swallowing [100]. One study in patients receiving concurrent chemoradiotherapy revealed that malnutrition was observed in 83.8% of patients, while 68.8% of patients developed severe dysphagia. Malnourished patients developed more treatment-related toxicities compared to those without malnutrition. Patients with impaired nutritional status presented severe dysphagia, anorexia, severe nausea/vomiting, and severe hematologic toxicities more frequently than those in a good nutrition status [17]. Although nutritionally related side effects occur frequently, nutritional assessment of patients with cancer receiving chemoradiotherapy is often omitted in the clinical setting. Scientific research has to focus on nutritional interventions during neoadjuvant chemoradiotherapy or postoperative adjuvant therapy that seems to improve patients' nutritional status, alleviate symptoms and increase tolerance to therapies.

4.2. Nutritional interventions during chemoradiotherapy

The type and timing of nutritional interventions during chemoradiotherapy challenge the caregivers, since a multidisciplinary approach seems more effective in managing treatment's side effects. Current literature emphasizes mainly on the immunomodulatory effects of some nutrients, on the impact of oral/tube administration of high-energy, and/or high protein supplements on the clinical outcome and on patients education about selecting an enriched diet. In cancer patients, it has been shown that the use of supplemental formulas and *n*-3 fatty acids, such as eicosapentaenoic acid (EPA) and docosahexaenoic acid (DHA), can improve body composition, preserve muscle mass, and possibly reverse or stop the development of cancer cachexia [101]. A controlled, randomized prospective, double-blind, multicenter study investigated the impact of enteral nutrition (via percutaneous endoscopic gastrostomy (PEG)) enriched with EPA and DHA on body composition, nutritional and functional status of esophageal and head and neck cancer patients undergoing concurrent chemoradiotherapy. There was a tendency toward improvement regarding loss of body cell mass and body weight following chemoradiotherapy, but did not reach statistical significance. However, Karnofsky score and subjective parameters, such as the NRS 2002 and the SGA score were significantly improved in the experimental group compared with the control group, indicating improved nutritional and functional status [102]. Similar results reported by another randomized double-blind clinical trial showed that administration of immunonutrition during chemoradiotherapy in head and neck and esophageal cancer patients was advantageous over standard enteral nutrition in terms of body weight, lean body mass, serum albumin levels, NRI assessment, plasma antioxidant capacity, and functional capacity [103].

Moreover, immunonutrition can modulate the immunological and inflammatory systems, thus reducing the risks of concurrent chemoradiotherapy. One randomized clinical trial examined the effects of immunonutrition on serum cytokine and inflammatory markers, and cellular immunity in locally advanced esophageal cancer patients undergoing chemoradiotherapy. The levels of C-Reactive Protein (CRP) and TNF increased more during treatment in the control group (standard enteral nutrition) than in the treatment group, whereas all other markers did not differ significantly between the two groups [104]. In addition, the impact of immunonutrients on immune system of head and neck and esophageal cancer patients during chemoradiotherapy was examined in another randomized clinical trial. Immune cells metabolism and functions were assessed at the initiation and at the completion of treatment. The experimental group had better adaptation to the systematic inflammation and oxidative stress, as indicated by $CD4^+/CD8^+$ T-lymphocyte counts ratio, CD3 membrane expression, polymorphonuclear cells CD62L and CD15 densities, reactive oxygen species (ROS) production, and peripheral blood mononuclear cells production of pro-inflammatory prostaglandin-E2 [105].

Another role of immunonutrition is the potential protection against chemotherapy-induced toxicities. Miyata et al. compared the effects between enteral nutrition rich in *n*-3 fatty acids (900 mg/d) and enteral nutrition poor in *n*-3 fatty acids (250 mg/d) on chemotherapy-related adverse events and inflammatory markers during neoadjuvant chemotherapy in esophageal cancer patients. This randomized control trial showed no significant difference in the incidence of grade 3/4 leukopenia and neutropenia, but stomatitis was observed less frequently in the *n*-3-rich group, than in the *n*-3-poor group. Grade 3/4 diarrhea was also observed less frequently in the *n*-3-rich group than in the *n*-3-poor group, but this was not statistically significant. Moreover, *n*-3-rich enteral nutrition seems to have hepatoprotective properties by preventing an increase of aspartate aminotransferase and alanine aminotransferase values [106].

Synbiotics seem also to mitigate chemotherapy-related side effects through adjustments to the intestinal microbiota. A randomized clinical trial investigated the effects of synbiotics in esophageal cancer patients undergoing neoadjuvant chemotherapy, on the intestinal microbiota, and the adverse events of treatment. Severe lymphopenia and diarrhea were less frequent in patients who received synbiotics than in the control group. Furthermore, febrile neutropenia occurred less in the synbiotics group compared to the control group [107]. Chemotherapy may disturb the intestinal microbiota, leading to reduced production of organic acids in the bowel, impaired mucosal integrity, and increased harmful bacteria. These, in turn, may induce chemotherapy-related toxicities, such as diarrhea and infectious complications [108]. Administration of synbiotics results in increased concentrations of short-chain fatty acids, such as acetate and propionate. These fatty acids are an important energy source of enterocytes, maintain intestinal environment acidity and intestinal motility. Synbiotics also maintain the number of beneficial bacteria and inhibit the overgrowth of possible diarrheal pathogens, thus reducing the incidence of diarrhea [109].

ESPEN guidelines on nutrition in cancer patients recommend the supplementation with long-chain *n*-3 fatty acids or fish oil to stabilize or improve appetite, food intake, lean body mass, and body weight in patients with advanced cancer undergoing chemotherapy and at risk of weight loss or malnourished [79]. It is therefore evident that immunonutrition enhances immune system and exerts anti-inflammatory properties, but the promising effects on clinical outcome during chemoradiotherapy in esophageal cancer are still under investigation. Additional clinical trials are needed to determine the preferred type, timing and duration of immunonutrition required to reduce inflammation and chemotherapy-induced toxicities, and maintain muscle mass.

Nutritional interventions, other than that examining the impact of specific immunonutrients on chemoradiotherapy-related outcomes, include nutritional counseling and/or enteral supplements in order to maintain stable body weight and cope with feeding difficulties (**Table 3**). A recent randomized controlled trial compared the effects of a walk-and-eat intervention versus conventional medical care for patients with esophageal cancer undergoing neoadjuvant chemoradiotherapy. This intervention consisted of a structured walking protocol and weekly nutritional advice including weight and intake evaluation, counseling to overcome feeding difficulties, supplementation, if necessary, with enteral formulas, and patient's education concerning food texture modification and oral care before and after eating. During chemoradiotherapy, the group that received the walk-and-eat intervention had 100-m less decline than controls in walk distance, 3 kg less decrease in handgrip strength, and 2.7 kg less reduction in body weight. Moreover, the experimental group had significantly reduced rates of intravenous nutritional support and wheel chair use [110]. Another randomized trial tested the effects of an interdisciplinary nutrition support team on clinical and hospitalized outcomes of esophageal cancer patients receiving concurrent chemoradiotherapy. Nutritional support included dietary counseling, oral nutritional supplements, enteral nutrition, and parenteral nutrition according to patient's needs. At the completion of treatment, nutritional status of patients in the interventional group was better compared to control group, as demonstrated by prealbumin, transferrin, and albumin levels. Bone marrow suppression and complications related to infections were significantly lower in the nutritional support group. Nutritional intervention was also associated with a lower average length of hospital stay and in-patient cost [111]. Furthermore, nutritional intervention improved survival of esophageal cancer patients treated with definitive chemoradiotherapy. It is noticeable that this effect was observed only if nutritional support was provided at baseline (dietary advice, oral supplementation, or major intervention), and not if provided later in the treatment course [10].

According to ESPEN, in patients receiving radiotherapy, especially radiotherapy of the head and neck, thorax, and gastrointestinal tract, an adequate nutritional intake should be ensured primarily by individualized nutritional counseling and/or with use of oral nutritional

Nutritional counseling
Oral supplementation
Immunonutrition
Synbiotics
Parenteral nutrition support

Table 3. Nutritional interventions during chemoradiotherapy.

supplements, in order to avoid nutritional deterioration, maintain intake, and avoid radiotherapy interruptions. In addition, for patients undergoing curative anticancer drug treatment who cannot meet their nutritional requirements despite counseling and oral nutritional supplements, ESPEN recommends supplemental enteral nutrition or, if this is not sufficient or possible, parenteral nutrition [79]. Therefore, assessment and maintenance of good nutritional status at baseline may be a simple and cost-effective intervention that improves clinical outcomes in esophageal cancer patients during chemoradiotherapy treatment.

4.3. Stent insertion

There are various types of stents available, such as self-expandable metallic stents, self-expandable plastic stents, and biodegradable stents. Esophageal stenting can be implemented to relieve dysphagia during preoperative chemotherapy and/or radiotherapy. A systematic review investigated the impact of stent insertion during neoadjuvant treatment on dysphagia improvement. Placement of an esophageal stent significantly improved overall dysphagia scores in all 12 studies reviewed. However, no consistent improvement in nutritional status was observed, defined by body weight and albumin levels. Moreover, stent insertion was associated with complications, such as migration and chest pain, frequently resulting in stent removal or replacement [112]. The European Society of Gastrointestinal Endoscopy (ESGE) does not recommend self-expandable metal stents placement as a bridge to surgery or prior to preoperative chemoradiotherapy, since it is associated with a high incidence of adverse events. Other options, such as feeding tube placement are preferable and should be considered in dysphagic or malnourished patients in the neoadjuvant setting [113].

5. Palliative care

Management of patients undergoing noncurative treatments due to advanced disease is difficult, since the goals are not to cure patients but to improve length and quality of remaining life. Nutritional support is a crucial part in the palliative care as long as its benefits outweigh its costs. Patients with metastatic disease present for the clinician not only clinical but ethical issues as well. Dysphagia is the main symptom in patients with unresectable disease which aggravates malnutrition and requires nutritional intervention [114]. Nutritional support of these patients includes intravenous fluids for hydration, feeding tubes, parenteral nutrition, and stent placement in order to supplement dietary and caloric intake. Various techniques have been proposed to manage dysphagia, such as brachytherapy, self-expanding metal stents, thermal laser therapy, and photodynamic therapy. Each one of them has specific advantages and risks that should be taken into consideration. The authors of a recent meta-analysis of 53 randomized controlled trials concluded that self-expanding metal stent insertion is safe, effective, and improves dysphagia faster compared to other modalities. High-dose intraluminal brachytherapy is a satisfactory alternative and might provide additional survival benefit with a better quality of life. Combinations of brachytherapy with self-expanding metal stent insertion or radiotherapy seem to be the preferable option addressed to inoperative patients [115]. ESGE recommends placement of partially or fully covered self-expandable metal stents for palliative treatment of malignant dysphagia over laser therapy, photodynamic therapy, and esophageal bypass [113].

Moreover, in esophageal cancer patients with short life expectancy unsuitable for esophageal stenting, percutaneous endoscopic gastrostomy (PEG) may be a suitable means in order to achieve nutritional support, while allowing patients to be at home [116]. Endoscopically assisted nasogastric tube feeding is also a feasible palliative option for nutritional support, with a low complication rate. Tube-feeding patients had significantly higher enteral calorie intake, higher serum albumin, shorter hospital stay, and longer median survival compared to those who received *nil per os*, according to a retrospective study of patients with malignant esophageal obstruction [117]. Palliative care in the terminal phase should be followed in an individualized manner. ESPEN recommends that in dying patients, artificial hydration and nutrition are unlikely to benefit patients. Nevertheless, in acute confusional states, patients might receive a short and limited hydration to rule out dehydration as precipitating cause [79].

6. Conclusion

Esophageal cancer patients suffer from malnutrition and cannot easily meet their nutritional needs. Nutritional assessment, in the perioperative phase, but also in patients undergoing chemoradiotherapy should be performed regularly, in order to identify undernourished patients. Regarding the perioperative management of these patients, early enteral nutrition support seems to be the method of choice in uncomplicated patients, especially as a part of ERAS programs. However, the impact of immunonutrition on clinical outcome is still under investigation. During chemoradiotherapy, prevention of weight loss is of great significance and might be achieved through close nutritional monitoring. Nutritional support mainly encompasses dietary counseling, oral supplementation, tube feeding, and combination of them and has promising results in ameliorating nutritional status and affecting the oncologic outcome. Moreover, patients with terminal-stage esophageal cancer might benefit from early stent insertion in order to reduce dysphagia. Individualized nutritional support should be addressed to every patient who is in need of nutritional intervention.

Author details

Dimitrios Schizas[1*], Irene Lidoriki[1], Demetrios Moris[2] and Theodore Liakakos[1]

*Address all correspondence to: schizasad@gmail.com

1 First Department of Surgery, Laikon General Hospital, National and Kapodistrian University of Athens, Athens, Greece

2 Department of Surgery, Division of Surgical Oncology, The Ohio State University Wexner Medical Center and James Cancer Hospital and Solove Research Institute, Columbus, OH, USA

References

[1] Global Burden of Disease Cancer Collaboration. The global burden of cancer 2013. JAMA Oncology. 2015;**1**(4):505-527. DOI: 10.1001/jamaoncol.2015.0735

[2] Yang CS, Chen X, Tu S. Etiology and prevention of esophageal cancer. Gastrointestinal Tumors. 2016;**3**(1):3-16. DOI: 10.1159/000443155

[3] Choi Y, Song S, Song Y, Lee JE. Consumption of red and processed meat and esophageal cancer risk: Meta-analysis. World Journal of Gastroenterology. 2013;**19**(7):1020-1029. DOI: 10.3748/wjg.v19.i7.1020

[4] Andrici J, Eslick G. Hot food and beverage consumption and the risk of esophageal cancer. American Journal of Preventive Medicine. 2015;**49**(6):952-960. DOI: 10.1016/j.amepre.2015.07.023

[5] Corley DA, Kubo A, Zhao W. Abdominal obesity and the risk of esophageal and gastric cardia carcinomas. Cancer Epidemiology, Biomarkers & Prevention: A Publication of the American Association for Cancer Research, Cosponsored by the American Society of Preventive Oncology. 2008;**17**(2):352-358. DOI: 10.1158/1055-9965.EPI-07-0748

[6] Cook MB, Corley DA, Murray LJ, et al. Gastroesophageal reflux in relation to adenocarcinomas of the esophagus: A pooled analysis from the Barrett's and Esophageal Adenocarcinoma Consortium (BEACON). Suzuki H, ed. PLoS One. 2014;**9**(7):e103508. DOI: 10.1371/journal.pone.0103508

[7] Kubo A, Block G, Quesenberry CP, et al. Effects of dietary fiber, fats, and meat intakes on the risk of Barrett's esophagus. Nutrition and Cancer. 2009;**61**(5):607-616. DOI: 10.1080/01635580902846585

[8] Anandavadivelan P, Lagergren P. Cachexia in patients with oesophageal cancer. Nature Reviews Clinical Oncology. 2016;**13**(3):185-198. DOI: 10.1038/nrclinonc.2015.200

[9] Llop-Talaveron JM, Farran-Teixidor L, Badia-Tahull MB, et al. Artificial nutritional support in cancer patients after esophagectomy: 11 years of experience. Nutrition and Cancer. 2014;**66**(6):1038-1046. DOI: 10.1080/01635581.2014.939292.

[10] Cox S, Powell C, Carter B, et al. Role of nutritional status and intervention in oesophageal cancer treated with definitive chemoradiotherapy: Outcomes from SCOPE1. British Journal of Cancer. 2016;**115**(2):172-177. DOI: 10.1038/bjc.2016.129

[11] Deans DAC, Tan BH, Wigmore SJ, et al. The influence of systemic inflammation, dietary intake and stage of disease on rate of weight loss in patients with gastro-oesophageal cancer. British Journal of Cancer. 2009;**100**(1):63-69. DOI: 10.1038/sj.bjc.6604828

[12] Riccardi D, Allen K. Nutritional management of patients with esophageal and esophagogastric junction cancer. Cancer Control. 1999;**6**(1):64-72

[13] Bailey SH, Bull DA, Harpole DH, et al. Outcomes after esophagectomy: A ten-year prospective cohort. The Annals of Thoracic Surgery. 2003;**75**(1):217-222

[14] Bower MR, Martin RC. Nutritional management during neoadjuvant therapy for esophageal cancer. Journal of Surgical Oncology. 2009;**100**(1):82-87. DOI: 10.1002/jso.21289

[15] Martin L, Lagergren P. Long-term weight change after oesophageal cancer surgery. British Journal of Surgery. 2009;**96**(11):1308-1314. DOI: 10.1002/bjs.6723

[16] Quyen TC, Angkatavanich J, Thuan TV, et al. Nutrition assessment and its relationship with performance and Glasgow prognostic scores in Vietnamese patients with esophageal cancer. Asia Pacific Journal of Clinical Nutrition. 2017;**26**(1):49-58. DOI: 10.6133/apjcn.122015.02

[17] Pan P, Tao G, Sun X. Subjective global assessment and prealbumin levels of esophageal cancer patients undergoing concurrent chemoradiotherapy. Nutricion Hospitalaria. 2015;**31**(5):2167-2173. DOI: 10.3305/nh.2015.31.5.8596

[18] Nitenberg G, Raynard B. Nutritional support of the cancer patient: Issues and dilemmas. Critical Reviews in Oncology/Hematology. 2000;**34**(3):137-168

[19] DiFiore F, Lecleire S, Pop D, et al. Baseline nutritional status is predictive of response to treatment and survival in patients treated by definitive chemoradiotherapy for a locally advanced esophageal cancer. American Journl of Gastroenterology. 2007;**102**(11):2557-2563. DOI: 10.1111/j.1572-0241.2007.01437.x

[20] National Collaborating Centre for Acute Care. Nutrition Support for Adults Oral Nutrition Support, Enteral Tube Feeding and Parenteral Nutrition Methods, Evidence and Guidance; 1e176. 2006. London: National Collaborating Centre for Acute Care at The Royal College of Surgeons of England; 2011

[21] Ryan AM, Hearty A, Prichard RS, et al. Association of hypoalbuminemia on the first postoperative day and complications following esophagectomy. Journal of Gastrointestinal Surgery. 2007;**11**(10):1355-1360

[22] Goh SL, De Silva RP, Dhital K, et al. Is low serum albumin associated with postoperative complications in patients undergoing oesophagectomy for oesophageal malignancies? Interactive CardioVascular and Thoracic Surgery. 2015;**20**(1):107-113. DOI: 10.1093/icvts/ivu324

[23] da Silva JB, Maurício SF, Bering T, Correia MI. The relationship between nutritional status and the Glasgow prognostic score in patients with cancer of the esophagus and stomach. Nutrition and Cancer. 2013;**65**(1):25-33. DOI: 10.1080/01635581.2013.741755

[24] Nozoe T, Kimura Y, Ishida M, et al. Correlation of pre-operative nutritional condition with post-operative complications in surgical treatment for oesophageal carcinoma. European Journal of Surgical Oncology. 2002;**28**(4):396-400. DOI: 10.1053/ejso.2002.1257

[25] Feng J-F, Chen Q-X. Significance of the prognostic nutritional index in patients with esophageal squamous cell carcinoma. Therapeutics and Clinical Risk Management. 2014;**10**:1-7. DOI: 10.2147/TCRM.S56159

[26] Filip B, Scarpa M, Cavallin F, et al. Postoperative outcome after oesophagectomy for cancer: Nutritional status is the missing ring in the current prognostic scores. European Journal of Surgical Oncology. 2015;**41**(6):787-794. DOI: 10.1016/j.ejso.2015.02.014

[27] Han-Geurts IJ, Hop WC, Tran TC, Tilanus HW. Nutritional status as a risk factor in esophageal surgery. Digestive Surgery. 2006;**23**(3):159-163. DOI: 10.1159/000093756

[28] Braga M, Ljungqvist O, Soeters P, et al. ESPEN guidelines on parenteral nutrition: Surgery. Clinical Nutrition. 2009;**28**(4):378-386. DOI: 10.1016/j.clnu.2009.04.002

[29] Ignacio de Ulibarri J, Gonzalez-Madrono A, de Villar NG, et al. CONUT: A tool for controlling nutritional status. First validation in a hospital population. Nutricion Hospitalaria. 2005;**20**(1):38-45

[30] Yoshida N, Baba Y, Shigaki H, et al. Preoperative nutritional assessment by controlling nutritional status (CONUT) is useful to estimate postoperative morbidity after esophagectomy for esophageal cancer. World Journal of Surgery. 2016;**40**(8):1910-1917. DOI: 10.1007/s00268-016-3549-3

[31] Hirahara N, Matsubara T, Hayashi H, et al. Prognostic importance of controlling nutritional status in patients undergoing curative thoracoscopic esophagectomy for esophageal cancer. American Journal of Therapeutics. 2016;**0**(0):1-9. DOI: 10.1097/MJT.0000000000000414

[32] Toyokawa T, Kubo N, Tamura T, et al. The pretreatment controlling nutritional status (CONUT) score is an independent prognostic factor in patients with resectable thoracic esophageal squamous cell carcinoma: Results from a retrospective study. BMC Cancer. 2016;**16**(1):722. DOI: 10.1186/s12885-016-2696-0

[33] Clavier JB, Antoni D, Atlani D, et al. Baseline nutritional status is prognostic factor after definitive radiochemotherapy for esophageal cancer. Diseases of the Esophagus. 2014;**27**(6):560-567. DOI: 10.1111/j.1442-2050.2012.01441.x

[34] Yamana I, Takeno S, Shibata R, et al. Is the geriatric nutritional risk index a significant predictor of postoperative complications in patients with esophageal cancer undergoing esophagectomy? European Surgical Research. 2015;**55**(1-2):35-42. DOI: 10.1159/000376610

[35] Cruz-Jentoft AJ, Baeyens JP, Bauer JM, et al. Sarcopenia: European consensus on definition and diagnosis—Report of the European Working Group on Sarcopenia in Older People. Age Ageing. 2010;**39**(4):412-423. DOI: 10.1093/ageing/afq034

[36] Muscaritoli M, Anker SD, Argiles J, et al. Consensus definition of sarcopenia, cachexia and pre-cachexia: Joint document elaborated by special interest groups (SIG) "cachexia-anorexia in chronic wasting diseases" and "nutrition in geriatrics". Clinical Nutrition. 2010;**29**(2):154-159. DOI: 10.1016/j.clnu.2009.12.004

[37] Fielding RA, Vellas B, Evans WJ, et al. Sarcopenia: An undiagnosed condition in older adults—Current consensus definition: Prevalence, etiology, and consequences. International working group on Sarcopenia. Journal of the American Medical Directors Association. 2011;**12**(4):249-256. DOI: 10.1016/j.jamda.2011.01.003

[38] Argilés JM, Olivan M, Busquets S, López-Soriano FJ. Optimal management of cancer anorexia–cachexia syndrome. Cancer Management and Research. 2010;**2**:27-38

[39] Sun L, Quan XQ, Yu S. An epidemiological survey of cachexia in advanced cancer patients and analysis on its diagnostic and treatment status. Nutrition and Cancer. 2015;**67**(7):1056-1062. DOI: 10.1080/01635581.2015.1073753

[40] Fearon K, Strasser F, Anker SD, et al. Definition and classification of cancer cachexia: An international consensus. Lancet Oncology. 2011;**12**(5):489-495. DOI: 10.1016/S1470-2045(10)70218-7

[41] Prado CM, Birdsell LA, Baracos VE. The emerging role of computerized tomography in assessing cancer cachexia. Current Opinion in Supportive and Palliative Care. 2009;**3**(4):269-275. DOI: 10.1097/SPC.0b013e328331124a

[42] Gibson DJ, Burden ST, Strauss BJ, et al. The role of computed tomography in evaluating body composition and the influence of reduced muscle mass on clinical outcome in abdominal malignancy: A systematic review. European Journal of Clinical Nutrition. 2015;**69**(10):1079-1086. DOI: 10.1038/ejcn.2015.32

[43] Chen CH, Ho-Chang, Huang YZ, Hung TT. Hand-grip strength is a simple and effective outcome predictor in esophageal cancer following esophagectomy with reconstruction: A prospective study. Journal of Cardiothoracic Surgery. 2011;**6**:98. DOI: 10.1186/1749-8090-6-98

[44] Levolger S, van Vugt JL, de Bruin RW, IJzermans JN. Systematic review of sarcopenia in patients operated on for gastrointestinal and hepatopancreatobiliary malignancies. British Journal of Surgery. 2015;**102**(12):1448-1458. DOI: 10.1002/bjs.9893

[45] Sheetz KH, Zhao L, Holcombe SA, et al. Decreased core muscle size is associated with worse patient survival following esophagectomy for cancer. Diseases of the Esophagus. 2013;**26**(7):716-722. DOI: 10.1111/dote.12020

[46] Tamandl D, Paireder M, Asari R, et al. Markers of sarcopenia quantified by computed tomography predict adverse long-term outcome in patients with resected oesophageal or gastro-oesophageal junction cancer. European Radiology. 2016;**26**(5):1359-1367. DOI: 10.1007/s00330-015-3963-1

[47] Ida S, Watanabe M, Yoshida N, et al. Sarcopenia is a predictor of postoperative respiratory complications in patients with esophageal cancer. Annals of Surgical Oncology. 2015;**22**(13):4432-4437. DOI: 10.1245/s10434-015-4559-3

[48] Nishigori T, Okabe H, Tanaka E, et al. Sarcopenia as a predictor of pulmonary complications after esophagectomy for thoracic esophageal cancer. Journal of Surgical Oncology. 2016;**113**(6):678-684. DOI: 10.1002/jso.24214

[49] Makiura D, Ono R, Inoue J, et al. Preoperative sarcopenia is a predictor of postoperative pulmonary complications in esophageal cancer following esophagectomy: A retrospective cohort study. Journal of Geriatric Oncology. 2016;**7**(6):430-436. DOI: 10.1016/j.jgo.2016.07.003

[50] Yip C, Goh V, Davies A, et al. Assessment of sarcopenia and changes in body composition after neoadjuvant chemotherapy and associations with clinical outcomes in oesophageal cancer. European Radiology. 2014;**24**(5):998-1005. DOI: 10.1007/s00330-014-3110-4

[51] Tan BH, Brammer K, Randhawa N, et al. Sarcopenia is associated with toxicity in patients undergoing neo-adjuvant chemotherapy for oesophago-gastric cancer. European Journal of Surgical Oncology. 2015;**41**(3):333-338. DOI: 10.1016/j.ejso.2014.11.040

[52] Anandavadivelan P, Brismar TB, Nilsson M, et al. Sarcopenic obesity: A probable risk factor for dose limiting toxicity during neo-adjuvant chemotherapy in oesophageal cancer patients. Clinical Nutrition. 2016;**35**(3):724-730. DOI: 10.1016/j.clnu.2015.05.011

[53] Aghajanzadeh M, Safarpour F, Koohsari MR, et al. Functional outcome of gastrointestinal tract and quality of life after esophageal reconstruction of esophagus cancer. Saudi Journal of Gastroenterology. 2008;**15**(1):24e8. DOI: 10.4103/1319-3767.45050

[54] Ginex P, Thom B, Jingeleski M, et al. Patterns of symptoms following surgery for esophageal cancer. Oncology Nursing Forum. 2013;**40**(3):E101-E107. DOI: 10.1188/13.ONF.E101-E107

[55] Greene CL, DeMeester SR, Worrell SG, et al. Alimentary satisfaction, gastrointestinal symptoms, and quality of life 10 or more years after esophagectomy with gastric pull-up. Journal of Thoracic and Cardiovascular Surgery. 2014;**147**(3):909-914. DOI: 10.1016/j.jtcvs.2013.11.004

[56] Mak RH, Mamon HJ, Ryan DP, et al. Toxicity and outcomes after chemoradiation for esophageal cancer in patients age 75 or older. Diseases of the Esophagus. 2010;**23**(4):316-323. DOI: 10.1111/j.1442-2050.2009.01014.x

[57] Sonti G, Ilyin SE, Plata-Salaman CR. Anorexia induced by cytokine interactions at pathophysiological concentrations. American Journal of Physiology. 1996;**270**(6 Pt 2):R1394-R402

[58] Zhou X, Wang JL, Lu J, et al. Reversal of cancer cachexia and muscle wasting by ActRIIB antagonism leads to prolonged survival. Cell. 2010;**142**(4):531-543. DOI: 10.1016/j.cell.2010.07.011

[59] Johns N, Stephens NA, Fearon KC. Muscle wasting in cancer. The International Journal of Biochemistry & Cell Biology. 2013;**45**(10):2215-2229. DOI: 10.1016/j.biocel.2013.05.032

[60] Mendes MC, Pimentel GD, Costa FO, Carvalheira JB. Molecular and neuroendocrine mechanisms of cancer cachexia. Journal of Endocrinology. 2015;**226**(3):R29-R43. DOI: 10.1530/JOE-15-0170

[61] Wu J, Huang C, Xiao H, et al. Weight loss and resting energy expenditure in male patients with newly diagnosed esophageal cancer. Nutrition. 2013;**29**(11-12):1310-1314. DOI: 10.1016/j.nut.2013.04.010

[62] Becker Veronese CB, Guerra LT, Souza Grigolleti S, et al. Basal energy expenditure measured by indirect calorimetry in patients with squamous cell carcinoma of the esophagus. Nutricion Hospitalaria. 2013;**28**(1):142-147. DOI: 10.3305/nh.2013.28.1.6152

[63] Cao DX, Wu GH, Zhang B, et al. Resting energy expenditure and body composition in patients with newly detected cancer. Clinical Nutrition. 2010;**29**(1):72-77. DOI: 10.1016/j.clnu.2009.07.001

[64] Dempsey DT, Feurer ID, Knox LS, et al. Energy expenditure in malnourished gastrointestinal cancer patients. Cancer. 1984;**53**(6):1265-1273

[65] Okamoto H, Sasaki M, Johtatsu T, et al. Resting energy expenditure and nutritional status in patients undergoing transthoracic esophagectomy for esophageal cancer. Journal of Clinical Biochemistry and Nutrition. 2011;**49**(3):169-173. DOI: 10.3164/jcbn.11-13

[66] Kobayashi K, Koyama Y, Kosugi S, et al. Is early enteral nutrition better for postoperative course in esophageal cancer patients? Nutrients. 2013;**5**(9):3461-3469. DOI: 10.3390/nu5093461

[67] Demeyer I, Bataillie K, Baute L. Long-term sedation in the ICU: Enteral versus parenteral feeding. Clinical Intensive Care. 1994;**5**(5 Suppl):13-16

[68] Takesue T, Takeuchi H, Ogura M, et al. A prospective randomized trial of enteral nutrition after thoracoscopic esophagectomy for esophageal cancer. Annals of Surgical Oncology. 2015;**22**(Suppl 3):S802-S809. DOI: 10.1245/s10434-015-4767-x

[69] Rajabi Mashhadi MT, Bagheri R, Ghayour-Mobarhan M, et al. Early postoperative enteral versus parenteral feeding after esophageal cancer surgery. Iranian Journal of Otorhinolaryngology. 2015;**27**(82):331-336

[70] Peng J, Cai J, Niu ZX, Chen LQ. Early enteral nutrition compared with parenteral nutrition for esophageal cancer patients after esophagectomy: A meta-analysis. Diseases of the Esophagus. 2016;**29**(4):333-341. DOI: 10.1111/dote.12337

[71] Lidder P, Flanagan D, Fleming S, et al. Combining enteral with parenteral nutrition to improve postoperative glucose control. British Journal of Nutrition. 2010;**103**(11):1635-1641. DOI: 10.1017/S0007114509993631

[72] Wu W, Zhong M, Zhu DM, et al. Effect of early Full-Calorie nutrition support following esophagectomy: A randomized controlled trial. Journal of Parenteral and Enteral Nutrition. 2016. pii: 0148607116651509. [Epub ahead of print]

[73] McClave SA, Taylor BE, Martindale RG, et al. Guidelines for the provision and assessment of nutrition support therapy in the adult critically ill patient: Society of Critical Care Medicine (SCCM) and American Society for Parenteral and Enteral Nutrition (A.S.P.E.N.). Journal of Parenteral and Enteral Nutrition. 2016;**40**(2):159-211. DOI: 10.1177/0148607115621863

[74] Wang G, Chen H, Liu J, et al. A comparison of postoperative early enteral nutrition with delayed enteral nutrition in patients with esophageal cancer. Nutrients. 2015;**7**(6):4308-4317. DOI: 10.3390/nu7064308

[75] Weijs TJ, Berkelmans GH, Nieuwenhuijzen GA, et al. Routes for early enteral nutrition after esophagectomy. A systematic review. Clinical Nutrition. 2015;**34**(1):1-6. DOI: 10.1016/j.clnu.2014.07.011

[76] Fujita T, Daiko H, Nishimura M. Early enteral nutrition reduces the rate of life-threatening complications after thoracic esophagectomy in patients with esophageal cancer. European Surgical Research. 2012;**48**(2):79-84. DOI: 10.1159/000336574

[77] Manba N, Koyama Y, Kosugi S, et al. Is early enteral nutrition initiated within 24 hours better for the postoperative course in esophageal cancer surgery? Journal of Clinical Medicine Research. 2014;**6**(1):53-58. DOI: 10.4021/jocmr1665w

[78] Langelotz C, Spies C, Müller JM, Schwenk W. "Fast-track"-rehabilitation in surgery, a multimodal concept. Acta Chirurgica Belgica. 2005;**105**:555-559

[79] Arends J, Bachmann P, Baracos V, et al. ESPEN guidelines on nutrition in cancer patients. Clinical Nutrition. 2017; **36**(1):11-48. DOI: 10.1016/j.clnu.2016.07.015

[80] Gustafsson UO and Ljungqvist O. Perioperative nutritional management in digestive tract surgery. Current Opinion in Clinical Nutrition and Metabolic Care. 2011;**14**(5):504-509. DOI: 10.1097/MCO.0b013e3283499ae1

[81] Markar SR, Karthikesalingam A, Low DE. Enhanced recovery pathways lead to an improvement in postoperative outcomes following esophagectomy: systematic review and pooled analysis. Diseases of the Esophagus. 2015;**28**(5):468-475. DOI: 10.1111/dote.12214

[82] Chen L, Sun L, Lang Y, et al. Fast-track surgery improves postoperative clinical recovery and cellular and humoral immunity after esophagectomy for esophageal cancer. BMC Cancer. 2016;**16**:449. DOI: 10.1186/s12885-016-2506-8

[83] Wang JY, Hong X, Chen GH, et al. Clinical application of the fast track surgery model based on preoperative nutritional risk screening in patients with esophageal cancer. Asia Pacific Journal of Clinical Nutrition. 2015;**24**(2):206-211. DOI: 10.6133/apjcn.2015.24.2.18

[84] Mabvuure NT, Roman A, Khan OA. Enteral immunonutrition versus standard enteral nutrition for patients undergoing oesophagogastric resection for cancer. International Journal of Surgery. 2013;**11**(2):122-127. DOI: 10.1016/j.ijsu.2012.12.012

[85] Kubota K, Kuroda J, Yoshida M, et al. Preoperative oral supplementation support in patients with esophageal cancer. The Journal of Nutrition Health and Aging. 2014;**18**(4):437-440. DOI: 10.1007/s12603-014-0018-2

[86] Wong CS, Aly EH. The effects of enteral immunonutrition in upper gastrointestinal surgery: A systematic review and meta-analysis. International Journal of Surgery. 2016;**29**:137-150. DOI: 10.1016/j.ijsu.2016.03.043

[87] dos Reis AM, Kabke GB, Fruchtenicht AVG, et al. Cost-effectiveness of perioperative immunonutrition in gastrointestinal oncologic surgery: A systematic review. Arquivos Brasileiros de Cirurgia Digestiva. 2016;**29**(2):121-125. DOI: 10.1590/0102-6720201600020014

[88] Tanaka K, Yano M, Motoori M, et al. Impact of perioperative administration of synbiotics in patients with esophageal cancer undergoing esophagectomy: A prospective randomized controlled trial. Surgery. 2012;**152**(5):832-842. DOI: 10.1016/j.surg.2012.02.021

[89] Yokoyama Y, Nishigaki E, Abe T, et al. Randomized clinical trial of the effect of perioperative synbiotics versus no synbiotics on bacterial translocation after oesophagectomy. British Journal of Surgery. 2014;**101**(3):189-199. DOI: 10.1002/bjs.9385

[90] Han-Geurts IJ, Hop WC, Verhoef C, et al. Randomized clinical trial comparing feeding jejunostomy with nasoduodenal tube placement in patients undergoing oesophagectomy. British Journal of Surgery. 2007;**94**(1):31-35. Doi: 10.1002/bjs.5283

[91] Wani ML, Ahangar AG, Lone GN, et al. Feeding jejunostomy: does the benefit overweight the risk (a retrospective study from a single centre). International Journal of Surgery. 2010;**8**(5):387-390. DOI: 10.1016/j.ijsu.2010.05.009

[92] Elshaer M, Gravante G, White J, et al. Routes of early enteral nutrition following oesophagectomy. Annals of the Royal College of Surgeons of England. 2016;**98**(7):461-467. DOI: 10.1308/rcsann.2016.0198

[93] Abdelgadir MA, Mahadi SE, Nasr AO, Ahmed ME. Role of jejunostomy feeding catheter as a model for nutritional support. International Journal of Surgery. 2010;**8**(6):439-443. DOI: 10.1016/j.ijsu.2010.05.006

[94] Torres Júnior LG, de Vasconcellos Santos FA, Correia MI. Randomized clinical trial: Nasoenteric tube or jejunostomy as a route for nutrition after major upper gastrointestinal operations. World Journal of Surgery. 2014;**38**(9):2241-2246. DOI: 10.1007/s00268-014-2589-9

[95] Weimann A, Braga M, Harsanyi L, et al. ESPEN Guidelines on Enteral Nutrition: Surgery including organ transplantation. Clinical Nutrition. 2006;**25**(2):224-244. DOI: 10.1016/j.clnu.2006.01.015

[96] Cunningham D, Allum WH, Stenning SP, et al. Perioperative chemotherapy versus surgery alone for resectable gastroesophageal cancer. New England Journal of Medicine. 2006;**355**(1):11-20. DOI: 10.1056/NEJMoa055531

[97] Ychou M, Boige V, Pignon JP, et al. Perioperative chemotherapy compared with surgery alone for resectable gastroesophageal adenocarcinoma: An FNCLCC and FFCD multicenter phase III trial. Journal of Clinical Oncology. 2011;**29**(13):1715-1721. DOI: 10.1200/JCO.2010.33.0597

[98] Sjoquist KM, Burmeister BH, Smithers BM, et al. Survival after neoadjuvant chemotherapy or chemoradiotherapy for resectable oesophageal carcinoma: an updated meta-analysis. Lancet Oncology. 2011;**12**(7):681-692. DOI: 10.1016/S1470-2045(11)70142-5

[99] Reisinger KW, Bosmans JW, Uittenbogaart M, et al. Loss of skeletal muscle mass during neoadjuvant chemoradiotherapy predicts postoperative mortality in esophageal cancer surgery. Annals of Surgical Oncology. 2015;**22**(13):4445-4452. DOI: 10.1245/s10434-015-4558-4

[100] Jiang N, Zhao JZ, Chen XC, et al. Clinical determinants of weight loss in patients with esophageal carcinoma during radiotherapy: A prospective longitudinal view. Asian Pacific Journal of Cancer Prevention. 2014;**15**(5):1943-1948

[101] Hardman WE. (n-3) fatty acids and cancer therapy. Journal of Nutrition. 2004;**134**(12): 3427S-3430S

[102] Fietkau R, Lewitzki V, Kuhnt T, et al. A disease-specific enteral nutrition formula improves nutritional status and functional performance in patients with head and neck and esophageal cancer undergoing chemoradiotherapy: results of a randomized, controlled, multicenter trial. Cancer. 2013;**119**(18):3343-3353. DOI: 10.1002/cncr.28197

[103] Vasson MP, Talvas J, Perche O, et al. Immunonutrition improves functional capacities in head and neck and esophageal cancer patients undergoing radiochemotherapy: A randomized clinical trial. Clinical Nutrition. 2014;**33**(2):204-210. DOI: 10.1016/j.clnu.2013.06.008

[104] Sunpaweravong S, Puttawibul P, Ruangsin S, et al. Randomized study of antiinflammatory and immune-modulatory effects of enteral immunonutrition during concurrent chemoradiotherapy for esophageal cancer. Nutrition and Cancer. 2014;**66**(1):1-5. DOI: 10.1080/01635581.2014.847473

[105] Talvas J, Garrait G, Goncalves-Mendes N, et al. Immunonutrition stimulates immune functions and antioxidant defense capacities of leukocytes in radiochemotherapy-treated head & neck and esophageal cancer patients: A double-blind randomized clinical trial. Clinical Nutrition. 2015;**34**(5):810-817. DOI: 10.1016/j.clnu.2014.12.002

[106] Miyata H, Yano M, Yasuda T, et al. Randomized study of the clinical effects of ω-3 fatty acid-containing enteral nutrition support during neoadjuvant chemotherapy on chemotherapy-related toxicity in patients with esophageal cancer. Nutrition. 2017;**33**:204-210. DOI: 10.1016/j.nut.2016.07.004

[107] Motoori M, Yano M, Miyata H, et al. Randomized study of the effect of synbiotics during neoadjuvant chemotherapy on adverse events in esophageal cancer patients. Clinical Nutrition. 2017; **36**(1):93-99. DOI: 10.1016/j.clnu.2015.11.008

[108] van Vliet MJ, Harmsen HJ, de Bont ES, Tissing WJ. The role of intestinal microbiota in the development and severity of chemotherapy-induced mucositis. PLoS Pathogens. 2010;**6**(5):e1000879. DOI: 10.1371/journal.ppat.1000879

[109] Bowen JM, Stringer AM, Gibson RJ, et al. VSL#3 probiotic treatment reduces chemotherapy-induced diarrhea and weight loss. Cancer Biology & Therapy. 2007;**6**(9):1449e54

[110] Xu Y-J, Cheng JC-H, Lee J-M, et al. A Walk-and-Eat intervention improves outcomes for patients with esophageal cancer undergoing neoadjuvant chemoradiotherapy. Oncologist. 2015;**20**(10):1216-1222. DOI: 10.1634/theoncologist.2015-0178

[111] Cong M-H, Li S-L, Cheng G-W, et al. An interdisciplinary nutrition support team improves clinical and hospitalized outcomes of esophageal cancer patients with concurrent chemoradiotherapy. Chinese Medical Journal (England). 2015;**128**(22):3003-3007. DOI: 10.4103/0366-6999.168963

[112] Jones CM, Griffiths EA. Should oesophageal stents be used before neo-adjuvant therapy to treat dysphagia in patients awaiting oesophagectomy? Best evidence topic (BET). International Journal of Surgery. 2014;**12**(11):1172-1180. DOI: 10.1016/j.ijsu.2014.09.008

[113] Spaander MC, Baron TH, Siersema PD, et al. Esophageal stenting for benign and malignant disease: European Society of Gastrointestinal Endoscopy (ESGE) Clinical Guideline. Endoscopy. 2016;**48**(10):939-948. DOI: 10.1055/s-0042-114210

[114] Gray RT, O'donnell ME, Scott RD, et al. Impact of nutritional factors on survival in patients with inoperable oesophageal cancer undergoing self-expanding metal stent insertion. European Journal of Gastroenterology & Hepatology. 2011;**23**(6):455-460. DOI: 10.1097/MEG.0b013e3283469761

[115] Dai Y, Li C, Xie Y, et al. Interventions for dysphagia in oesophageal cancer. The Cochrane Database of Systematic Reviews. 2014;(10):CD005048. DOI: 10.1002/14651858.CD005048.pub4

[116] Grilo A, Santos CA, Fonseca J. Percutaneous endoscopic gastrostomy for nutritional palliation of upper esophageal cancer unsuitable foresophageal stenting. Arquivos de Gastroenterologia. 2012;**49**(3):227-231

[117] Yang C, Lin H, Hsieh T, Chang W. Palliative enteral feeding for patients with malignant esophageal obstruction: A retrospective study. BMC Palliative Care. 2015;**14**:58. DOI: 10.1186/s12904-015-0056-5

Permissions

All chapters in this book were first published in EA, by InTech Open; hereby published with permission under the Creative Commons Attribution License or equivalent. Every chapter published in this book has been scrutinized by our experts. Their significance has been extensively debated. The topics covered herein carry significant findings which will fuel the growth of the discipline. They may even be implemented as practical applications or may be referred to as a beginning point for another development.

The contributors of this book come from diverse backgrounds, making this book a truly international effort. This book will bring forth new frontiers with its revolutionizing research information and detailed analysis of the nascent developments around the world.

We would like to thank all the contributing authors for lending their expertise to make the book truly unique. They have played a crucial role in the development of this book. Without their invaluable contributions this book wouldn't have been possible. They have made vital efforts to compile up to date information on the varied aspects of this subject to make this book a valuable addition to the collection of many professionals and students.

This book was conceptualized with the vision of imparting up-to-date information and advanced data in this field. To ensure the same, a matchless editorial board was set up. Every individual on the board went through rigorous rounds of assessment to prove their worth. After which they invested a large part of their time researching and compiling the most relevant data for our readers.

The editorial board has been involved in producing this book since its inception. They have spent rigorous hours researching and exploring the diverse topics which have resulted in the successful publishing of this book. They have passed on their knowledge of decades through this book. To expedite this challenging task, the publisher supported the team at every step. A small team of assistant editors was also appointed to further simplify the editing procedure and attain best results for the readers.

Apart from the editorial board, the designing team has also invested a significant amount of their time in understanding the subject and creating the most relevant covers. They scrutinized every image to scout for the most suitable representation of the subject and create an appropriate cover for the book.

The publishing team has been an ardent support to the editorial, designing and production team. Their endless efforts to recruit the best for this project, has resulted in the accomplishment of this book. They are a veteran in the field of academics and their pool of knowledge is as vast as their experience in printing. Their expertise and guidance has proved useful at every step. Their uncompromising quality standards have made this book an exceptional effort. Their encouragement from time to time has been an inspiration for everyone.

The publisher and the editorial board hope that this book will prove to be a valuable piece of knowledge for researchers, students, practitioners and scholars across the globe.

List of Contributors

Ivan M. Buzurovic, Desmond A. O'Farrell, Mandar S. Bhagwat and Phillip M. Devlin
Department of Radiation Oncology, Dana-Farber/Brigham and Women's Cancer Center, Harvard Medical School, Boston, MA, USA

Borbala Daroczi
Department of Radiology, Brigham and Women's Hospital, Harvard Medical School, Boston, MA, USA

Mona Boudabous, Héla Gdoura, Leila Mnif, Lassad Chtourou, Amal Grati, Ali Amouri and Nabil Tahri
Gastroenterology Department, Hedi Chaker Hospital, Sfax, Tunisia

Tian Wang and Yi Zhang
Biotherapy Center, The First Affiliated Hospital of Zhengzhou University, Zhengzhou, Henan, China

Rafael Cholvi Calduch, Isabel Mora Oliver, Fernando Lopez Mozos and Roberto Martí Obiol
Division of Oesophageal and Upper Gastrointestinal Surgery, Department of Surgery, Hospital Clínico Universitario de Valencia, Valencia, Spain

Yabin Zhu, Mi Zhou and Ruixia Hou
The Medical School of Ningbo University, Ningbo, China

Mauricio Canals Lambarri
Programa de Salud Ambiental, Escuela de Salud Pública, Facultad de Medicina, Universidad de Chile, Chile
Departamento de Medicina, Facultad de Medicina, Universidad de Chile, Chile

Andrea Canals Cifuentes
Programa de Bioestadística, Escuela de Salud Pública, Facultad de Medicina, Universidad de Chile, Chile
Dirección Académica, Clínica santa María, Chile

Salvador Ayala
Departamento de Asuntos Científicos, Instituto de Salud Pública, Chile

Valentina Tapia-Garay and Dante Cáceres Lillo
Programa de Salud Ambiental, Escuela de Salud Pública, Facultad de Medicina, Universidad de Chile, Chile

Lucian Mocan, Cornel Iancu and Furcea Luminita
Regional Institute of Gastroenterology and Hepatology, "Prof. Dr. Octavian Fodor", Cluj-Napoca, Romania
Department of Surgery, University of Medicine and Pharmacy, "Iuliu Hatieganu", Cluj-Napoca, Romania

Ofelia Mosteanu and Teodora Pop
Regional Institute of Gastroenterology and Hepatology, "Prof. Dr. Octavian Fodor", Cluj-Napoca, Romania
Department of Gastroenterology, University of Medicine and Pharmacy, "Iuliu Hatieganu", Cluj-Napoca, Romania

Lucia Agoston-Coldea
Department of Internal Medicine, University of Medicine and Pharmacy, "Iuliu Hatieganu", Cluj-Napoca, Romania

Teodora Mocan
Regional Institute of Gastroenterology and Hepatology, "Prof. Dr. Octavian Fodor", Cluj-Napoca, Romania
Department of Physiology, University of Medicine and Pharmacy, "Iuliu Hatieganu", Cluj-Napoca, Romania

Alfredo Larrosa-Haro
Servicio de Gastroenterología y Nutrición, UMAE Hospital de Pediatría, Centro Médico Nacional de Occidente, Instituto Mexicano del Seguro Socia, Guadañajara, México
Instituto de Nutrición Humana, Departamento de Clínicas de la Reproducción Humana Crecimiento y Desarrollo Infantil, Centro Universitario de Ciencias de la Salud, Universidad de Guadalajara, Guadalajara, México

Carmen A Sánchez-Ramírez
Servicio de Gastroenterología y Nutrición, UMAE Hospital de Pediatría, Centro Médico Nacional de Occidente, Instituto Mexicano del Seguro Socia, Guadañajara, México
Instituto de Nutrición Humana, Departamento de Clínicas de la Reproducción Humana Crecimiento y Desarrollo Infantil, Centro Universitario de Ciencias de la Salud, Universidad de Guadalajara, Guadalajara, México
Facultad de Medicina, Universidad de Colima, Colima, México

Johnatan M Mesa-Magaña
Servicio de Gastroenterología y Nutrición, UMAE Hospital de Pediatría, Centro Médico Nacional de Occidente, Instituto Mexicano del Seguro Socia, Guadañajara, México

Edgar M Vasquez-Garibay
Instituto de Nutrición Humana, Departamento de Clínicas de la Reproducción Humana Crecimiento y Desarrollo Infantil, Centro Universitario de Ciencias de la Salud, Universidad de Guadalajara, Guadalajara, México

Murat Ferhat Ferhatoglu and Taner Kıvılcım
General Surgery Department, Okan University, Istanbul, Turkey

Hiroshi Makino and Hiroshi Yoshida
Department of Surgery, Nippon Medical School, Tama-Nagayama Hospital, Tama, Japan

Eiji Uchida
Department of Gastrointestinal and Hepato-Biliary-Pancreatic Surgery, Nippon Medical School, Tama, Japan

Jacqueline Oxenberg
Geisinger Wyoming Valley, Wilkes-Barre, PA, USA

Mehrdad Hosseinpour and Bahareh Ahmadi
Imam Hossein Children Hospital, Isfahan University of Medical Sciences, Isfahan, Iran

Dane Christina Daoud and Mickael Bouin
University of Montreal, Saint-Luc Hospital, Montréal, Canada

Dimitrios Schiza, Irene Lidoriki and Theodore Liakakos
First Department of Surgery, Laikon General Hospital, National and Kapodistrian University of Athens, Athens, Greece

Demetrios Moris
Department of Surgery, Division of Surgical Oncology, The Ohio State University Wexner Medical Center and James Cancer Hospital and Solove Research Institute, Columbus, OH, USA

Index

O

P

R

S

T

Lightning Source UK Ltd.
Milton Keynes UK
UKHW050328310822
408102UK00002B/17

9 781639 872794